Inflammation in Parkinson's Disease

Madhavi Thomas
Editor

Inflammation in Parkinson's Disease

Scientific and Clinical Aspects

Springer

Editor
Madhavi Thomas
North Texas Movement Disorders Institute, Inc.
Bedford, TX, USA

ISBN 978-3-319-08045-1 ISBN 978-3-319-08046-8 (eBook)
DOI 10.1007/978-3-319-08046-8
Springer Cham Heidelberg New York Dordrecht London

Library of Congress Control Number: 2014945339

Printed on acid-free paper

Springer is part of Springer Science+Business Media (www.springer.com)

I would like to dedicate this volume to my mentors, Stanley H. Appel, Joseph Jankovic, and Thomas N. Chase.

Foreword

Neuroinflammation is a prominent pathological hallmark of Parkinson's disease (PD), but, more often than not, neuroinflammation has been considered the consequence rather than the cause of PD. The many timely chapters in this book expand our understanding of the role of neuroinflammation in the pathogenesis of neuronal injury in PD, and strengthen the evidence that neuroinflammation is not merely the consequence but can actively mediate neuronal injury. In PD as in other neurodegenerative diseases, including Alzheimer disease and amyotrophic lateral sclerosis, neuroinflammation fans the flames of neurodegeneration. These neurodegenerative diseases present predominantly as sporadic and, to a lesser extent, inheritable disorders. The etiology of the sporadic forms of disease is largely unknown, but discovery of specific mutations responsible for inheritable forms of each of these disorders has revealed the central role of misfolded proteins in sporadic as well as familial disease. Dysfunction in multiple molecular pathways has been implicated in neurodegeneration, including autophagy and ubiquitin-proteasomal pathways, mitochondrial function, production of reactive oxygen species (ROS), alterations in axonal transport, and impaired RNA metabolism. All are key events that can initiate and promote neurodegeneration. The heterogeneity of the clinical phenotypes might be attributable at least in part to the multiplicity of these compromised pathways. The key question is whether compromise of any or all of these perturbations within neurons is sufficient to cause neuronal death. Data from ALS transgenic mouse models suggest that expression of a genetic defect in superoxide dismutase (mSOD1) solely in motor neurons does not lead to clinical disease. Furthermore, expression solely in microglia also does not cause motor neuron injury or give rise to disease, nor does expression solely in astrocytes. Expression of the mutant gene and misfolded proteins must be present in motor neurons and be communicated to glia to cause motor neuron injury, progressive disease, and shortened survival. Thus, in the animal model of ALS, dysfunction of the multiple compromised pathways within neurons is not sufficient to cause neuronal cell death; motor neuron injury is non-cell autonomous and disease progression depends on a well-orchestrated involvement of motor neurons and glia, and subsequently T lymphocytes.

A similar scenario appears relevant to PD. Ever since the report that a mutation in α-synuclein gave rise to familial PD, there has been an explosion of evidence documenting the central role of misfolded α-synuclein in the pathophysiology of both motor and non-motor signs as well as dopaminergic and non-dopaminergic systems in PD, prompting the delineation of PD as an α-synuclein proteinopathy. The pathological hallmark of PD is the Lewy body, an α-synuclein-containing intraneuronal cytoplasmic inclusion; a central role for misfolded α-synuclein has also been reinforced by reports that increased copy number of the α-synuclein gene can cause familial parkinsonism. In PD as in ALS, non-cell autonomous pathways can be implicated, which means that signaling between neurons and glia may be required to promote progressive neuronal injury and accelerated death. Regardless whether intraneuronal accumulation of misfolded and aggregated α-synuclein proteins leading to mitochondrial dysfunction, increased ROS, and altered RNA processing are early events in neuronal injury, cell death depends on the well-orchestrated participation of non-neuronal cells including microglia and astrocytes. Neuroinflammation is the hallmark of this non-cell autonomous process and depends on neuron-glial-T lymphocyte signaling, fostered and initiated by the compromised intra-neuronal pathways. In experimental models signals from injured neurons are initially communicated to microglia, members of the innate immune system, and subsequently to astrocytes, thereby coordinating a communal response to neuronal injury. In response to alterations in the activation states of the innate immune microglia and astrocytes, T lymphocytes, as members of the adaptive immune system, join the process by infiltrating the CNS at sites of neuronal injury.

The potential contribution of neuroinflammation to the pathogenesis of PD is supported by a number of reports. A genome-wide association study (GWAS) associated PD with a highly polymorphic region of HLA-DR, previously reported with numerous inflammatory disorders. HLA-DR immunoreactive microglia are prominent in the SN of PD patients, and are known to interact with T lymphocytes. Degeneration of the ventral midbrain DA neurons in PD is accompanied by the presence of activated microglia with increased inducible nitric oxide synthase (iNOS), TNF-α, IL-1β, IFN-γ, and nuclear translocation of NF-κB. In PD, activated microglia exhibit a pro-inflammatory M1 phenotype. Increased lipid peroxidation, as well as carbonyl- and nitrotyrosine-modified proteins, is also observed in CNS nigral tissue. Activated microglia that surround DA neurons are noted in postmortem tissues of human subjects that have previously developed symptoms and signs of parkinsonism following exposure to the neurotoxin MPTP.

In vitro and experimental in vivo studies provide evidence that misfolded α-synuclein itself may contribute to the neuronal-glial signaling that promotes neurodegeneration. Normal monomeric and aggregated forms of α-synuclein secreted from DA neurons can convert M2 anti-inflammatory microglia to M1 pro-inflammatory microglia, enhancing secretion of ROS and cytokines and leading to neuronal cell death, while inhibitors of these ROS attenuate in vitro DA neurotoxicity. Following expression of the human α-synuclein protein in transgenic mice, insoluble α-synuclein aggregates accumulate in nigral neurons, and render DA neurons more vulnerable to LPS-induced microglia-mediated neurotoxicity.

DA neurons exposed to MPP+ have increased accumulation and secretion of misfolded and aggregated α-synuclein, but the MPP+-mediated DA neuronal injury was not sufficient to cause neuronal death; microglia are necessary to deliver the coup de grace by releasing free radicals and pro-inflammatory cytokines. The increased release of misfolded and aggregated α-synuclein from injured DA neurons has a self-propagating effect causing further oxidation and further release of α-synuclein from DA neurons, and further amplifying DA neurodegeneration. In addition, intracerebral inoculation of preformed α-synuclein fibrils in non-transgenic mice spreads in a prion-like fashion, spreading severe dopaminergic cell injury.

T lymphocytes also participate in the ongoing inflammatory process. Both CD4+ and CD8+ T lymphocytes are present in the SN of PD patients. Although end-stage autopsy tissue cannot define the functional role of T lymphocytes, experimental animal models have provided meaningful insights. In MPTP-treated mice, T lymphocytes enhance cytotoxicity. SCID, Rag1−/−, or TCR−/− mice lacking T lymphocytes are relatively resistant to MPTP-induced SN dopaminergic cell degeneration; in mice lacking CD4+ T lymphocytes, MPTP caused significantly less DA cell death. Thus, MPTP-mediated DA cell killing requires CD4+ T lymphocytes as well as microglia.

T lymphocytes can be neuroprotective as well; transplantation of T lymphocytes from mice immunized with the immunomodulatory drug glatiramer acetate (GA) attenuated the MPTP-induced SN cell loss. IL-4 provided neuroprotection from toxicity mediated by activated microglia, and studies in ALS animal models suggest that Th2 lymphocytes as well as Tregs release IL-4 and modulate the pro-inflammatory M1 phenotype, suggesting that a similar mechanism may be relevant to PD. Several studies of the MPTP model suggest that increased Tregs mediate neuroprotection and Th17 lymphocytes promote neurotoxicity. Adoptive transfer of CD3-activated Tregs to MPTP-intoxicated mice provides greater than 90 % protection of the nigrostriatal system. The response is dose-dependent and parallels modulation of microglial responses and up-regulation of GDNF and TGF-β. Transplantation of Teffs provided no significant neuroprotective activities. The ratio of neuroprotective to cytotoxic T lymphocytes (Th2/Tregs to Th1/Th17) appears to be a relevant parameter in mediating neuroprotection versus neurotoxicity. Tregs were found to mediate neuroprotection possibly through suppression of microglial responses to aggregated and nitrated α-synuclein. In vitro, Tregs suppress microglial release of ROS induced by misfolded α-synuclein, whereas Teffs exacerbate microglial release of ROS. Thus, neuroprotection can be achieved through modulation of microglial oxidative stress and inflammation. Taken together, these results demonstrate that Tregs can suppress nitrated α-synuclein-induced cytotoxic neuroinflammation.

The cumulative data from in vitro and experimental studies of PD models suggest that both microglia and T lymphocytes can serve protective as well as cytotoxic functions. The combination of M2 monocyte/microglia and Tregs/Th2 lymphocytes are neuroprotective and actively suppress M1/Th1/Th17-mediated toxicity; the combination of M1 monocyte/microglia and Th1/Th17 lymphocytes are cytotoxic. However, the timing of protection and cytotoxicity remains to be determined.

Is the milieu protective early in the course of experimental models of PD as well as in PD patients, and toxic later in disease, as noted in models of ALS? The answers are not available. What is needed is a better understanding of how to limit populations of cells mediating cytotoxic immunomodulation and how to expand populations of cells mediating neuroprotective immunomodulation.

More critical is whether the experimental data are truly applicable to patients with PD, and whether neuroinflammation can mediate neurodegeneration in patients. Biomarkers specific for neuroinflammatory pathways that effectively monitor the evolution of disease and potential responses to immunomodulatory therapy would provide important support for the relevance of neuroinflammation to the pathogenesis of disease. As an approach, neuroimaging, as delineated in this book, may well function as a biomarker to monitor microglial activation, especially in concert with immune/inflammatory blood markers. Dr Thomas is to be congratulated for assembling these first-rate authors and chapters that detail the inflammatory responses and their contribution to neurodegeneration; novel pathways are defined that could potentially lead to meaningful therapies that promote effective neuroprotection.

Houston, TX, USA Stanley H. Appel, M.D.

Preface

Inflammation in Parkinson's disease (PD) has always been a subject of great interest. Chronic inflammation in the brain can be induced in a primate model even with a single injection of MPTP. Many genetic and environmental factors contribute to onset of PD. There is much to learn from recent developments in systems biology including study of proteomics and metabolomics in developing future biologic markers. Of great interest is whether inflammation is a co-contributor or an independent driving process for cell death in PD. Arguments can be made for both. However, PD is a heterogeneous disease. Based on familial risk factors for PD, one can hypothesize that PD can be due to pathways of pure apoptosis, inflammation, vascular risk factors, presence of oncogenes, and multifactorial etiology. One needs to review this carefully and perhaps develop biological markers based on familial risk factors, and these pathways need to be clarified further. There could be isolated subtype of PD, with predominant inflammatory pathology, and therapeutic targets can be developed in the future. The focus of this publication is to bring together basic laboratory advances as well as currently available clinical literature to support this concept of inflammation as being an important process in PD. In this maiden venture I have sought help from many of my learned colleagues, who have kindly agreed to work on bringing this volume together. I am hoping this volume will help students, researchers, and clinicians alike in developing novel concepts in research in the future.

Bedford, TX, USA — Madhavi Thomas, M.D.

Contents

Parkinson's Disease: An Overview of Etiology, Clinical Manifestations, and Treatment 1
Arif Dalvi, Kelly E. Lyons, and Rajesh Pahwa

Neuropathology of Parkinson's Disease 25
Kurt A. Jellinger

Role of the Innate and Adaptive Immune System in the Pathogenesis of PD 75
George T. Kannarkat and Malú G. Tansey

"Good" and "Bad" Microglia in Parkinson's Disease: An Understanding of Homeostatic Mechanisms in Immunomodulation 105
Yu Tang and Weidong Le

The Role of Astrocytes in Parkinson's Disease 127
Claire Stevens and Glenda Halliday

Proinflammatory Chemical Signaling: Cytokines 145
Kumi Nagamoto-Combs and Colin K. Combs

Cell Culture Models of Inflammation in Parkinson's Disease 175
Patrick Flood

Clinical Aspects of Inflammation in Parkinson's Disease 189
Madhavi Thomas and Christopher Adams

PET Imaging in Neuroinflammation 205
David J. Brooks

Index 217

Contributors

Christopher Adams, M.S. North Texas Movement Disorders Institute, Inc., Bedford, TX, USA

Stanley H. Appel, M.D. Houston Methodist Neurological Institute, Houston, TX, USA

Edwards Distinguished Endowed Chair for ALS Research, Houston, TX, USA

Department of Neurology, Houston Methodist Hospital, Houston, TX, USA

David J. Brooks, M.D., D.Sc., F.R.C.P. (UK) Imperial College London, London, UK

Aarhus University, Aarhus, Denmark

Medicine ICL, Nuclear Medicine AU, Hammermsith Hospital, London, UK

Colin K. Combs, Ph.D. Department of Basic Sciences, University of North Dakota School of Medicine and Health Sciences, Grand Forks, ND, USA

Arif Dalvi, M.D., M.B.A. Parkinson's Disease and Movement Disorders Program, Methodist Hospital Neuroscience Institute, Merrillville, IN, USA

Patrick Flood, Ph.D. Department of Faculty of Medicine and Dentistry, Katz Group Centre for Pharmacy and Health Research, University of Alberta, Edmonton, AB, Canada

Glenda Halliday, B.Sc. (Hons), Ph.D. Department of Medicine, and Neuroscience Research Australia, University of New South Wales, Randwick, NSW, Australia

Kurt A. Jellinger, M.D. Institute of Clinical Neurobiology, Vienna, Austria

George T. Kannarkat, M.D., Ph.D. Department of Physiology, Emory University School of Medicine, Atlanta, GA, USA

Weidong Le, M.D., Ph.D. Institute of Health Sciences, Shanghai Institutes for Biological Sciences, Chinese Academy of Sciences, Shanghai, China

The First Affiliated Hospital of Dalian Medical University, Translational Research Institutes of Medicine, Dalian, China

Kelly E. Lyons, Ph.D. Department of Neurology, University of Kansas Medical Center, Kansas City, KS, USA

Kumi Nagamoto-Combs, Ph.D. Department of Basic Sciences, University of North Dakota School of Medicine and Health Sciences, Grand Forks, ND, USA

Rajesh Pahwa, M.D. Department of Neurology, University of Kansas Medical Center, Kansas City, KS, USA

Claire Stevens, B.Med.Sci. (Hons), Ph.D. Department of Medicine, and Neuroscience Research Australia, University of New South Wales, Randwick, NSW, Australia

Yu Tang, Ph.D. Institute of Health Sciences, Shanghai Institutes for Biological Sciences, Chinese Academy of Sciences, Shanghai, China

Malú G. Tansey, Ph.D. Department of Physiology, Emory University School of Medicine, Atlanta, GA, USA

Madhavi Thomas, M.D. North Texas Movement Disorders Institute, Inc., Bedford, TX, USA

Department of Neurology, Baylor University Medical Center, Dallas, TX, USA

Parkinson's Disease: An Overview of Etiology, Clinical Manifestations, and Treatment

Arif Dalvi, Kelly E. Lyons, and Rajesh Pahwa

Parkinson syndrome is an umbrella term grouping together clinical syndromes that share the cardinal symptoms of bradykinesia, rigidity, and rest tremor. By far the largest occupant of this umbrella is idiopathic Parkinson's disease (PD), with degeneration of the nigrostriatal dopaminergic system and the presence of Lewy bodies in the substantia nigra as its pathological hallmarks [1].

A number of other neurodegenerative diseases share this space with distinct clinical features and pathological mechanisms. The combination of the cardinal features of Parkinson syndrome with additional manifestations such as ophthalmoplegia, dysautonomia, cortical and cerebellar signs, or dementia is referred to by the rubric parkinson-plus syndrome that includes disorders such as progressive supranuclear palsy (PSP), multiple system atrophy (MSA), corticobasal degeneration (CBD), and dementia with Lewy bodies (DLB). Other well-defined heredodegenerative diseases such as Wilson's disease and Huntington's disease can also mimic PD. Finally, structural lesions in the brain such as normal pressure hydrocephalus and small vessel ischemic disease can resemble PD [2].

Clinical Features

The diagnosis of PD is primarily based on clinical criteria. The United Kingdom Parkinson's Disease Society Brain Bank criteria are most often used, with positive diagnostic features including the presence of bradykinesia, and at least one of muscular rigidity, tremor at rest, or postural instability not explained by other etiologies.

A. Dalvi, M.D., M.B.A. (✉)
Parkinson's Disease and Movement Disorders Program, Methodist Hospital Neuroscience Institute, Merrillville, IN, USA
e-mail: dalvi.md@gmail.com

K.E. Lyons, Ph.D. • R. Pahwa, M.D.
Department of Neurology, University of Kansas Medical Center, Kansas City, KS, USA

M. Thomas (ed.), *Inflammation in Parkinson's Disease: Scientific and Clinical Aspects*, DOI 10.1007/978-3-319-08046-8_1,

Exclusionary criteria include history of strokes, repeated head injury, or definite encephalitis, oculogyric crisis, neuroleptic treatment at symptom onset, sustained remission, unilateral symptoms after 3 years, supranuclear gaze palsy, cerebellar signs, early, severe autonomic features or dementia, Babinski sign, cerebral tumor or hydrocephalus, or no response to high doses of levodopa. Supportive features include at least three of the following: unilateral onset, rest tremor, progression, persistent asymmetry with side of onset most affected, good response to levodopa, levodopa-induced dyskinesia, and clinical course of at least 10 years [3].

The clinical syndrome of PD is not limited to these cardinal symptoms. Other motor manifestations include postural instability, stooped posture, a shuffling, festinating or freezing gait, and dystonic posturing, particularly in the lower extremities. In addition, long-term treatment, particularly with levodopa is associated with the development of dyskinesia and a fluctuating response to medical treatment described as the "on–off" phenomenon [4].

There is an increasing recognition of non-motor symptoms in PD, some of which may precede the onset of motor symptoms by many decades. An altered sense of smell and constipation can occur in PD and have also been examined as potential predictors of the onset of PD. Depression and anxiety are common comorbid symptoms. Changes in the sleep–wake cycle and REM behavior disorder may also be seen. Dysautonomia usually becomes more prominent in the later stages of the disease, unlike in MSA, where it may be a presenting feature. Autonomic symptoms include orthostatic hypotension, urinary frequency and incontinence, delayed gastric emptying and sialorrhea, erectile dysfunction, and loss of libido [5]. Dementia is part of the natural history of PD, although, in contrast to DLB, it occurs relatively late in the course. A global dementia, such as is seen in Alzheimer's disease, is less commonly observed. Instead an executive dysfunction is seen with retrieval being affected more than memory and short-term memory loss more common than that of long-term memory. Long-standing PD may also be complicated by the development of hallucinations and psychosis [6].

Laboratory Studies

The diagnosis of PD remains a clinical diagnosis. However, judicious use of imaging and laboratory studies helps exclude diseases that may resemble PD but have a significantly different treatment and prognosis. In younger patients it is important to screen for Wilson's disease with serum ceruloplasmin, 24-h urine copper, and liver function studies. Imaging studies in the form of CT or MRI of the brain help rule out structural etiologies such as normal pressure hydrocephalus and vascular parkinsonism. Brain MRI also detects changes in the basal ganglia or thalamus in Wilson's disease and may reveal caudate atrophy in Huntington's disease [1].

Where diagnostic uncertainty exists, for example, between essential tremor (ET) and PD, the use of DaTscan SPECT imaging can be useful. Dopamine transporter (DaT) levels in the striatum are lower in parkinsonism due to loss of dopaminergic cells but are normal in other etiologies of tremor such as ET. Labeling the dopamine transporter with ioflupane (a radioactive iodine-labeled cocaine derivative) and measuring the levels with SPECT imaging can help distinguish ET from parkinsonism including PD. It is important to note that DaTscan is unable to distinguish PD from other forms of parkinsonism [7].

Etiology of PD

In his seminal *An Essay on the Shaking Palsy* Sir James Parkinson considered "indulgence in spirituous liquors" and "long lying on the damp ground" as possible etiologies of PD [8]. Seventy years later Gower reported that about 15 % of his patients with PD had a family history [9]. A twin study on WWII veterans showed genetic factors in patients with typical or older age of onset played a lesser role, as similar concordance rates were observed in monozygotic and dizygotic twins. In contrast, in patients with an onset prior to age 50, there was a more substantial genetic contribution [10]. Following the discovery of the α-synuclein (SNCA) gene [11] and the subsequent discovery of a number of additional PARK genes the debate between supporters of genetic and environmental causes has been renewed. The assumptions of Parkinson regarding the etiology of PD have not held up, but a number of alternative environmental factors have been proposed. Current understanding of the etiology of PD points to a multifactorial disorder with gene–environment interactions leading to neuronal cell death (Fig. 1).

Selective Vulnerability of the Nigrostriatal Tract

The reason for selective vulnerability of the substantia nigra pars compacta (SNc) in the pathogenesis of PD is an area of active study. A number of hypotheses have been proposed as an explanation. Oxidative stress involving mitochondrial dysfunction may be more prominent in the SNc relative to other brain regions, primarily due to reactive oxygen species produced during dopamine storage and breakdown [12]. Models of endoplasmic reticulum stress show age-dependent selective vulnerability of dopaminergic neurons, also related to the oxidative by-products of dopamine metabolism. Dopamine metabolites, especially the monoamine oxidase (MAO) metabolite 3,4-dihydroxyphenylacetaldehyde (DOPAL), can trigger SNCA aggregation in SNc neurons [13].

Accumulation of SNCA in cultured human dopaminergic neurons results in apoptotic cell death. This mechanism requires endogenous dopamine production and is mediated by reactive oxygen species. In contrast, SNCA is neuroprotective in non-dopaminergic human cortical neurons. Thus, accumulation of soluble SNCA protein complexes can render endogenous dopamine toxic, suggesting a potential

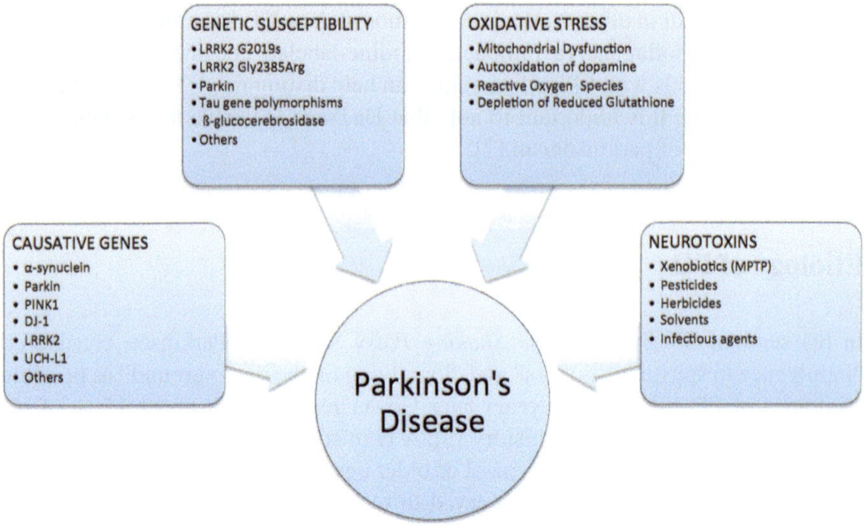

Fig. 1 The multifactorial etiology of Parkinson's disease. Causative genes and genetic susceptibility factors interact with environmental triggers and endogenous causes of oxidative stress. Misfolding and aggregation of proteins together with mitochondrial dysfunction provide the framework for neuronal cell death leading to Parkinson's disease. © Arif Dalvi 2007. Reprinted from Dalvi A, Walsh R. Etiology of Parkinson's disease. In: Simuni T, Pahwa R, editors. Parkinson's Disease. New York: Oxford University Press; 2009: 51–62, Figure 5.1. By permission of Oxford University Press, USA

mechanism for the selectivity of neuronal loss in PD [14]. Inflammatory mechanisms may also play a role, especially in the context of activated microglial cells. Patients with PD have selective degeneration of neurons in the SNc accompanied by microglial activation and a challenged immune system [15].

Environmental Factors

Environmental factors have always been considered to play a significant role in the etiology of PD. One of the most commonly identified is exposure to herbicides and pesticides. In a multifactorial model based on a study of rural populations, years of rural living and groundwater use were predictive of PD. Pesticide exposure was found to be a risk factor independent of rural living [16]. However, not all studies support rural living as a risk factor. In China drinking well water was associated with a reduced risk of PD, while living in proximity to rubber plants or drinking river water was associated with a higher risk [17]. In a large serial cross-sectional study of Medicare beneficiaries, two geographic belts with high predisposition to PD were found. This series of over 450,000 PD cases revealed a higher concentration of PD cases in the Midwest and Northeast regions. Prevalence in urban counties was greater than in rural ones [18]. Epidemiologic studies investigating potential links between solvents and PD have yielded mostly null or weak associations [19]. However, a study of 99 twin pairs from the World War II Veterans Twin Cohort suggested possible etiologic relations with trichloroethylene (TCE) and other chlorinated solvents, although the sample size was small and dose–response gradients were not observed. It should be noted that TCE is the most common organic contaminant in groundwater [20]. Welding and manganese exposure have been suggested as risk factors for PD [21]. However, a meta-analysis that pooled data from 13 studies for welding and 3 studies for manganese exposure failed to support this hypothesis [22].

Genetic Factors

A first-degree relative of an affected individual is approximately twice as likely to develop PD compared to someone with no family history of PD [23]. While concordance rates in monozygotic and dizygotic twins are equal in late-onset PD, they are much higher in monozygotic (~100 %) than in dizygotic twins (~17 %) in early-onset PD, consistent with early-onset PD having a strong genetic determinant [24]. Several genes have been definitively linked with familial PD, along with other candidate genes whose association with PD is less established.

α-Synuclein

Three mutations of this gene as well as duplication and triplication of the gene region have been described in familial PD. The pathological role of SNCA in PD is also not definitively known, but SNCA is a major component of Lewy bodies observed in post-mortem studies of PD brains [12]. Autosomal-dominant inheritance of familial PD is observed with mutations of α-synuclein. The clinical course of affected individuals is similar to sporadic PD, but with an earlier mean age of onset, higher rate of dementia, and some neuropathological features not common in sporadic PD including more tau-positive extra-perikaryal spheroid-like and thread-like lesions and more marked neuronal loss. The physiological role of SNCA is unclear, but it may be involved in synaptic vesicle recycling particularly involving dopamine storage [25].

Parkin

This gene is the most common autosomal-recessive PD gene mutation, and a wide variety of parkin mutations have been found in familial PD. Parkin is mutated in ~50 % of autosomal-recessive early-onset PD and in ~70 % of juvenile PD with onset less than 20 years. The clinical course of affected individuals is typically characterized by early onset, slow progression, and good response to dopamine [26]. The physiological role of parkin is thought to relate to its function as an ubiquitin ligase important in normal cellular protein degradation pathways. Deficiency in this function may underlie the pathology associated with mutant parkin, including possible disruption of microtubule and mitochondrial function, proteasomal degradation, and neuroprotection [27].

PINK1

Mutations of this gene are thought to result in loss of kinase function consistent with the observed autosomal-recessive inheritance pattern. The clinical course in affected individuals typically demonstrates disease onset at less than 50 years with otherwise mostly classical features of sporadic PD [28]. The physiological role of PINK1 is thought to involve regulation of the electron transport chain and maintenance of mitochondrial membrane potential, and the pathology resulting from mutations of PINK1 may relate to mitochondrial dysfunction in response to oxidative stress, possibly involving parkin [29].

DJ-1

Multiple types of DJ-1 mutations have been identified, and inheritance is autosomal-recessive. Affected individuals typically have age of onset around 20–40 years with mostly classical Parkinsonian symptoms and usually respond well to dopaminergic therapy. Focal dystonia and blepharospasm may present early in the course of the disease [30]. DJ-1 is thought to play a role as an antioxidant and sensor of oxidative stress, but may also be involved in protein degradation pathways and apoptotic signaling possibly in conjunction with parkin and PINK1. Furthermore, dysfunction of DJ-1 may affect these pathways in a manner that preferentially involves dopaminergic neurons [31].

LRRK2

LRRK2 mutations are found throughout this gene's functional domains with the most common mutant being relatively frequent in both familial autosomal-dominant PD (~4 %) and in sporadic PD (~1 %) [32]. In certain populations, such as North African Arabs and Ashkenazi Jews, the prevalence of LRRK2 mutations may account for up to 40 % of all PD cases [33, 34]. LRRK2 mutations result in parkinsonism very similar to classical PD, and penetrance of symptoms is very tightly linked with aging, also similar to idiopathic PD. Despite the relatively uniform classic parkinsonism seen with LRRK2 mutations, the neuropathology is quite diverse suggesting that LRRK2 dysfunction may be important in the initiation of altered function of multiple cellular systems with a final common pathway resulting in dopaminergic cell death [35]. The physiologic role of LRRK2 is thought to involve its putative kinase and GTPase activity, and mutant forms have shown increased kinase activity consistent with a gain of function seen often in autosomal-dominant diseases [36]. PD-causing LRRK2 mutations deregulate the autophagy–lysosomal pathway. G2019S mutant LRRK2 can lead to abnormal accumulation of autophagic and lysosomal structures in primary cortical neurons and neuronal cell lines in culture [37].

UCH-L1

It is unclear if mutations of UCH-L1 identified in several families are truly involved in PD due to the failure of the mutation to segregate with disease in one family and the failure of other mutations to be identified despite extensive screening [38]. It is intriguing, however, that a polymorphism in this gene may protect against development of PD, possibly through alteration of interaction of UCH-L1 with SNCA [39]. UCH-L1 accumulation is likely to play a pathological role in inclusion formation in PD through a malfunction of the ubiquitin/proteasome system that leads to an inability to clear aggresomes [40].

Gene–Environment Interactions

The ultimate etiology of PD may be based on multiple factors including genetics, environmental exposures and aging-related apoptotic processes. The complex interaction between these factors may serve as an explanation for the heterogeneity observed in clinical presentations. Various animal models have attempted to examine the interplay of these interactions.

DJ-1 mutations have been associated with autosomal-recessive early-onset PD. In a DJ-1 knockout transgenic mouse model the susceptibility of nigrostriatal deficits was found to increase following exposure to MPTP (1-methyl-4-phenyl-1,2,3,6-tetrahydropyridine). In addition, in wild-type mice adenoviral-mediated overexpression of DJ-1 was found to block MPTP induced neuronal loss and neurodegeneration in the substantia nigra. Thus, DJ-1 may play a significant role in the protection of neurons against oxidative stress and environmental neurotoxins [41]. Lymphoblast cells derived from DJ-1 patients display aberrant mitochondrial morphology. These DJ-1-dependent mitochondrial defects contribute to oxidative stress-induced sensitivity to cell death. The aberrant mitochondrial phenotype can be rescued by the expression of Pink1 and Parkin, two PD-linked genes involved with mitochondrial function. Thus a complex interplay between genetic factors can lead to a differential response to oxidative stress produced by environmental toxins [42].

Infectious Etiologies for PD

In 1916–1927 an epidemic of an influenza-like illness ravaged Europe and North America. Mortality was up to 40 % in those affected, and most survivors developed parkinsonism over the next 10 years [43]. The specific agent causing this pandemic of encephalitis lethargica was never isolated. However, it drew attention to an infectious etiology as a contributor to PD. Of note, the possibility that an encephalitis lethargica syndrome is still prevalent has been raised with the suggested mechanism being autoimmunity against deep grey matter neurons [44].

Antibodies to the Epstein–Barr virus have shown cross reactivity with SNCA in the brains of patients with PD [45]. Although no evidence of ongoing viral infection in PD has been reported, immunohistochemistry shows reactive microglia and activated complement components suggestive of chronic inflammation occur in affected brain regions in PD [46]. The viral hypothesis has also been invoked to explain the observation of the higher incidence of PD in teachers, medical workers, loggers, and miners [47]. In monozygotic twins discordant for PD a significantly increased risk was noted in the twin working as a teacher or health care worker [24].

PD as a Prion-Like Disease

SNCA has been determined to be the major component of Lewy bodies, which are the pathological hallmark of PD [48]. Three missense mutations in the SNCA gene have been associated with autosomal-dominant PD, and genome-wide association studies have linked single-nucleotide polymorphisms in this gene to sporadic PD [49]. The spread of SNCA pathology in the brain has been implicated in the progression of PD and in the caudal to rostral spread of Lewy bodies in PD that forms the basis of Braak staging in PD [50]. This has led to the recognition that SNCA has attributes that are common to prion-like proteins, including multiple conformations and the ability to transfer from cell to cell. The physiological form of SNCA has an unstructured α-helical conformation that changes to oligomers and fibrils rich in β-sheets in the mutant pathological form [51]. In vivo studies have also documented the ability of SNCA to transfer and propagate from cell to cell [52]. Support for the prion-like spread of PD was furthered by observations in autopsied brains of individuals who underwent embryonic stem cell implants in the 1980–1990s. Of note SNCA pathology was found not only in the patient's own brain tissue but also in the grafted neurons. These grafted neurons were found to show SNCA and ubiquitin immunoreactivity and showed the typical morphology of Lewy bodies with a dense core and a lighter halo. Given that the grafted cells were only 10–15 years old, it was felt that an independent autonomic process could not be implicated but rather the possibility of spread through a prion-like mechanism was raised [53]. However, in contrast to prion diseases like Creutzfeldt–Jakob disease there is no evidence that misfolded SNCA can be transmitted from one individual to another; thus, it is best described as a prion-like protein.

Inflammation and PD

Inflammation has been increasingly studied as part of the pathophysiology of neurodegenerative diseases. In PD an increase in microglial activation has been shown in the substantia nigra cells that may be a marker of neurotoxicity [54]. Microglia have multiple roles, including immune surveillance and mediating immune responses to pathogens by secreting cytokines, chemokines, prostaglandins, reactive oxygen and nitrogen species, and growth factors. Some of these factors have neuroprotective effects, while others enhance oxidative stress and can trigger apoptosis. Chronic neuroinflammation may reduce the levels of neuroprotective factors, increasing the vulnerability to inflammation induced cell death of substantia nigra neurons [55].

In a rat model created by injecting an adeno-associated virus vector for SNCA into the substantia nigra the control arm showed a significant loss of tyrosine hydroxylase positive (TH+) neurons. However, in rats that were fed a diet rich in spirulina, a blue-green algae, a significantly greater number of TH + cells were preserved. A neuroprotective effect from reducing the inflammatory component associated with microglial association was hypothesized as the mechanism [56]. Telmisartan, an angiotensin I receptor blocker has been shown in animal models to inhibit the microglial inflammatory response and thereby reduce dopaminergic cell death. The neuroprotective effect is believed to be mediated, at least in part, by the activation of peroxisome proliferator-activated receptor gamma (PPAR-γ) [57]. Oral antidiabetic thiazolidinediones have also been shown to exert neuroprotective effects in models of PD. Their antidiabetic effect is due to activation of PPAR-γ, and this may also reduce inflammation and apoptosis, thereby leading to a neuroprotective effect [58]. Pioglitazone and retinoic acid were tested in a rotenone-induced model of PD in rats. Rotenone significantly reduced locomotor activity of the rats and also significantly reduced dopamine levels in the striatum and hippocampus. Pioglitazone, but not retinoic acid, significantly reversed the reduced striatal dopamine level [59]. Isradipine, a dihydropyridine calcium channel blocker (DiCCB), has also been shown to be neuroprotective in preclinical models of parkinsonism. It was suggested that with increasing age, dopaminergic neurons relied more on L-type voltage-gated calcium channels with a pore-forming Cav1.3 (caveolin.3) subunit, making them more vulnerable to toxin-induced injury. Neurons of younger animals used sodium-dependent channels. If Cav1.3 channels in older animals were blocked by isradipine, their neurons reverted to the juvenile form of the channels rendering them less prone to injury [60].

Oxidative Stress and PD

The discovery that MPTP is toxic to nigral dopaminergic cells led to research into the environmental causes of PD and oxidative stress as an underlying mechanism [61]. A higher incidence of PD had been reported in those living in rural areas, and the observation that paraquat, a weed killer, had structural resemblance to MPTP lent further credence to this hypothesis [62]. Oxidative stress remains a key concept in understanding the pathophysiology of PD [63]. It is believed that free radical production resulting from the enzymatic oxidation of dopamine as well as exposure to external toxins that cause oxidative stress play a role in the causation of the disease and disease progression [64]. In contrast, the observation of a negative correlation between plasma urate levels and disease progression in PD may represent altered antioxidant activity through reduced glutathione levels or the antioxidant and metal complexing properties of urate [65].

Both neuronal and glial sources have been implicated in oxidative stress. The most likely contributor of oxidative stress is believed to be increased free radical formation from the mitochondria. Neurotoxicity of MPTP through its metabolite MPP^+ occurs through the inhibition of complex 1 in the electron transport chain [66]. Mutations in SNCA, parkin, PINK1, DJ-1, and possibly LRRK2 have been associated with altered mitochondrial function. Thus the mitochondria may represent a common target for both genetic and environmental etiologies of PD [67].

Mechanism of Action of PD Medications

Arvid Carlsson in 1957 discovered that depleting dopamine from the brains of rabbits by using reserpine caused them to become slow and rigid, similar to the symptoms of PD. He also found that injecting the rabbits with L-Dopa reversed these symptoms. This eventually led to the acceptance of levodopa as a medication for treating PD [68]. Levodopa is a dopamine precursor that unlike dopamine crosses the blood–brain barrier and is enzymatically converted into dopamine within the brain. This dopamine replacement offers significant symptomatic relief compared to untreated patients with PD. Cotzias was the first to use levodopa successfully in clinical practice. He countered the severe nausea experienced when using levodopa by starting with very small doses and gradually building up the dose. However, even in his initial series of patients dyskinesia was reported to be present and dose failures and motor fluctuations were also reported [69]. The addition of a dopa-decarboxylase inhibitor allowed considerably lower doses of levodopa to be used for the same clinical effect, allowing for reduced peripheral conversion of levodopa to dopamine and thus reducing nausea and other side effects thus cementing the role of levodopa as the mainstay of PD therapy [70]. However, the short half-life of levodopa is associated with long-term side effects including motor fluctuations and dyskinesia. Stimulating the dopamine receptors with long-acting dopamine agonists could potentially alleviate these side effects [71].

The pharmacotherapeutic basis of treatment of the motor symptoms is correction of the underlying dopamine deficit. The gold standard remains levodopa, which has the highest efficacy [72]. The bioavailability of levodopa is increased by combining it with a dopa decarboxylase inhibitor and/or with a catechol-O-methyltransferase (COMT) inhibitor [73]. Dopamine agonists may be used as an alternative and have a significantly longer half-life but lower efficacy. In early stages the antiviral amantadine may provide adequate symptomatic benefit. Monoamine oxidase type B (MAO-B) inhibitors extend the duration of dopamine in the synaptic cleft and may also be used in early PD as monotherapy. Anticholinergics have been used based on the idea that there is a relative excess of acetylcholine, but their propensity to cause cognitive side effects limits their use [74].

Levodopa

Dopamine does not adequately cross the blood–brain barrier; hence, direct replacement is not possible. However, the dopamine precursor levodopa can cross the blood–brain barrier where it is enzymatically converted into dopamine. A significant amount of levodopa is metabolized in the periphery to dopamine. Carbidopa reduces this peripheral conversion, improving levodopa delivery to the brain and reducing peripheral side effects of dopamine such as nausea and orthostatic hypotension. The half-life of levodopa is increased from approximately 50 to 90 min by this combination. Thus, levodopa is rarely prescribed by itself but is used in the form of a combination tablet of carbidopa/levodopa (CD/LD) or Sinemet [75].

CD/LD is available in dosages of 10/100, 25/100, and 25/250 mg tablets. The initial target dose of CD/LD is generally one 25/100 mg tablet three times per day. It is advisable to initiate CD/LD slowly, starting with one-half of a 25/100 mg tablet twice a day for 1 week and then increasing by one-half tablet daily until symptoms are well controlled.

A controlled-release formulation of CD/LD (Sinemet-CR) is available in doses of 25/100 and 50/200 mg. This formulation is generally started with 25/100 mg/day and increased to 25/100 mg three times per day or 50/200 mg twice a day. Controlled-release preparations are not as well absorbed, and the bioavailability is 20–30 % lower than standard preparations [76]. CD/LD is also available in an orally disintegrating tablet (Parcopa). This formulation is available in the same strengths as immediate-release CD/LD and has similar bioavailability, safety, and efficacy. It is particularly useful in patients with swallowing difficulties [77].

Common acute adverse effects with CD/LD include nausea, vomiting, drowsiness, and orthostatic hypotension. Other side effects include diaphoresis, cardiac arrhythmias, and pedal edema. Cognitive side effects include confusion, vivid dreams, and hallucinations. The long-term use of CD/LD is associated with the development of dyskinesia and motor fluctuations, which are discussed below [78].

Dopamine Agonists

Pramipexole (Mirapex) and ropinirole (Requip) are the nonergot dopamine agonists in current use as oral agents. Older ergot derivatives such as bromocriptine and pergolide have long-term side effects such as cardiac valve damage and retroperitoneal fibrosis and have fallen out of use. Apomorphine (Apokyn) is a post-synaptic nonergot dopamine agonist available as an injectable preparation mainly used as rescue therapy during "off" episodes. Rotigotine (Neupro) is a nonergot dopamine agonist formulated as a transdermal patch.

Unlike the direct replacement of dopamine by levodopa, dopamine agonists work by stimulation of the post-synaptic dopamine receptors. The oral agents have a significantly longer half-life than levodopa of around 6–8 h. This more continuous stimulation of the dopaminergic receptors may play a role in reducing the incidence of dyskinesia and motor fluctuations compared to levodopa [79]. However, while improvement in motor symptoms is based on their effect on D2 receptors in the basal ganglia, there is a relatively high affinity for D3 receptors as well, increasing the tendency to cause cognitive side effects such as excessive daytime somnolence (EDS), hallucinations, and compulsive behavior including gambling [80].

Pramipexole (Mirapex) is approved for use as monotherapy and adjunctive therapy in PD. Pramipexole acts on the D2, D3, and D4 dopamine receptors and has a half-life of 8–12 h. It reaches peak drug plasma concentration in approximately 2 h. It is excreted mostly unchanged in the urine. Pramipexole is initiated at 0.125 mg three times per day and increased over several weeks to a maximum dose of 1.5 mg three times per day [81]. An extended-release form of pramipexole (Mirapex ER) is also available that allows once-daily dosing [82].

Ropinirole (Requip) is approved for both monotherapy and adjunctive therapy in PD. It has affinity for the D2 dopamine receptors and no effect on the D1 or D5 dopaminergic receptors. The plasma half-life of ropinirole is approximately 6 h, with peak drug plasma concentrations occurring in 1–2 h. Ropinirole is initiated at 0.25 mg three times per day and increased over several weeks to a maximum dose of 8 mg three times per day [83]. An extended-release formulation, ropinirole (Requip XL), is also available, allowing once-daily dosing [84].

Rotigotine (Neupro) is a dopamine agonist that is available as a transdermal preparation and is approved both as monotherapy and as an adjunct to levodopa. Rotigotine for monotherapy is initiated at 2 mg/24 h and titrated weekly up to 6 mg/24 h [85]. When used as an adjunct to levodopa in patients with motor fluctuations, rotigotine may be started at 4 mg/24 h and titrated weekly up to 8 mg/24 h [86]. Rotigotine is generally well tolerated, with the most common adverse events being application-site reactions, gastrointestinal disturbances, somnolence, and headache. Application-site reactions are generally mild to moderate in severity. However, up to 3 % of patients had severe skin reactions [87].

Apomorphine (Apokyn) is approved for advanced PD as a rescue therapy for severe off periods and is available as a subcutaneous injection. It is a fast-acting, injectable dopamine agonist. It is rapidly absorbed in 10–60 min. However, the half-life of approximately 40 min results in an effect that lasts for only up to 90 min. It can be given every 2 h up to five times per day. A test dose of 2 mg (0.2 mL) is given in the physician's office, and the dose is titrated by 0.1-mL increments up to a maximum single dose of 0.6 mL [88]. Premedication with an anti-nausea medication, usually trimethobenzamide (Tigan), is required because apomorphine can cause severe nausea.

MAO Inhibitors

Metabolism of dopamine within dopaminergic terminals by MAO-B shortens the effect of dopamine. In addition, this metabolic pathway creates oxygen radicals including O_2^- and H_2O_2 that may potentially accelerate the death of dopaminergic neurons. MAO-B inhibitors are a treatment option for PD.

Selegiline (Eldepryl) is approved as an adjunct treatment to levodopa; however, it may also be used as monotherapy in early disease. The typical dose is 5 mg with breakfast and lunch. An orally disintegrating form of selegiline (Zelapar) is available in the strength of 1.25 mg. It is approved for use in advanced PD with motor fluctuations. The initial dose is 1.25 mg a day, which can be increased to 2.5 mg per day if clinically indicated. By the avoidance of first-pass metabolism, it results in higher concentrations of selegiline and lower concentrations of its metabolites compared with the 5-mg swallowed selegiline tablet [89].

Selegiline is generally well tolerated. The most common adverse effects include nausea, dizziness, insomnia, confusion, hallucinations, dry mouth, and orthostatic hypotension. It can lead to increased dyskinesia when used as an adjunct to levodopa therapy. As the dose of selegiline is increased, its selectivity to inhibit MAO-B is decreased, and inhibition of MAO-A can also occur; thus, it is important to not to increase the dose beyond 5 mg twice a day [90].

Rasagiline is an irreversible MAO-B inhibitor. It reaches peak plasma concentrations in approximately 1 h and has a half-life of approximately 3 h. However, since it irreversibly inhibits MAO-B, its therapeutic benefit is independent of its half-life. It is approved as monotherapy [91] in early disease at a dose of 1 mg/day, and in PD patients with motor fluctuations on levodopa starting at 0.5 mg/day, which can be increased to 1 mg/day [92].

Commonly observed adverse events with rasagiline monotherapy are arthralgia, depression, and gastrointestinal side effects. As an adjunct to levodopa, the common adverse effects included worsening of dyskinesia, weight loss, postural hypotension, arthralgia, gastrointestinal side effects, somnolence, and paresthesia. Unlike selegiline, rasagiline does not have amphetamine metabolites [93].

COMT Inhibitors

COMT inhibitors inhibit the action of catechol-O-methyl transferase, one of the metabolic pathways for the metabolism of levodopa. Tolcapone and entacapone are two COMT inhibitors used in the treatment of PD. The COMT inhibitor entacapone when given with CD/LD increases the area under the curve of levodopa by about 35 % and prolongs the half-life of levodopa to about 2.4 h while leaving the average peak levodopa plasma concentration unaffected, thus reducing the risk of peak-dose side effects [94].

Entacapone (Comtan) is approved for the management of motor fluctuations in PD. Its half-life is 0.4–0.7 h. It reduces the peripheral metabolism of levodopa, thereby increasing the half-life of levodopa to about 2.4 h. It is initiated at 200 mg with each dose of levodopa for a maximum of eight doses per day [95]. The common side effects of COMT-inhibitors are mostly related to increased dopaminergic stimulation. Dyskinesia, nausea, vomiting, and hallucinations are the most commonly seen dopaminergic adverse effects. These may be reduced by decreasing the levodopa dose. There is no known hepatotoxicity associated with entacapone and liver enzyme monitoring is not required. Diarrhea as an adverse effect usually begins at 6–12 weeks but can appear as early as 2 weeks after entacapone is started. If the diarrhea is bothersome, therapy must be discontinued. Urine discoloration is a harmless side effect that occurs in less than 10 % of patients [96].

The triple combination of carbidopa/levodopa/entacapone (Stalevo) is available in six different combinations: Stalevo 50 (carbidopa 12.5 mg/levodopa 50 mg/entacapone 200 mg), Stalevo 75 (carbidopa 18.75 mg/levodopa 75 mg/entacapone 200 mg), Stalevo 100 (carbidopa 25 mg/levodopa 100 mg/entacapone 200 mg), Stalevo 125 (carbidopa 31.25 mg/levodopa 125 mg/entacapone 200 mg), Stalevo 150 (carbidopa 37.5 mg/levodopa 150 mg/entacapone 200 mg), and Stalevo 200 (carbidopa 50 mg/levodopa 200 mg/entacapone 200 mg). This triple combination is indicated in PD patients as a substitute for immediate-release carbidopa/levodopa and entacapone previously administered separately [97].

Tolcapone (Tasmar) has a half-life of approximately 2–3 h with maximum plasma concentrations occurring in approximately 2 h. It is initiated at 100 mg three times a day and increased to 200 mg three times a day if needed [98]. Tolcapone should always be used with levodopa. Due to the risk of fatal hepatotoxicity, it may only be used in PD patients who have tried all other antiparkinsonian medications, and serum ALT and AST should be tested at baseline, every 2–4 weeks for the first 6 months, and then as clinically indicated. Tolcapone should be discontinued if the patient does not have a response or in the event of a two times increase in the upper limit of ALT and AST [99].

Anticholinergics and Amantadine

Anticholinergics were used in the treatment of PD before the discovery of levodopa. The basis for using these drugs is that in PD the nigral dopaminergic neurons that inhibit the GABAergic output from the striatum are lost. This allows cholinergic neurons in the striatum to exert an unopposed excitatory effect on these GABAergic neurons with resulting inhibition of the motor system. Anticholinergic drugs can reduce this effect. However, they are poorly tolerated by elderly patients due to their cognitive side effects. Other antimuscarinic side effects such as dry mouth, constipation, and reduced bladder outflow may also occur. Their use is mostly restricted to patients with tremor that is intractable to levodopa treatment [100].

Anticholinergics are generally well absorbed orally and usually require dosing two or three times a day. Anticholinergics most commonly used in the treatment of PD include trihexyphenidyl (Artane) and benztropine (Cogentin). Anticholinergics should be started at low doses and increased very slowly. Contraindications include narrow-angle glaucoma, tachycardia, prostate hypertrophy, gastrointestinal obstruction, and megacolon. Common side effects include blurring of vision, nausea, constipation, urinary retention, and dry mouth. Confusion, hallucinations, psychosis, and sedation may also occur. Central side effects occur more often in the elderly and in patients with impaired cognitive function [101].

Amantadine is a glutamate antagonist that increases release of dopamine at the nerve terminals and has anticholinergic properties. It may be used in early PD, but cognitive side effects may occur due to its anticholinergic properties. Due to its glutamate antagonist properties, it has a role as an anti-dyskinetic agent in later stages of PD [102]. Amantadine is well absorbed orally, with peak blood levels occurring in 2–4 h. It should be avoided in patients with renal failure. The usual dose is 200–300 mg/day in divided doses. Side effects of amantadine include dizziness, anxiety, impaired coordination, insomnia, and nervousness. Nausea and vomiting occur in 5–10 % of patients. In some patients, pedal edema and a type of skin rash called livedo reticularis can require discontinuation of therapy [103].

Management of Motor Fluctuations and Dyskinesia

While the immediate response to levodopa is often dramatic, the long-term use is limited by the development of motor fluctuations. The most common of these are an end-of-dose wearing off with a return of symptoms before the next dose is due, also called the wearing-off effect. The duration of response becomes increasingly shorter and patients who were previously well controlled on three to four doses a day may need a higher frequency of dosing. Some 40–50 % of patients on levodopa monotherapy will experience a degree of motor fluctuations at the 5-year mark [104]. Over time the fluctuations may occur at random with respect to the timing of medications described as the on–off effect. Dose-failures may occur, and the latency to clinical effect may be prolonged [105]. The addition of a COMT inhibitor or a MAO-B inhibitor can increase the duration of action of levodopa, thus allowing for a smoother therapeutic effect. Adding a dopamine agonist as an adjunct therapy may also reduce wearing off, as these drugs have a longer half-life than levodopa [106].

Dyskinesia is another limiting factor in the long-term use of levodopa. These occur in the form of involuntary choreiform movements, usually at the peak of the levodopa dose. However, other forms, including end-of-dose dyskinesia and diphasic dyskinesia, are also seen [107]. The incidence of dyskinesia in patients on CD/LD monotherapy was approximately 40 % at the 5-year mark compared with an incidence of approximately 10 % on ropinirole or pramipexole. Most dyskinesias represent a peak-dose response to levodopa, thus reducing individual doses, and administering doses more frequently can help reduce dyskinesia. In patients who have dyskinesia, switching from sustained-release formulations of levodopa to regular formulations may reduce the duration of the dyskinesia after any given dose. Amantadine also has a role as an anti-dyskinetic agent [108].

Management of Cognitive and Psychiatric Symptoms

Anxiety and depression are common comorbid symptoms of PD and may even precede the onset of motor symptoms. A wide variety of selective serotonin uptake inhibitors (SSRIs) have been successfully used in the treatment of PD. These drugs must be used with caution when patients are on MAO-B inhibitors. Benzodiazepines may be used in the treatment of anxiety, but long-term use should be avoided if possible [109].

Dementia is a common finding in later stages of PD. Rivastigmine showed a beneficial effect in PD-associated dementia both as an oral preparation and as a transdermal patch. GI side effects are less common with the patch, but skin irritation may be a limiting factor in some cases [110]. PD is also associated with hallucinations, paranoid symptoms, and psychosis in later stages. The dopamine agonists are more likely to have these side effects because they have a relatively high affinity for D3 dopamine receptors present in the limbic system. Traditional neuroleptics such as haloperidol should be avoided because they can cause a marked worsening of motor symptoms of PD due to their dopamine antagonist effects. Of the novel neuroleptics, clozapine and quetiapine have been used with some degree of success, but clozapine requires frequent monitoring for agranulocytosis [111].

Treatment of Nonmotor Symptoms

While PD has been recognized as a movement disorder, its nonmotor symptoms have been generally less well recognized though documented in the literature. James Parkinson himself described sleep disorders, constipation, urinary incontinence, and delirium in his seminal essay. Nonmotor symptoms can occur at any stage of the disease including early PD and can even be a marker of the disease state prior to development of motor symptoms, the so-called premotor phase of the disease [112].

In addition to the cognitive and psychiatric symptoms discussed above, hyposmia, disturbances of sleep–wake cycle regulation, and features of autonomic dysfunction, including orthostatic hypotension, urogenital dysfunction, and constipation, are commonly seen [113]. There is no specific treatment for hyposmia. Sleep–wake cycle disorders in PD include insomnia, EDS, and REM sleep behavior disorder (RBD) [114]. Modafinil was shown to be helpful in treating EDS in a small clinical trial [115]. Attention to good sleep hygiene is important in addressing insomnia. Quetiapine can be helpful in insomnia in the setting of PD; however, long-term use should be approached with caution [116]. Treatment options for RBD include benzodiazepines and melatonin. Clonazepam is the preferred benzodiazepine as it is long-acting and lasts through the night. It can also help reduce off-state dystonia that may occur through the night as the dopaminergic medications wear off. The mechanism of action of clonazepam may include controlling phasic locomotor activity at the brainstem level and modifying dream content in REM sleep [117].

Orthostatic hypotension when occurring soon after diagnosis raises suspicion of a parkinson-plus syndrome such as MSA. However, it is common and can have a significant adverse impact on the quality of life in the later stages of PD [118]. Management includes non-pharmacological measures such as increasing salt in the diet and pressure stockings. Fludrocortisone can also be helpful in this setting [119]. Midodrine has been shown to be helpful in neurogenic orthostatic hypotension and can also be helpful in the PD setting [120]. Botulinum toxin for sialorrhea, sildenafil for erectile dysfunction, and lubiprostone and probiotics for constipation are other suggestions for the management of these troubling non-motor symptoms. There is a great need for well-designed clinical trials to allow firm evidence-based recommendations for non-motor PD symptoms [121].

Neuroprotective Strategies

There is no drug with a proven neuroprotective effect in PD. Neuroprotective strategies are generally aimed at reducing oxidative stress or improving handling of free radicals through the use of antioxidant molecules. The DATATOP trial, one of the earliest studies of neuroprotection, compared selegiline with high-dose vitamin E in PD. The endpoint was the delay in the need for symptomatic treatment with levodopa. While vitamin E was no better than placebo, patients on selegiline required levodopa about 6 months later. Subsequent studies, however, indicated that this was due to a mild symptomatic benefit of selegiline rather than a true neuroprotective effect [72]. The ADAGIO trial used a delayed start design with placebo compared to patients started on rasagiline immediately or 9 months after the baseline visit. All groups were followed for a total of 18 months from the baseline visit. While the 1 mg dose of rasagiline met the hierarchical statistical criteria, the 2 mg dose failed to do so. Possible explanations for failure of the 2-mg doses that were proposed include a U-shaped dose–response effect and the presence of a "floor effect" on the rating scale used in the study, with patients with the mildest disease failing to show benefit. A post-hoc analysis did reveal a statistically significant difference in the most severely affected quartile even on the 2-mg dose [122]. Coenzyme Q10 was hypothesized to have a neuroprotective effect due to its role as an antioxidant and free radical scavenger. However, clinical trials have failed to support any neuroprotective role for Coenzyme Q10 in PD [123].

Surgical Treatment of Parkinson's Disease

With the advent of levodopa, the surgical treatment of PD receded into the background for some years. However, with time the limitations of levodopa treatment in the long-term, including motor fluctuations and dyskinesia, led to the recognition that surgical treatment could play a role in selected cases. Thalamotomy helped control intractable tremor, and pallidotomy helped reduce severe dyskinesia. The discovery that high-frequency stimulation of the surgical targets could control symptoms while offering a relative degree of reversibility in case of suboptimal target localization led to a resurgence of surgical treatment for PD. Deep brain stimulation (DBS) has become part of standard of care in selected patients in the later stages of PD [124].

The initial targets for DBS surgery were based on the experience of lesioning techniques of thalamotomy and pallidotomy. The corresponding targets included the ViM nucleus of the thalamus and the internal segment of the globus pallidus (GPi). The ViM was found to be an excellent target for control of tremor from PD; however, its impact on other features was limited. The GPi was found to be a good target in patients with troublesome dyskinesias [124]. The subthalamic nucleus (STN) was also explored as a surgical target and was found to be of benefit in control of overall symptoms of PD as well as allowing for a reduction in medication dosing to a somewhat greater extent than with GPi DBS. The current consensus appears to be that both GPi and STN are viable targets for overall control of PD symptoms including tremor. The choice of target is usually determined by institutional preferences. Alterative targets have included the pedunculopontine nucleus for patients with prominent freezing of gait. However, clinical experience is limited for alternative targets [125].

Appropriate patient selection is critical with respect to both the type of parkinsonism and duration and severity of the disease. Only patients with idiopathic PD are suitable candidates and those with parkinson-plus syndromes should be excluded. Appendicular symptoms such as tremor and dyskinesia improve more than axial symptoms such as gait and balance. In general, it is difficult to improve symptoms beyond the level seen in the patient's best "on-state" prior to surgery. There is approximately a 2 % risk of hemorrhage that can lead to greater disability or even death. Hence, surgery should only be offered to patients who have either significant motor fluctuations or specific symptoms such as tremor or dyskinesia that are intractable to medication adjustments. On the other hand, surgery should not be offered too late in the course of the disease when both physical debilitation and cognitive symptoms can play a limiting role preventing a successful outcome [125]. Alternative surgical therapies such as stem cell implantation, nerve growth factor infusion, and gene therapy are not part of current clinical practice, although research is ongoing both at the basic science level and in the form of early clinical trials [126].

References

1. Dalvi A. Parkinsonism. In: Bope E, Kellerman R, editors. Conn's current therapy. Philadelphia: Saunders Elsevier; 2013.
2. Dalvi A. Parkinsonism. Dis Mon. 2012;58:690–707.
3. Bhidayasiri R, Reichmann H. Different diagnostic criteria for Parkinson disease: what are the pitfalls? J Neural Transm. 2013;120:619–25.
4. Khan TS. Off spells and dyskinesias: pharmacologic management of motor complications. Cleve Clin J Med. 2012;79 Suppl 2:S8–13.
5. Pandya M, Kubu CS, Giroux ML. Parkinson disease: not just a movement disorder. Cleve Clin J Med. 2008;75:856–64.
6. Watson GS, Leverenz JB. Profile of cognitive impairment in Parkinson's disease. Brain Pathol. 2010;20:640–5.
7. Cummings JL, Henchcliffe C, Schaier S, Simuni T, Waxman A, Kemp P. The role of dopaminergic imaging in patients with symptoms of dopaminergic system neurodegeneration. Brain. 2011;134:3146–66.
8. Parkinson J. An essay on the shaking palsy. London: Sherwood, Neeley and Jones; 1817.
9. Gower W. A manual of diseases of the nervous system. Philadelphia: P. Blakiston; 1888.
10. Tanner CM, Ottman R, Goldman SM, Ellenberg J, Chan P, Mayeux R, et al. Parkinson disease in twins: an etiologic study. JAMA. 1999;281:341–6.
11. Polymeropoulos MH, Lavedan C, Leroy E, Ide SE, Dehejia A, Dutra A, et al. Mutation in the alpha-synuclein gene identified in families with Parkinson's disease. Science. 1997;276: 2045–7.
12. Moore DJ, West AB, Dawson VL, Dawson TM. Molecular pathophysiology of Parkinson's disease. Annu Rev Neurosci. 2005;28:57–87.
13. Burke WJ, Kumar VB, Pandey N, Panneton WM, Gan Q, Franko MW, et al. Aggregation of alpha-synuclein by DOPAL, the monoamine oxidase metabolite of dopamine. Acta Neuropathol. 2008;115:193–203.
14. Xu J, Kao SY, Lee FJ, Song W, Jin LW, Yankner BA. Dopamine-dependent neurotoxicity of alpha-synuclein: a mechanism for selective neurodegeneration in Parkinson disease. Nat Med. 2002;8:600–6.
15. Orr CF, Rowe DB, Halliday GM. An inflammatory review of Parkinson's disease. Prog Neurobiol. 2002;68:325–40.
16. Hubble JP, Cao T, Hassanein RE, Neuberger JS, Koller WC. Risk factors for Parkinson's disease. Neurology. 1993;43:1693–7.
17. Wang WZ, Fang XH, Cheng XM, Jiang DH, Lin ZJ. A case-control study on the environmental risk factors of Parkinson's disease in Tianjin, China. Neuroepidemiology. 1993;12: 209–18.
18. Wright Willis A, Evanoff BA, Lian M, Criswell SR, Racette BA. Geographic and ethnic variation in Parkinson disease: a population-based study of US Medicare beneficiaries. Neuroepidemiology. 2010;34:143–51.
19. Lock EA, Zhang J, Checkoway H. Solvents and Parkinson disease: a systematic review of toxicological and epidemiological evidence. Toxicol Appl Pharmacol. 2013;266:345–55.
20. Goldman SM, Quinlan PJ, Ross GW, Marras C, Meng C, Bhudhikanok GS, et al. Solvent exposures and Parkinson disease risk in twins. Ann Neurol. 2012;71:776–84.
21. Racette BA, Criswell SR, Lundin JI, Hobson A, Seixas N, Kotzbauer PT, et al. Increased risk of parkinsonism associated with welding exposure. Neurotoxicology. 2012;33:1356–61.
22. Mortimer JA, Borenstein AR, Nelson LM. Associations of welding and manganese exposure with Parkinson disease: review and meta-analysis. Neurology. 2012;79:1174–80.
23. Tan EK, Skipper LM. Pathogenic mutations in Parkinson disease. Hum Mutat. 2007;28: 641–53.
24. Tanner CM. Is the cause of Parkinson's disease environmental or hereditary? Evidence from twin studies. Adv Neurol. 2003;91:133–42.

25. Wood-Kaczmar A, Gandhi S, Wood NW. Understanding the molecular causes of Parkinson's disease. Trends Mol Med. 2006;12:521–8.
26. Gosal D, Ross OA, Toft M. Parkinson's disease: the genetics of a heterogeneous disorder. Eur J Neurol. 2006;13:616–27.
27. Spratt DE, Martinez-Torres RJ, Noh YJ, Mercier P, Manczyk N, Barber KR, et al. A molecular explanation for the recessive nature of parkin-linked Parkinson's disease. Nat Commun. 2013;4:1983.
28. Rango M, Arighi A, Marotta G, Ronchi D, Bresolin N. PINK1 parkinsonism and Parkinson disease: distinguishable brain mitochondrial function and metabolomics. Mitochondrion. 2013;13:59–61.
29. Johnson BN, Charan RA, LaVoie MJ. Recognizing the cooperative and independent mitochondrial functions of Parkin and PINK1. Cell Cycle. 2012;11:2775–6.
30. Abou-Sleiman PM, Healy DG, Wood NW. Causes of Parkinson's disease: genetics of DJ-1. Cell Tissue Res. 2004;318:185–8.
31. Miyazaki S, Yanagida T, Nunome K, Ishikawa S, Inden M, Kitamura Y, et al. DJ-1-binding compounds prevent oxidative stress-induced cell death and movement defect in Parkinson's disease model rats. J Neurochem. 2008;105:2418–34.
32. Healy DG, Falchi M, O'Sullivan SS, Bonifati V, Durr A, Bressman S, et al. International LRRK2 consortium. Phenotype, genotype, and worldwide genetic penetrance of LRRK2-associated Parkinson's disease: a case-control study. Lancet Neurol. 2008;7:583–90.
33. Ozelius LJ, Senthil G, Saunders-Pullman R, Ohmann E, Deligtisch A, Tagliati M, et al. LRRK2 G2019S as a cause of Parkinson's disease in Ashkenazi Jews. N Engl J Med. 2006;354:424–5.
34. Lesage S, Dürr A, Tazir M, Lohmann E, Leutenegger AL, Janin S, et al. French Parkinson's Disease Genetics Study Group. LRRK2 G2019S as a cause of Parkinson's disease in North African Arabs. N Engl J Med. 2006;354:422–3.
35. Puschmann A. Monogenic Parkinson's disease and parkinsonism: clinical phenotypes and frequencies of known mutations. Parkinsonism Relat Disord. 2013;19:407–15.
36. West AB, Moore DJ, Biskup S, Bugayenko A, Smith WW, Ross CA, et al. Parkinson's disease-associated mutations in leucine-rich repeat kinase 2 augment kinase activity. Proc Natl Acad Sci U S A. 2005;102:16842–7.
37. Góomez-Suaga P, Fdez E, Blanca Ramírez M, Hilfiker S. A link between autophagy and the pathophysiology of LRRK2 in Parkinson's disease. Parkinsons Dis. 2012;2012:324521.
38. Zhang ZJ, Burgunder JM, An XK, Wu Y, Chen WJ, Zhang JH, et al. Lack of evidence for association of a UCH-L1 S18Y polymorphism with Parkinson's disease in a Han-Chinese population. Neurosci Lett. 2008;442:200–2.
39. Liu Y, Fallon L, Lashuel HA, Liu Z, Lansbury Jr PT. The UCH-L1 gene encodes two opposing enzymatic activities that affect alpha-synuclein degradation and Parkinson's disease susceptibility. Cell. 2002;111:209–18.
40. Ardley HC, Scott GB, Rose SA, Tan NG, Robinson PA. UCH-L1 aggresome formation in response to proteasome impairment indicates a role in inclusion formation in Parkinson's disease. J Neurochem. 2004;90:379–91.
41. Kim RH, Smith PD, Aleyasin H, Hayley S, Mount MP, Pownall S, et al. Hypersensitivity of DJ-1-deficient mice to 1-methyl-4-phenyl-1,2,3,6-tetrahydropyridine (MPTP) and oxidative stress. Proc Natl Acad Sci U S A. 2005;102:5215–20.
42. Irrcher I, Aleyasin H, Seifert EL, Hewitt SJ, Chhabra S, Phillips M, et al. Loss of the Parkinson's disease-linked gene DJ-1 perturbs mitochondrial dynamics. Hum Mol Genet. 2010;19:3734–46.
43. Ransmayr G. Constantin von Economo's contribution to the understanding of movement disorders. Mov Disord. 2007;22:469–75.
44. Dale RC, Webster R, Gill D. Contemporary encephalitis lethargica presenting with agitated catatonia, stereotypy, and dystonia-parkinsonism. Mov Disord. 2007;22:2281–4.
45. Woulfe J, Hoogendoorn H, Tarnopolsky M, Muñoz DG. Monoclonal antibodies against Epstein–Barr virus cross-react with alpha-synuclein in human brain. Neurology. 2000;55: 1398–401.

46. McGeer PL, Yasojima K, McGeer EG. Inflammation in Parkinson's disease. Adv Neurol. 2001;86:83–9.
47. Kumar A, Calne SM, Schulzer M, Mak E, Wszolek Z, Van Netten C, et al. Clustering of Parkinson disease: shared cause or coincidence? Arch Neurol. 2004;61:1057–60.
48. Spillantini MG, Schmidt ML, Lee VM, Trojanowski JQ, Jakes R, Goedert M. Alpha-synuclein in Lewy bodies. Nature. 1997;388:839–40.
49. Marques O, Outeiro TF. Alpha-synuclein: from secretion to dysfunction and death. Cell Death Dis. 2012;3:e350.
50. Goedert M, Spillantini MG, Del Tredici K, Braak H. 100 years of Lewy pathology. Nat Rev Neurol. 2013;9:13–24.
51. Dunning CJ, Reyes JF, Steiner JA, Brundin P. Can Parkinson's disease pathology be propagated from one neuron to another? Prog Neurobiol. 2012;97:205–19.
52. George S, Rey NL, Reichenbach N, Steiner JA, Brundin P. α-Synuclein: the long distance runner. Brain Pathol. 2013;23:350–7.
53. Kordower JH, Brundin P. Lewy body pathology in long-term fetal nigral transplants: is Parkinson's disease transmitted from one neural system to another? Neuropsychopharmacology. 2009;34:254.
54. McGeer PL, McGeer EG. Glial reactions in Parkinson's disease. Mov Disord. 2008;23: 474–83.
55. Schwab C, McGeer PL. Inflammatory aspects of Alzheimer disease and other neurodegenerative disorders. J Alzheimers Dis. 2008;13:359–69.
56. Pabon MM, Jernberg JN, Morganti J, Contreras J, Hudson CE, Klein RL, et al. A spirulina-enhanced diet provides neuroprotection in an α-synuclein model of Parkinson's disease. PLoS One. 2012;7:e45256.
57. Garrido-Gil P, Joglar B, Rodriguez-Perez AI, Guerra MJ, Labandeira-Garcia JL. Involvement of PPAR-γ in the neuroprotective and anti-inflammatory effects of angiotensin type 1 receptor inhibition: effects of the receptor antagonist telmisartan and receptor deletion in a mouse MPTP model of Parkinson's disease. J Neuroinflammation. 2012;9:38.
58. Ridder DA, Schwaninger M. In search of the neuroprotective mechanism of thiazolidinediones in Parkinson's disease. Exp Neurol. 2012;238:133–7.
59. Ulusoy GK, Celik T, Kayir H, Gürsoy M, Isik AT, Uzbay TI. Effects of pioglitazone and retinoic acid in a rotenone model of Parkinson's disease. Brain Res Bull. 2011;85:380–4.
60. Chan CS, Gertler TS, Surmeier DJ. A molecular basis for the increased vulnerability of substantia nigra dopamine neurons in aging and Parkinson's disease. Mov Disord. 2010;25 Suppl 1:S63–70.
61. Langston JW, Ballard P, Tetrud JW, Irwin I. Chronic Parkinsonism in humans due to a product of meperidine-analog synthesis. Science. 1983;219:979–80.
62. McCormack AL, Thiruchelvam M, Manning-Bog AB, Thiffault C, Langston JW, Cory-Slechta DA, et al. Environmental risk factors and Parkinson's disease: selective degeneration of nigral dopaminergic neurons caused by the herbicide paraquat. Neurobiol Dis. 2002;10: 119–27.
63. Jenner P. Oxidative stress and Parkinson's disease. Handb Clin Neurol. 2007;83:507–20.
64. Jenner P, Olanow CW. The pathogenesis of cell death in Parkinson's disease. Neurology. 2006;66:S24–36.
65. Cipriani S, Chen X, Schwarzschild MA. Urate: a novel biomarker of Parkinson's disease risk, diagnosis and prognosis. Biomark Med. 2010;4:701–12.
66. Schapira AH. Evidence for mitochondrial dysfunction in Parkinson's disease—a critical appraisal. Mov Disord. 1994;9:125–38.
67. McInnes J. Insights on altered mitochondrial function and dynamics in the pathogenesis of neurodegeneration. Transl Neurodegener. 2013;2:12.
68. Carlsson A. Thirty years of dopamine research. Adv Neurol. 1993;60:1–10.
69. Cotzias GC, Van Woert MH, Schiffer LM. Aromatic amino acids and modification of parkinsonism. N Engl J Med. 1967;276:374–9.

70. Rao SK, Vakil SD, Calne DB, Hilson A. Augmenting the action of levodopa. Postgrad Med J. 1972;48:653–6.
71. Tambasco N, Simoni S, Marsili E, Sacchini E, Murasecco D, Cardaioli G, et al. Clinical aspects and management of levodopa-induced dyskinesia. Parkinsons Dis. 2012;2012:745947.
72. Rascol O, Lozano A, Stern M, Poewe W. Milestones in Parkinson's disease therapeutics. Mov Disord. 2011;26:1072–82.
73. Merello M, Lees AJ, Webster R, Bovingdon M, Gordin A. Effect of entacapone, a peripherally acting catechol-O-methyltransferase inhibitor, on the motor response to acute treatment with levodopa in patients with Parkinson's disease. J Neurol Neurosurg Psychiatry. 1994;57:186–9.
74. Schapira AH. Present and future drug treatment for Parkinson's disease. J Neurol Neurosurg Psychiatry. 2005;76:1472–8.
75. Markham C, Diamond SG, Treciokas LJ. Carbidopa in Parkinson disease and in nausea and vomiting of levodopa. Arch Neurol. 1974;31:128–33.
76. LeWitt PA, Nelson MV, Berchou RC, Galloway MP, Kesaree N, Kareti D, et al. Controlled-release carbidopa/levodopa (Sinemet 50/200 CR4): clinical and pharmacokinetic studies. Neurology. 1989;39:45–53. discussion 59.
77. Parcopa: a rapidly dissolving formulation of carbidopa/levodopa. Med Lett Drugs Ther. 2005;47(1201):12. PubMed PMID: 15706700.
78. Poewe W, Antonini A, Zijlmans JC, Burkhard PR, Vingerhoets F. Levodopa in the treatment of Parkinson's disease: an old drug still going strong. Clin Interv Aging. 2010;5:229–38.
79. Watts RL. The role of dopamine agonists in early Parkinson's disease. Neurology. 1997;49:S34–48.
80. Voon V, Mehta AR, Hallett M. Impulse control disorders in Parkinson's disease: recent advances. Curr Opin Neurol. 2011;24:324–30.
81. Shannon KM, Bennett Jr JP, Friedman JH. Efficacy of pramipexole, a novel dopamine agonist, as monotherapy in mild to moderate Parkinson's disease. The Pramipexole Study Group. Neurology. 1997;49:724–8.
82. Hametner EM, Seppi K, Poewe W. Role and clinical utility of pramipexole extended release in the treatment of early Parkinson's disease. Clin Interv Aging. 2012;7:83–8.
83. Rascol O, Brooks DJ, Korczyn AD, De Deyn PP, Clarke CE, Lang AE. A five-year study of the incidence of dyskinesia in patients with early Parkinson's disease who were treated with ropinirole or levodopa. 056 Study Group. N Engl J Med. 2000;342:1484–91.
84. Nashatizadeh MM, Lyons KE, Pahwa R. A review of ropinirole prolonged release in Parkinson's disease. Clin Interv Aging. 2009;4:179–86.
85. Watts RL, Jankovic J, Waters C, Rajput A, Boroojerdi B, Rao J. Randomized, blind, controlled trial of transdermal rotigotine in early Parkinson disease. Neurology. 2007;68:272–6.
86. LeWitt PA, Lyons KE, Pahwa R, SP 650 Study Group. Advanced Parkinson disease treated with rotigotine transdermal system: PREFER Study. Neurology. 2007;68:1262–7.
87. Sanford M, Scott LJ. Rotigotine transdermal patch: a review of its use in the treatment of Parkinson's disease. CNS Drugs. 2011;2:699–719.
88. Stacy M, Silver D. Apomorphine for the acute treatment of "off" episodes in Parkinson's disease. Parkinsonism Relat Disord. 2008;14:85–92.
89. Elmer LW, Bertoni JM. The increasing role of monoamine oxidase type B inhibitors in Parkinson's disease therapy. Expert Opin Pharmacother. 2008;9:2759–72.
90. Olanow CW, Mytilineou C, Tatton W. Current status of selegiline as a neuroprotective agent in Parkinson's disease. Mov Disord. 1998;13 Suppl 1:55–8.
91. Stern MB, Marek KL, Friedman J, Hauser RA, LeWitt PA, Tarsy D, et al. Double-blind, randomized, controlled trial of rasagiline as monotherapy in early Parkinson's disease patients. Mov Disord. 2004;19:916–23.
92. Stocchi F, Rabey JM. Effect of rasagiline as adjunct therapy to levodopa on severity of OFF in Parkinson's disease. Eur J Neurol. 2011;18:1373–8.
93. Perez-Lloret S, Rascol O. Safety of rasagiline for the treatment of Parkinson's disease. Expert Opin Drug Saf. 2011;10:633–43.

94. Marsala SZ, Gioulis M, Ceravolo R, Tinazzi M. A systematic review of catechol-O-methyltransferase inhibitors: efficacy and safety in clinical practice. Clin Neuropharmacol. 2012;35:185–90.
95. Rinne UK, Larsen JP, Siden A, Worm-Petersen J. Entacapone enhances the response to levodopa in Parkinsonian patients with motor fluctuations. Nomecomt Study Group. Neurology. 1998;51:1309–14.
96. Brooks DJ. Safety and tolerability of COMT inhibitors. Neurology. 2004;62:S39–46.
97. Hauser RA. Levodopa/carbidopa/entacapone (Stalevo). Neurology. 2004;62:S64–71.
98. Kurth MC, Adler CH, Hilaire MS, Singer C, Waters C, LeWitt P, et al. Tolcapone improves motor function and reduces levodopa requirement in patients with Parkinson's disease experiencing motor fluctuations: a multicenter, double-blind, randomized, placebo-controlled trial. Tolcapone Fluctuator Study Group I. Neurology. 1997;48:81–7.
99. Truong DD. Tolcapone: review of its pharmacology and use as adjunctive therapy in patients with Parkinson's disease. Clin Interv Aging. 2009;4:109–13.
100. Brocks DR. Anticholinergic drugs used in Parkinson's disease: an overlooked class of drugs from a pharmacokinetic perspective. J Pharm Pharm Sci. 1999;2:39–46.
101. Fahn S, Burke R, Stern Y. Antimuscarinic drugs in the treatment of movement disorders. Prog Brain Res. 1990;84:389–97.
102. Blanchet PJ, Metman LV, Chase TN. Renaissance of amantadine in the treatment of Parkinson's disease. Adv Neurol. 2003;91:251–7.
103. Crosby N, Deane KH, Clarke CE. Amantadine in Parkinson's disease. Cochrane Database Syst Rev. 2003;1:CD003468.
104. Stocchi F, Jenner P, Obeso JA. When do levodopa motor fluctuations first appear in Parkinson's disease? Eur Neurol. 2010;63:257–66.
105. Melamed E, Ziv I, Djaldetti R. Management of motor complications in advanced Parkinson's disease. Mov Disord. 2007;22:S379–84.
106. Pahwa R, Lyons KE. Levodopa-related wearing-off in Parkinson's disease: identification and management. Curr Med Res Opin. 2009;25:841–9.
107. Fahn S. The spectrum of levodopa-induced dyskinesias. Ann Neurol. 2000;47:S2–9.
108. Pahwa R, Lyons KE. Early diagnosis of Parkinson's disease: recommendations from diagnostic clinical guidelines. Am J Manag Care. 2010;16:S94–9.
109. Weintraub D, Burn DJ. Parkinson's disease: the quintessential neuropsychiatric disorder. Mov Disord. 2011;26:1022–31.
110. Svenningsson P, Westman E, Ballard C, Aarsland D. Cognitive impairment in patients with Parkinson's disease: diagnosis, biomarkers, and treatment. Lancet Neurol. 2012;11:697–707.
111. Starkstein SE, Brockman S, Hayhow BD. Psychiatric syndromes in Parkinson's disease. Curr Opin Psychiatry. 2012;25:468–72.
112. Dalvi A. Premotor symptoms. In: Pahwa R, Lyons KE, editors. Handbook of Parkinson's disease. New York: Informa; 2013.
113. Poewe W. Non-motor symptoms in Parkinson's disease. Eur J Neurol. 2008;15:S14–20.
114. Comella CL. Sleep disorders in Parkinson's disease: an overview. Mov Disord. 2007;22:S367–73.
115. Högl B, Saletu M, Brandauer E, Glatzl S, Frauscher B, Seppi K, et al. Modafinil for the treatment of daytime sleepiness in Parkinson's disease: a double-blind, randomized, crossover, placebo-controlled polygraphic trial. Sleep. 2002;25:905–9.
116. Juri C, Chaná P, Tapia J, Kunstmann C, Parrao T. Quetiapine for insomnia in Parkinson disease: results from an open-label trial. Clin Neuropharmacol. 2005;28:185–7.
117. Lapierre O, Montplaisir J. Polysomnographic features of REM sleep behavior disorder: development of a scoring method. Neurology. 1992;42:1371–4.
118. Sánchez-Ferro A, Benito-León J, Gómez-Esteban JC. The management of orthostatic hypotension in Parkinson's disease. Front Neurol. 2013;4:64.
119. Schoffer KL, Henderson RD, O'Maley K, O'Sullivan JD. Nonpharmacological treatment, fludrocortisone, and domperidone for orthostatic hypotension in Parkinson's disease. Mov Disord. 2007;22:1543–9.

120. Low PA, Gilden JL, Freeman R, Sheng KN, McElligott MA. Efficacy of midodrine vs placebo in neurogenic orthostatic hypotension. A randomized, double-blind multicenter study. Midodrine Study Group. JAMA. 1997;277:1046–51.
121. Perez-Lloret S, Rey MV, Pavy-Le Traon A, Rascol O. Emerging drugs for autonomic dysfunction in Parkinson's disease. Expert Opin Emerg Drugs. 2013;18:39–53.
122. Schapira AH. Monoamine oxidase B inhibitors for the treatment of Parkinson's disease: a review of symptomatic and potential disease-modifying effects. CNS Drugs. 2011;25:1061–71.
123. Storch A, Jost WH, Vieregge P, Spiegel J, Greulich W, Durner J, et al. German Coenzyme Q(10) Study Group. Randomized, double-blind, placebo-controlled trial on symptomatic effects of coenzyme Q(10) in Parkinson disease. Arch Neurol. 2007;64:938–44.
124. Rodriguez-Oroz MC, Moro E, Krack P. Long-term outcomes of surgical therapies for Parkinson's disease. Mov Disord. 2012;27:1718–28.
125. Bronstein JM, Tagliati M, Alterman RL, Lozano AM, Volkmann J, Stefani A, et al. Deep brain stimulation for Parkinson disease: an expert consensus and review of key issues. Arch Neurol. 2011;68:165.
126. Hickey P, Stacy M. Available and emerging treatments for Parkinson's disease: a review. Drug Des Devel Ther. 2011;5:241–54.

Neuropathology of Parkinson's Disease

Kurt A. Jellinger

Introduction

Parkinson's disease (PD) (OMIN 168600), or "brain stem type of Lewy body disease," is the most frequent neurodegenerative movement disorder in advanced age, affecting 1–3 % of the population over 65 years and an estimated seven to ten million people worldwide [1], which will considerably increase in the future [2]. It is characterized by progressive degeneration of the dopaminergic nigrostriatal system, responsible for the core motor symptoms, and by involvement of many other neuronal networks and extraneuronal organs. These lesions are associated with widespread deposition of phosphorylated α-synuclein (α-syn), the major protein marker and biological hallmark of PD and other synucleinopathies [3, 4], as well as intracytoplasmic Lewy bodies (LB), dystrophic neurites (LN) in cell processes, and other inclusions. Multifocal neurodegenerative lesions are affecting the central, peripheral, and autonomic nervous system and many other organs (e.g., adrenals, retina, heart, skin) [5–11]. Recent studies have confirmed the multiorgan distribution of α-syn and Lewy pathologies [5, 12–15]. There is early involvement of the peripheral autonomic system, spinal cord, and adrenal medulla in neurologically unimpaired subjects (incidental Lewy body disease, or ILBD) considered as initial or preclinical stage of PD [16, 17]. In sporadic PD, the pathologic process initially involves preganglionic neurons, plexuses, and nerves, particularly in the gastrointestinal system [18–23] and is suggested to advance caudo-rostrally from there along the neuraxis [15, 24, 25]. The resulting biochemical deficits cause the heterogeneous clinical picture of PD including the core features—tremor at rest, rigidity, akinesia (or bradykinesia), and postural instability (TRAP)—and often early presenting nonmotor deficits [26–31]. However, PD can present with a variety of additional clinical features and complications in advanced stages [32].

K.A. Jellinger, M.D. (✉)
Institute of Clinical Neurobiology, Vienna, Austria
e-mail: kurt.jellinger@univie.ac.at

M. Thomas (ed.), *Inflammation in Parkinson's Disease: Scientific and Clinical Aspects*, DOI 10.1007/978-3-319-08046-8_2, © Springer International Publishing Switzerland 2014

Various clinical phases and subtypes have been described [33–35], and the neuropathology underlying clinical variability in PD and other synucleinopathies has been reviewed [13, 36, 37].

Recent research has improved the clinical diagnostic criteria of PD [38–40] for which histopathological confirmation following new criteria using standardized methods of assessment of lesions by a semiquantitative grading system and immunohistochemical methods for the detection of α-syn/Lewy pathology are required [36, 41–43].

The etiology and pathogenesis of PD and other synucleinopathies are poorly understood, but the majority of PD cases may result from complex interactions between environmental factors and genetic background [44]. There is increasing evidence that the neurodegenerative process in PD is caused by a combination of complex mechanisms including dysregulation of mitochondrial bioenergetics and of calcium homeostasis, impaired protein turnover control, prion-like behavior of misfolded proteins, oxidative and nitritive stress, neuroinflammation and their complex interaction (for review, see [45, 46]).

This chapter will critically update the neuropathology of "sporadic" PD, formation and development of Lewy pathology including new guidelines, its relations with α-syn deposition, and their clinical relevance. Furthermore, it will discuss the spreading and grading of α-syn and its interaction with other pathologic proteins, clinicopathologic subtypes of PD, and major factors in the pathogenesis of PD. Several recent reviews of the neuropathology of sporadic PD [13, 47–49] and of genetic PD are available [50, 51].

Basic Neuropathology of PD

Degeneration of the Nigrostriatal System

The brain is usually grossly unremarkable or shows mild frontal atrophy and enlargement of the ventricles. There is no significant atrophy of the brain stem, which differs from progressive supranuclear palsy (PSP) and multisystem atrophy (MSA). The brain stem usually shows loss of the normally dark black pigment in the substantia nigra (SN) and locus coeruleus (LC).

Histopathology of PD is featured by widespread α-syn-immunoreactive deposits in neurons (Lewy bodies [LBs]) and dystrophic neurites (LNs) in nerve processes, as well as within the synaptic compartment, enriched in the presynaptic terminals [52, 53] throughout the CNS. It is associated with variable neuron loss in many subcortical nuclei, in particular the substantia nigra compacta (SNc), LC, nucleus basalis of Meynert (NBM), and dorsal motor nucleus of vagus (dmX), but also affecting many other neuronal systems. Severe depletion of melanized and dopaminergic neurons immunoreactive for tyrosine hydroxylase (TH), the key enzyme of dopamine synthesis, affects the A-9 group of SNc. It is most severe in the caudal and ventrolateral tier (about 98 %), projecting to the striatum, than in the matrix, and spreading along a caudorostral, lateromedial, and ventrodorsal progression [54].

This temporospatial disorder corresponds to a somatotopic pattern of dopaminergic terminal loss in the striatum that is more severe in the dorsal and caudal putamen, with later involvement of the ventral putamen and caudate nucleus [55].

Degeneration of the nigrostriatal system causes denervation of the striatum with dopamine loss, ranging from 44 to 98 % [56]. In earlier disease stages, dopamine depletion provokes an increased number of striatal dopaminergic neurons [57], which may be the result of a phenotypic shift and not neurogenesis [58]. Similar changes in the olfactory bulb could reflect a compensatory mechanism [59] that may be more efficient in younger PD patients [60], while MRI studies showed early volume changes in the striatum [61]. Higher nigrostriatal dopaminergic neuron loss occurs in early-onset than in late-onset PD [62]. Longitudinal PET studies identified dopamine dysfunction approximately 10 years before disease onset in older PD patients, which may be present for as long as 25 years in younger ones. Preclinical intervals thus vary depending on the age of onset. Younger PD patients are able to endure more damage to the dopaminergic system before the onset of motor symptoms.

The degree of area A-9 SNc cell loss and the resulting progression of striatal dopaminergic hypofunction (reduction of dopa uptake, TH and dopamine transporter [DAT] immunoreactivity), indicating the extent of loss of dopaminergic neurons and terminals in the striatum, are strongly correlated with disease duration and the severity of motor dysfunction [63–65]. Relative preservation of F-DOPA (fluorodopa) uptake in the anterior striatum may reflect a delay in pathologic involvement of the striatonigral projections, while loss of monoaminergic function in extranigral regions is delayed and occurs independently from striatonigral dysfunction in PD [64]. SN volume loss has been observed before basal forebrain degeneration in early PD [66]. Patients with end-stage PD showed a massive loss of SN neurons with significant atrophy of the remaining cells (20 % of controls) [67]. However, recent SPECT studies indicated that degeneration of the dopaminergic system is not total, even after many years of illness, the loss being more prominent in the putamen than in the caudate nucleus [68]. DAT immunoreactivity in the striatum is inversely correlated with the total α-syn burden but not with LB counts in the SN [69], which supports the concept of synaptic dysfunction or impairment of axonal transport of α-syn aggregation. Alterations in axonal transport proteins in sporadic and experimental PD have been confirmed [70].

Morphometric studies have shown a 35–40 % reduction in pigmented SN cells, with severe loss of DAT-immunoreactive neurons in older persons, with an estimated SN cell loss between 4.3 % and almost 10 % per decade [71, 72]. Stereologic studies of the human SN revealed a significant loss of pigmented (28.3 %) and TH+neurons (36.2 %) in older versus younger controls, with hypertrophy of cells in older subjects as a compensatory mechanism to allow normal motor function despite cell loss [72]. SN cell degeneration is preceded by loss of neurofilament proteins, neurofilament mRNA, neuronal TH and DAT immunoreactivity, and cyclooxygenase (COX) indicative of functional neuronal damage [73]. Neuronal loss is accompanied by extracellular release of neuromelanin with uptake by macrophages, rare neuronophagia, and astroglial reaction [74]. Microglial activation and corresponding dopaminergic terminal loss in the affected nigrostriatal system suggest that neuroinflammatory reactions contribute to the progressive degenerative process [75–80]. α-Syn has an important role in the initiation and maintenance of inflammation in PD [81], which is a double-edged sword that is protective in the early stage but becomes detrimental with disease progression [76].

Lewy pathology first appears in the ventrolateral parts of the SN and spreads to the paranigral nucleus, to the medial part, and, finally, to the dorsal tier of the SNc [82]. The proportion of LB-bearing and α-syn-positive SN neurons does not correlate with disease duration and is apparently stable over time, with 3.6 % of the neurons being involved on average, suggesting that during the course of the disease, the destruction of LBs may be equal to their production and that they are destroyed together with the afflicted neurons. With LB-bearing neurons having an estimated life span of around 6.2 months (15.9 months for any type of α-syn inclusion), neuronal loss of 71 %, necessary for the manifestation of motor symptoms, would be reached after about 20 years [83], which is in line with estimated standard progression of the disease. At the time of motor symptom onset, the extent of striatal dopamine marker loss exceeds that of dopaminergic SN neurons. Of note, the previous concept that PD motor symptoms first appear which more than 50 % of dopaminergic SN neurons are lost [65] has recently been changed by the finding that at the time of first diagnosis of PD, only around 30 % of dopaminergic SN neurons, but 50–60 % of their axon terminals have been lost [84]. This is preceded by substantial loss of dopamine markers in the nigrostriatal terminals in early phases of PD, while melanin-containing SN neurons more than TH+ cells may persist for a longer time [85].

Neuronal Vulnerability

That multiple neuronal systems are affected by α-syn/Lewy pathology is largely undiscussed. How these multiple systems become involved over time and the reasons for only certain neurons within different brain regions becoming affected is still a matter of conjecture and has been discussed [15, 86].

The neurodegenerative lesions in PD show a selective vulnerability of midbrain neurons rich in neuromelanin located in the densely populated ventral tier of the SNc, which are rich in DAT but poor in glycolytic enzymes and calbindin, a calcium-binding protein, which has a neuroprotective role by buffering effects of Ca^{2+} influx into cells. All are projection neurons with a long, thin axon that is unmyelinized or poorly myelinated. The selective vulnerability of A-9 nigral neurons may be related to increased iron content, making them susceptible to oxidative stress [87–92]. In later stages of degeneration, SN neurons show a significant reduction in intracellular pigment, whereas those of normal morphologic appearance exhibit increased pigment density associated with higher concentrations of α-syn. No such changes have been observed in other melanin-containing neurons in the A-10 areas in early PD, which emphasizes the selectivity of early neuromelanin changes in A-9 neurons [93]. Iron regulates α-syn expression at the translational level [94] and promotes α-syn aggregation [95]. Overexpression of α-syn by cells increases iron (II) levels [96], leading to their selective loss [97]. Increased concentrations of α-syn around pigment-associated lipid under oxidative conditions may trigger a cascade of events leading to intracellular aggregates of α-syn and dispersal of protective pigments to precipitate cell death [89, 93, 98].

SNc neurons in PD show reduced expression of brain-derived neurotrophic factor (BDNF) and reduced numbers of TrkB mRNA (a high-affinity BDNF-receptor) without a decrease in the remaining cells [99]. While biochemistry reveals no reduction of glial cell line-derived neurotrophic factor (GDNF) in the nigrostriatal regions in PD [100], immunohistochemistry showed a 20 % reduction of GDNF and loss of BDNF in both neurons and neuropil [101], but increased numbers of BDNF- and neurotrophin-3 (NT-3)-immunoreactive microglia around damaged neurons [102].

Selective increase of mitochondrial DNA deletions/rearrangements involves the SN but also other regions of the PD brain compared with age-matched controls, indicating that mitochondrial dysfunction is not limited to the SN [103]. This suggests that dopaminergic SN neurons are more dependent on mitochondrial energy metabolism and oxidative phosphorylation than other brain stem populations. Reduction of cerebral mitochondrial metabolism occurs early in PD, but whether it is a primary or secondary event remains to be elucidated [104].

Conversely, most dopaminergic neurons that resist degeneration in PD are located in the scantly populated dorsal tier of SNc and contain calbindin and glycolytic enzymes but are poor in DAT, therefore being involved only in terminal stages of PD [105, 106]. The A-10 group of dopaminergic neurons—ventral tegmental area, nucleus parabrachialis, and nucleus parabrachialis pigmentosus—projecting to the striatal matrix, thalamus, cortical, and limbic areas (mesocorticolimbic system), shows less severe involvement (40–50 % cell loss) [89], whereas the retrorubral A-8 region, which contains only a few dopaminergic but calbindin-rich neurons, and the central periventricular gray matter show little or no degeneration [107]. Cell depletion in these nuclei does not correlate with the duration of disease. The minor vulnerability of other populations, e.g., dopaminergic hypothalamic neurons [108], has now been confirmed by recent findings of increased hypocretin (orexin) cell loss in PD [109, 110].

Other neurons that remain unaffected by Lewy pathology such as the large Betz cells of the motor cortex, the large Meynert cells of the visual cortex, the relay nuclei of the thalamus and subthalamus, brain stem, and spinal neuronal groups (motor neurons of the medulla oblongata and dorsal column nuclei) have heavy myelinated axons [86], but whether such neurons have susceptibility factors [105, 111] remains to be determinated. Of note, the neuronal populations susceptible to PD are similar to those involved in DLB, with Lewy pathology more restricted to the amygdala in many patients with AD [36, 112]. Such different regional susceptibility to similar pathological processes needs to be answered.

Multiorgan Distribution of α-Synuclein and Lewy Pathologies

It has been known for many years that LBs in PD extend well beyond the SN [113]. α-Syn pathology is not restricted to specific dopaminergic brain stem nuclei but involves non-nigral nuclei [113–116], the olfactory bulb, and related olfactory nuclei in the brain (amygdala, perirhinal cortex), suggesting that olfactory dysfunction frequently occurring in PD is related to involvement of the central olfactory pathways rather than from peripheral sensory nerve fibers [117, 118]. α-Syn pathology further involves parts of the spinal cord [19, 86, 119, 120] and multiple areas of the autonomic and peripheral nervous system, sympathetic and parasympathetic ganglia and plexuses, the intramural enteric nervous system, the skin, the retina, the submandibular gland, the cardiac nervous system, and other visceral organs [6–8, 10, 11, 22, 23, 117, 121–128]. The greatest densities and frequencies of α-syn pathology occur in the spinal cord, followed by the paraspinal sympathetic ganglia, vagus nerve, gastrointestinal tract, and endocrine organs, with negative involvement of the musculoskeletal system and major parts of sensory components of the nervous system including the sciatic nerve [36, 43, 129]. Despite early involvement of the enteric nervous system, there is no gastrointestinal myenteric or ganglion cell loss in PD [130]. Early involvement is seen in the peripheral autonomic system and adrenal medulla in neurologically unimpaired subjects (ILBD) [16, 17, 131, 132], as well as in cutaneous nerves [132a]. Diminished TH-immunoreactivity is seen in the cardiac conduction system and myocardium in both ILBD and PD [17, 125]. Early involvement of the olfactory system related with local inflammation leads to olfactory neuronal dysfunctions causing early olfactory impairment, α-syn aggregation, and spreading through the olfactory network to the brain that may contribute to PD initiation and progression [133]. Since α-syn internalized by neurons can be transported in neurons, but not by trans-synaptic transfer [134], affection of the autonomic nervous system and gastrointestinal tract before involvement of the CNS has forwarded the hypothesis of another possible route for spreading α-syn via the vagus nerve to the brain [6, 25].

Development of α-Synuclein/Lewy Pathology

Biochemical increase of phospho-α-syn precedes α-syn aggregation, which is followed by the formation of LBs and LNs [14, 135], but it does not necessarily correlate with Lewy pathology [135, 136], the latter showing an inconsistent relationship to clinical disease progression [137]. Loosely packed α-syn filaments as premature "pale neurites" are initiated at axon collaterals and extend centripetally into proximal segments [138]. These changes and the formation of "pale bodies," rounded areas of granular, pale-staining eosinophilic material displacing neuromelanin, in brain stem neurons precede the development of LBs [139]. The early intra-axonal aggregation of α-syn could damage the parental neurons by interfering with axonal transport [138, 140], but it is still unclear why some types of neurons seem more predisposed to developing axonal inclusions compared with perikaryal LBs.

Recent studies showed lower neuron densities in the SN before LB deposition in the nigrostriatal system, suggesting that neurodegeneration and cellular dysfunction precede Lewy pathology and supporting a dying-back mechanisms in neuronal α-syn pathology, in which dysfunction starts at the synapse and leads to axonopathy as the hallmark of presymptomatic and early-stage PD followed by neuronal degeneration [70, 141]. More than 90 % of α-syn aggregates are present as small deposits in presynaptic terminals of the affected neurons. This is considered a key event in the pathogenesis of synucleinopathies, but the responsible mechanisms are poorly understood. Dysfunction of the soluble N-ethylmaleimide-sensitive factor activating protein receptor (SNARE) leading to accumulation of α-syn in nerve terminals is suggested to occur in an early stage of neurodegenerative changes in the nigrostriatal system [141a], which appears to be a downstream event associated with abnormal accumulation of α-syn.

A BAC (Bacterial Artificial Chromosome) mouse model, created with the most frequent disease-causing human mutant (LRRK2/R1441G/) recapitulating cardinal features of human PD, showed no loss of mesencephalic dopaminergic neurons, but diminished dopamine release and axonal pathology of nigrostriatal projections [142]. Another autosomal recessive rat model featured by overexpression of α-syn and neuronal loss in the SN, degeneration of the striatonigral dopaminergic pathway, and reduced dopamine in the striatum revealed neuronal degeneration of the "dying-back" type, providing a naturally occurring animal model for PD [143]. Enlarged vGlut1-positive nerve cells of SNAP-25 mice showed concomitant accumulation of α-syn and p-α-syn triggered by presynaptic dysfunction [143a]. Assessment of the relationship between TH immunoreactivity as marker of nigral dysfunction and LB burden in the SN of ILBD cases suggests that Lewy pathology is not the first sign of degeneration in vulnerable neurons in PD and ILBD [144]. This data and the demonstration of small α-syn aggregates in presynaptic terminals in PD and DLB suggest that synaptic dysfunction and axon degeneration, not nerve cell loss, may be the primary determinant of progression of the neurodegeneration in PD [85, 145]. Loss of neurons might be an epiphenomenon after the loss of synapses, defining PD as a "synaptopathy" [53, 145].

The presence or absence of abnormal immunostaining for α-syn cannot be interpreted as evidence that the cell suffers from or is free of dysfunction related to abnormal protein deposition [69]; immunostaining for α-syn in pigmented SN neurons could also reflect a successful response to proteolytic stress. Reduced TH immunoreactivity in neurons early associated with α-syn accumulation may represent a cytoprotective mechanism [146], decrease of dopamine synthesis causing a reduction of cytotoxic α-syn oligomers [147], but it can also be preserved in neurons with α-syn accumulation [46, 69]. Evidence for the formation of soluble pathologic forms of α-syn in the regions with progressive neuronal loss in PD is currently lacking, since normal levels in the cytosolic fraction and no correlations with nigral LB intensity have been found. No widespread extranigral α-syn accumulation as suggested by immunohistochemical reports has been confirmed by neurochemical methods demonstrating only mildly increased α-syn in putamen [148, 149]. However, PD brains show a significant increase in soluble and lipid-associated phospho-α-syn over the disease course, with progressive decrease of soluble α-syn but no corresponding decrease in α-syn mRNA levels [150].

The mechanism that causes conformational changes of α-syn includes phosphorylation at Ser 129 (promoting fibril formation in vitro [151], C-terminal truncation, and ubiquitination [152, 153]). Changes in properties of serine 129 phosphorylated α-syn occur with progression of Lewy pathology in human brains [153a]. In PD brain, tissue transglutaminase (tTG)-induced cross-links have been identified in α-syn monomers, oligomers, and aggregates, suggesting an interaction between α-syn and tTg [154], and α-syn aggregation is promoted by increased calcium [155]. Reduction of proteasome activity may be involved as a cellular defense mechanism against dopaminergic neuronal death [156]. The presence of numerous α-syn deposits in younger-onset patients with long disease duration and LB distribution consistent with Braak staging [157] suggests that neurons harboring inclusions may remain viable in the tissue for a long time. On the other hand, serine 129 phosphorylation of α-syn as its dominant modification in LB disorders induces unfolded protein-mediated cell death [158]. Although the duration and severity of motor dysfunction and the corresponding decrease of dopamine, DAT, and vesicular monoamine transporter-2 (VMAT2) in the striatum are negatively correlated with total SN α-syn burden and neuronal loss [65, 159, 160], the latter shows no correlation with LB formation [69]. No relationship between LB stage and both clinical severity of PD (Hoehn and Yahr score) and age at death was found [137]. On the other hand, many studies have shown higher LB densities in PD patients with later disease onset and shorter disease duration [36, 43, 48, 161–163], consistent with a more rapid disease course with aging. This may be associated with an increased amount of normal cellular α-syn with age [164].

Structure and Molecular Components of Lewy Bodies

Lewy bodies occur in two types. *Classic LBs* are spherical cytoplasmic intraneuronal inclusions 8–30 ym in diameter with a hyaline eosinophilic core, concentric lamellar bands, and a narrow pale-stained halo, forming single or multiple inclusions (Fig. 1a). In some brain regions, such as the dmX, similar inclusions within neural processes are intraneuritic LBs. They can be detected in routine histological preparations and should be distinguished from LNs, which are not visible on routine histology. Ultrastructurally, LBs are non-membrane-bound, granulofilamentous structures composed of radially arranged 7–20 nm intermediate filaments associated with electron-dense granule material and vesicular structures, with the core showing densely packed filaments and dense granular material and the periphery having radially arranged 10 nm filaments (see Fig. 1b) [165]. *Cortical LBs* are eosinophilic, rounded, angular, or reniform structures without a halo (see Fig. 1c). They present invariable numbers in almost all cases of PD [157]. Ultrastructurally, they are poorly organized granulofibrillary structures with a feltlike arrangement composed of 7–27 nm wide filaments, mostly devoid of a central core [166, 167]. They are found in small nonpyramidal neurons in the lower cortical layers, with densest accumulation in the insular cortex, amygdala, and parahippocampal and cingulate gyri [168].

α-Syn as the best marker to decorate LBs and LNs has replaced that for ubiquitin as the preferred method for detecting these inclusions. Antibodies that preferentially recognized N-terminal epitopes (Syn 505, 506, and 514) selectively detect α-syn, consistent with the conformational changes associated with its polymerization into amyloid fibrils that form pathologic inclusions [169]. α-Syn adopts a three-

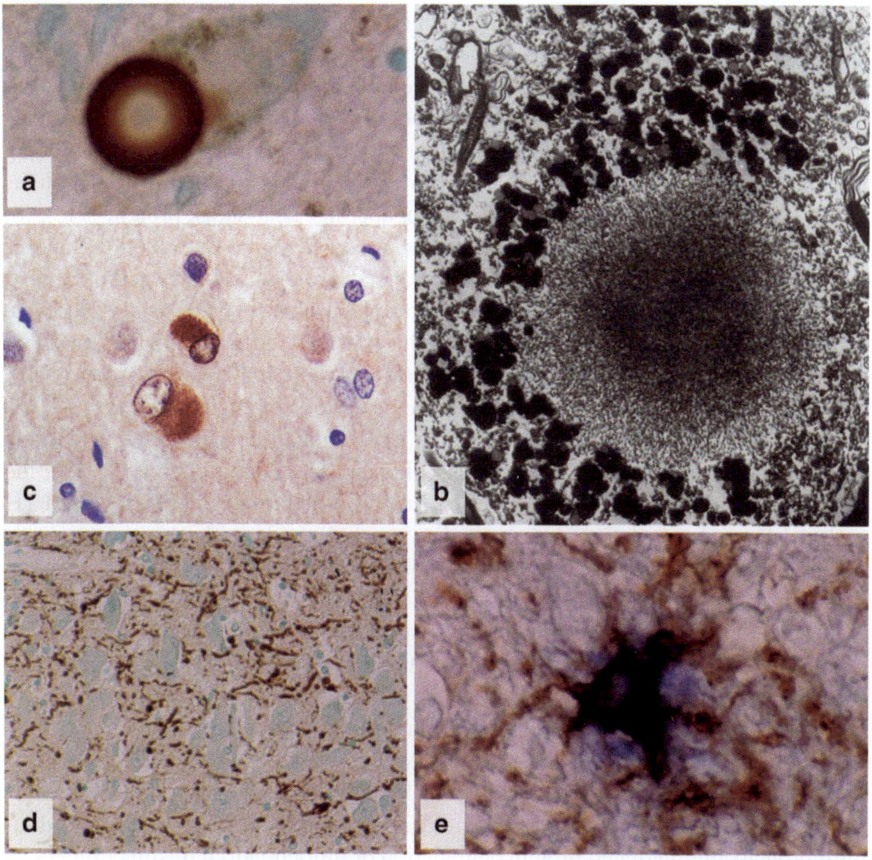

Fig. 1 (**a**) Lewy body (LB) in substantia nigra whose peripheral rim is stained with anti-α-synuclein × 300. (**b**) Electron microscopy of nigral LB showing a central electron-dense filamentous core with a loosely fibrillary rim (× 2.500). (**c**) Cortical Lewy bodies (anti-α-synuclein, × 150). (**d**) Dystrophic Lewy neurites in the hippocampal C2/3 region, anti-α-synuclein × 150. (**e**) Astrocytic inclusion in substantia nigra of Parkinson's disease brain labeled with anti-α-synuclein (*black*) and glial fibrillary acidic protein (GFAP; *gray*; × 900). Reprinted with permission from Jellinger KA. Neuropathology of sporadic Parkinson's disease: Evaluation and changes of concepts. Mov Disord 2012; 27: 8–30. Copyright © 2011 Movement Disorder Society

dimensional structure and undergoes N-terminal ubiquitination [170]. The mechanisms of its aggregation that may serve as a nidus for LB formation in vivo have not yet been fully elucidated. Mutant and wild-type α-syn interact with the mitochondrial complex IV enzyme and cytochrome C oxidase (COX), suggesting that α-syn aggregation may contribute to enhancing mitochondrial dysfunction, a key factor in the pathogenesis of PD [171].

Both classic and cortical LBs share immunochemical and biochemical characteristics, the major components being α-syn, ubiquitin, and phosphorylated ubiquitin associated with many other substances (see [14]). The molecular components can be divided into several groups: (1) structural elements of the LB fibril (α-syn, neurofilaments); (2) α-syn-binding proteins (microtubule-associated protein [MAP], synphilin-1, tau, 14-3.3 protein); (3) synphilin-1-binding proteins (α-syn, dorfin, parkin, etc.), (4) proteins implicated in the ubiquitin–proteasome system (UPS) (ubiquitin, proteasome subunits, and related enzymes and proteins); (5) proteins implicated in the autophagosome–lysosome system (NUB1, a synphilin-1-binding protein, glucocerebrosidase); (6) aggresome-related proteins (γ-tubulin); (7) proteins implicated in cellular responses (molecular chaperons, heat-shock proteins, etc); (8) molecules associated with protein phosphorylation and signal transduction (kinases and other enzymes or proteins); (9) cytoskeletal proteins (MAPs, neurofilament, tubulin); (10) mitochondria-related proteins (cytochrome C, COX); (11) cell cycle proteins (cyclin B, etc.); (12) cytosolic proteins passively diffused into LBs (amyloid precursor protein, calbindin, choline acetyltransferase [ChAT], synaptophysin, TH, VMT 2);, and (13) others (complement proteins, lipids, immunoglobulin).

Double-labeling revealed TH and ChAT co-localization with α-syn in cortical LBs, whereas brain stem LBs had intense TH and ChAT immunoreactivity in the core surrounded by a peripheral rim of α-syn [172]. Sequestration of ChAT and TH within LBs suggested that they may disrupt cholinergic and catecholaminergic transmitter production [168]. Demonstration of the autophagy adapter protein NBR1 in LBs [173, 174] and ubiquitin-1 (UBQLN1) in cytoplasmic and nuclear inclusions in several proteinopathies suggests that they are involved in their formation [175]. Co-localization of α-syn, synphilin, and parkin within LBs suggests that parkin plays a role in posttranslational modification of α-syn, which results in changes in protein size and structure-enhancing fibrillation and formation of LBs [176]. These modifications and alternative splicing have been suggested to trigger neurodegeneration in PD [152]. Pathogenic mutants of α-syn promoting toxic interactions between α-syn oligomers and lipids may interact with liposomal and ubiquitin/proteasome-mediated protein degradation or mitochondrial dysfunction [177]. LBs further contain 14-3-3 proteins that are involved in numerous signal transduction pathways and interact with α-syn and torsin A, a novel protein that may serve as a chaperon for misfolded proteins that require refielding or degradation [168].

Proteomic analysis of cortical LBs revealed 296 proteins related to multiple or unknown functions. In brain stem LBs, more than 90 proteins were identified [178], whereas another study identified 1,263 proteins in PD SN [179]. The proteome of LC in PD is of some relevance for pathogenesis [180].

The formation of LBs runs through several stages. Classic LBs show an initial intraneuronal appearance of dustlike particles related to neuromelanin or lipofuscin that are cross-linked with α-syn, with homogenous deposition of α-syn and ubiquitin in the center, with diffuse, pale, or fine granular cytoplasmic staining [153, 181]. Follows a stepwise condensation of ubiquitinated dense filamentous inclusions, forming "early LBs" that later develop into classical LBs, that are finally degraded to extraneuronal LBs after disappearance of the involved neuron. The development of cortical LBs has been divided into six stages [140]. They first show diffuse α-syn and ubiquitin labeling, whereas subcortical LBs have a distinct, central ubiquitin domain with α-syn occurring primarily in the periphery and ubiquitination being the later event. Initial granular accumulation of α-syn in the neuronal cytoplasm is followed by stepwise accumulation of dense filaments, spreading to dendrites, formation of LBs, and final degradation by astroglial processes. Glutathione peroxidase (GPX-1)-positive microglia, an important antioxidant enzyme, may be involved in neuroprotection of LB-containing neurons [182]. LBs are accompanied by coarse dystrophic neurites and also contain α-syn and ubiquitin as inclusions in axonal processes (see Fig. 1d), which, according to three-dimensional studies, may evolve into LBs, with ubiquitin at the core and neurofilaments at the outermost layer [183].

About 10 % of pigmented SN neurons contain abnormal α-syn aggregates, with diffuse cytoplasmic staining and less often pale bodies, while in the LC, 55 % of pigmented neurons contain α-syn aggregates; diffuse cytoplasmic staining is more frequent than pale bodies or LBs [146].

The absence of TH immunoreactivity suggests that many of the neuritic processes are not derived from dopaminergic neurons, although non-dopaminergic neurons partly expressing a similar phenotype are widely distributed throughout the brain [184]. α-Syn-immunoreactive glial cells (see Fig. 1e) are suggested to be responsive for the progression of PD degeneration and to play an important role in initiating early tissue response by causing recruitment of phagocytic microglia and attacking selected neurons in specific brain areas responsible for clinical symptoms [185]. Such glial inclusions are found in wide brain regions; they are also composed of abnormal filaments [186].

Although LBs are not specific to PD and may occur in a variety of conditions as a secondary pathology, a positive diagnosis of PD can usually be made by inspecting two unilateral sections from the mid-part of the SN and finding LBs. If no such inclusions are found, two further sections should be examined. If LBs are not seen in either the SN or LC, then the diagnosis of PD of the LB type could be excluded. In case of cell loss from the SN and LC in the absence of LBs, an alternative cause for parkinsonism should be pursued [17, 42].

Intranuclear inclusions, referred to as Marinesco bodies, are found in higher frequency in elderly individuals in the pigmented neurons of the SN and LC that contain LBs than in those without such inclusions, and their frequency appears to have an inverse relationship with striatal concentration of DAT and TG [187].

Pathobiological Role of Lewy Bodies

The significance of these insoluble proteinaceous cytoplasmic inclusions and their impact on promoting neurodegeneration or neuroprotection are poorly understood. Similar to other inclusions such as Pick bodies, neurofibrillary tangles, or Rosenthal fibers, LBs may represent end products or reactions to unknown neuronal degenerative processes [188]. Inhibition of complex I (reduced nicotinamide adenine dinucleotide ubiquinone oxidoreductase), a central factor in the pathogenesis of PD, causes aggregation of α-syn, which contributes to the impairment in protein handling and detoxification, whereas mitochondrial accumulation of α-syn may interact with complex I and interfere with its function [189], producing neuronal death due to mitochondrial energy deficit, oxidative stress, and impaired regulation of protein turnover [190, 191]. α-Syn mutants are prone to formation of oligomeric and prefibrillar structures, being the consequence of abnormal membrane changes, alterations in vesicle traffic, and involvement of mitochondria or lysosomal membranes [171, 192, 193]. This may be a result of the action of substances produced during early phases of protein misfolding, induced by oligomeric species of α-syn and activated in nigral dopaminergic neurons in PD and experimental models [194, 195]. Recent evidence indicates that early oligomeric forms of α-syn and not the final protein aggregates are responsible for its toxicity [196]. Small intermediates termed "soluble oligomers" in the aggregation process might lead to synaptic dysfunction and neuronal death, whereas insoluble fibrillary aggregates may function as a reservoir for bioactive oligomers [197].

Oligomerization of α-syn at the initial stage of PD is well documented [198–200], and initiation of α-syn oligomers may induce protein aggregation, disrupt cellular function, and eventually lead to neuronal death [198, 201]. Although α-syn aggregates are related to neuronal loss and LBs are considered markers of an ongoing neuronal damage, they might even be harmless end products of sequestration of toxic molecules as a type of cellular protective mechanism rather than a cause of neuronal cell death [14, 188]. LBs and pale bodies are immunoreactive for autophagic adaptor proteins p62 and NBRI [153, 175, 202], which may sequester the soluble proteins containing oligomeric α-syn into inclusions. The UPS and autophagy–lysosomal pathway (ALP) render mutated or damaged proteins less toxic than their soluble forms. They are suggested to contribute to α-syn turnover, while alterations in these major proteolytic pathways may result in α-syn accumulation due to impaired clearance [203]. Conversely, increased α-syn protein burden promotes the generation of aberrant species that impair further UPS and ALP function, thus generating a bidirectional positive-feedback loop leading to neuronal death [201, 203]. This suggests that the ubiquitinated proteins in LBs may be a manifestation of a cytoprotective response designed to eliminate damaged cellular components and to delay the onset of neuronal degeneration. However, the ultimate mechanisms for the regulation of the machinery that handles toxic waste by segregating it into insoluble aggregates is still poorly understood.

Fragmentation of the Golgi apparatus, seen in 5 % of PD nigral neurons with LBs and 3 % in those without them but in 19 % of neurons containing pale bodies, suggests that the cytotoxicity of α-syn is reduced by the process of LB formation [204], whereas SN neurons showing DNA fragmentation have no somal LBs. Mitochondrial DNA deletion was highest in LB-positive neurons in PD brains, followed by LB-negative neurons and controls, suggesting increased mitochondrial damage in LB-positive neurons in PD [205].

Lewy Pathology Staging

There are three current major staging system in use for LB disorders, one for PD [24, 206], another one for DLB [207], and revised guidelines for LB disease [208].

Based on semiquantitative assessment of LBs in a large autopsy series, a staging of the chronological spread of Lewy pathology was proposed to designate the predictable sequence of lesions in the nervous system [6, 24, 206, 209] (Fig. 2).

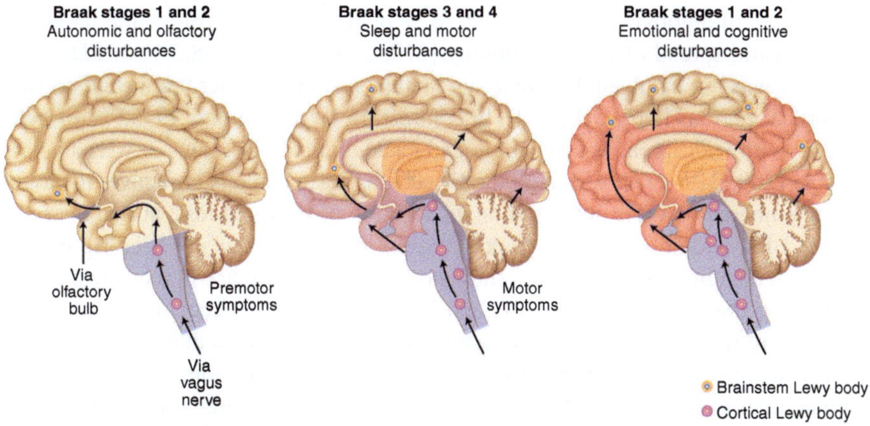

Fig. 2 Stylized representation of the Braak staging for Parkinson's disease showing the initiation sites in the medulla oblongata and olfactory bulb through to the later infiltration of Lewy pathology into the cortical regions

LB pathology is suggested to begin in the lower brain stem and involve the dmX, intermediate reticular zone, and anterior olfactory nucleus, with NBM and midbrain regions being preserved (stage 1). It extends to the caudal raphe nuclei, gigantocellular reticular nucleus, and coeruleus–subcoeruleus complex (stage 2). These initial stages are considered asymptomatic or presymptomatic and may explain the early nonmotor (autonomic and olfactory) symptoms that precede somatomotor dysfunctions [27, 31, 116, 210]. In stage 3, the LC, the central nucleus of the amygdala, and the posterolateral and posteromedial SNc are the focus of cytoskeletal changes and neuronal depletion, whereas the allocortex and isocortex are preserved. In stage 4, the anteromedial temporal limbic cortex, neocortex, and amygdala are affected. Stages 3 and 4 have been correlated with clinical motor symptoms. In terminal stages 5 and 6, the pathologic process reaches the neocortex, with the high-order sensory association cortex and prefrontal areas affected first, later progressing to the primary sensory and motor areas or involving the entire neocortex [86, 123, 209]. Metabolic and functional abnormalities already occur in brain regions in early stages of PD, which are not accompanied by Lewy pathology [16, 131, 190, 211].

Cases with severe Lewy pathology (stages 5 and 6) that show overlap or transition between PD and dementia with Lewy bodies (DLB) frequently are associated with cognitive impairment that may increase with neuropathologic stages [6].

The validity of the Braak staging scheme, which corresponds roughly to the classification of Lewy body disorders into three phenotypes—brain stem predominant, limbic/transitional, and diffuse neocortical [211]—has gained acceptance [212–215] but has also been a matter of vigorous debate [15, 42, 137, 217–220]. It often, but not consistently, shows acceptable correlations between morphological findings and clinical data, mainly in a subgroup with early onset and prolonged duration [157].

However, retrospective clinicopathologic studies have shown that at least 15 % of PD patients did not conform to this pattern [218, 219, 220]. Between 6.3 and 47 %

of all cases of autopsy-proven PD and 18 % of ILBD did not follow the predicted caudo-rostral spread of Lewy pathology [217, 219, 220]. In 7–8.3 % of PD cases, the dmX was not involved despite α-syn inclusions in the higher brain stem or even in cortical regions [216, 218, 219]. In contrast, in large samples, 49–55 % of individuals with widespread α-syn pathology lacked clinical symptoms or were unclassifiable [208, 219–221]. Although the Braak staging scheme is attractive, it should be remembered that it is not based on distribution of neuronal loss, but on distribution of LBs, and how it relates to progression of cell loss has not been rigorously studied. The numbers of LB cases show no age-related increase in incidence [208], suggesting that both prodromal PD and DLB are likely to occur in a continuum. While there will probably always be a number of outlying cases that do not conform to any staging scheme, the numbers with alternate distributions of LBs may be greater than expected for PD but may also reflect the different types of cohorts examined [15]. Thus, the proposed staging should be interpreted cautiously.

Incidental Lewy Body Disease

This term is used when LBs are found in the nervous system of individuals without clinically documented Parkinsonian symptoms. The distribution of LBs is similar to that in definite PD, with one or multiple brain areas involved and some sparing of LBs in the limbic or temporal cortex (average Braak PD stage 2.7), whereas in definite PD, more numerous LBs are found and the Braak stages significantly higher (average 4.4). Decreased TH immunoreactivity was shown in the striatum and epicardial nerve fibers compared with normal controls, but not to the same extent as in PD [17, 131]. Lewy pathology was also seen in the spinal cords of many ILBD cases [119]. Based on these and other findings, ILBD is considered as a precursor of PD, in which the lack of definite symptoms is due to subthreshold pathology. These studies support the concept that dopamine deficits begin preclinically, although the loss of dopaminergic nigral neurons is also common in DLB and differentiates LB disorders from AD [222, 223].

Initial diffuse Lewy pathology (stages 5 and 6) without clinical PD symptoms could represent a precursor to DLB, suggesting a dichotomy in the distribution of ILBD [132].

Lipoxidative damage and advanced glycation end products (AGEs) indicating oxidative damage in the cerebral cortex have been demonstrated in ILBD with none or only mild neurologic symptoms [190]. Single clinicopathological case reports suggested that REM sleep behavior disorder (RBD) may represent ILBD or an early clinical manifestation of PD [224], and that the lack of symptoms is due to subthreshold pathology [225]. The time interval between RBD and the onset of Parkinsonian symptoms ranged up to 50 years with a median of 25 years [226], while others reported that olfaction and color vision identify early-stage α-syn-mediated neurodegeneration at least 5 years before disease onset [227].

An explanation for the relatively high prevalence of asymptomatic pathologic phenotypes is threshold effect, that is, pathology in the absence of lethal comorbidities would continue to accumulate until it reached the threshold for onset of clinical disease [17, 132].

Many studies have reported that between 5 and 24 % of clinically unremarkable elderly people showed abundant Lewy pathology [16, 18, 228–233], often not related to cognitive status [234]. The distribution pattern of LBs was similar to that seen in PD, but the pigmented SN neurons were relatively well preserved. Some elderly individuals have LBs confined to the olfactory bulb [129, 235] or the amygdala, the latter particularly true if associated with concurrent Alzheimer-type pathology [112]. Moreover, some neurologically unremarkable subjects have sparse but widespread Lewy pathology even involving the cortex [132, 236], which would seem to violate the theory of progression from the brain stem and perhaps fit better with a multicentric disease progress from the onset [42]. Clearly, the observed distribution of LBs is dependent on case selection [231].

New Guidelines for Lewy Pathology

The revised guidelines for the pathologic diagnosis of Lewy body diseases with semiquantitative assessment of LB density in the brain stem, limbic system, and five cortical regions [220] distinguish three phenotypes—brain stem predominant, limbic/transitional, and diffuse neocortical (Table 1)—taking into account

Table 1 Neuropathological staging of Lewy body disease[a]

Kosaka LBD stage	Braak PD stage	Anatomical distribution of Lewy bodies
		Enteric nervous system, peripheral autonomic system, anterior olfactory nucleus
Brain stem-predominant type	1	Medulla oblongata: dorsal IX/X motor nucleus, intermediate reticular zone; lower raphe nuclei; spinal cord
	2	Medulla oblongata and pontine tegmentum: caudal raphe nuclei, gigantocellular reticular nucleus, and coeruleus–subcoeruleus complex; olfactory bulb
	3	Midbrain: pathology of stage 2 plus midbrain lesions, substantia nigra compacta (!)
Transitional (limbic) type	4	Basal prosencephalon and mesocortex: stage 3 plus prosencephalic lesions, amygdala, intralaminar thalamus. Cortical involvement confined to the temporal mesocortex (transentorhinal region) and allocortex (CA2 sector)
Diffuse cortical type	5	Neocortex: stage 4 plus lesions in high-order sensory association areas and the prefrontal neocortex
	6	Advanced neocortex: stage 5 plus first-order sensory association areas of the neocortex and premotor areas; occasionally, mild changes in primary sensory areas and the primary motor field

[a]Metabolic and functional abnormalities already occur in brain regions at early stages of PD that are not accompanied by Lewy pathology

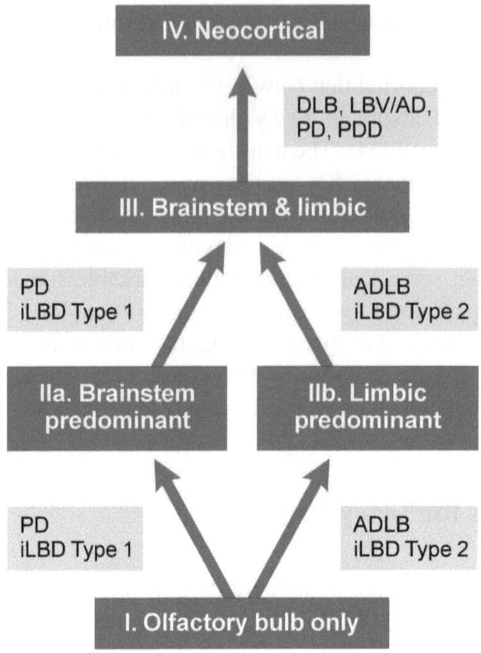

Fig. 3 Scheme of the hypothetic progression pathways and stages of Lewy body (LB) disorders. The pathway for Parkinson's disease (PD) is suggested to proceed through stage IIa (brain stem predominant), and those for dementia with Lewy bodies (DLB) and Alzheimer's disease (AD) with LBs probably pass through stage IIb. For incidental LB disease (iLBD), both pathways seem possible, whereas only PD/PD dementia (PDD), DLB, and the LB variant of AD (LBV/AD) progress to the neocortical stage. Reprinted with permission from Jellinger KA. Neuropathology of sporadic Parkinson's disease: Evaluation and changes of concepts. Mov Disord 2012; 27: 8–30. Copyright Â© 2011 Movement Disorder Society

Alzheimer-type pathology. However, the stage of AD-related lesions is usually not associated with the pattern of Lewy pathology [208]. A recently proposed unifying system correlates α-syn pathology with nigrostriatal degeneration, cognitive impairment, and motor dysfunction [129]. Whereas the old classification left 45–50 % of elderly individuals unclassified, all were classified into one of four stages (Fig. 3). Progression through these stages was accompanied by stepwise deterioration in terms of striatal TH concentration, SN pigmented cell loss, Mini-Mental State score, and the Unified Parkinson's disease Rating Scale. There were significant correlations between these measures and α-syn pathology. This is supported by an increase of phosphorylated α-syn restricted to the olfactory bulb and brain stem in early stages of Lewy pathology [5, 129]. This staging system would allow a better classification of Lewy disorders but it needs validation in a greater proportion of patients. However, despite several limitations, the brain pathology for most patients with typical PD can be predicted using Braak's scheme [15, 208]. The relationship between age and late progression of PD has been studied recently [215].

Interaction Between α-Syn and Other Proteins

Considerable overlap between synucleinopathies and other protein-misfolding diseases suggests interactions of pathological proteins engaging common downstream pathways [13, 49, 188, 237, 238]. The co-occurrence of α-syn, tau, and other proteins in various neurodegenerative disorders highlights the interface between these misfolded proteins, which may be co-aggregated in the same brain, in the same region, or even in the same cell in human brain and transgenic mice [239–241].

Accumulated α-syn (promoted by oxidative stress) has a stimulatory effect on tau phosphorylation by glycogen synthase kinase-3β (GSK-3β), a major kinase that hyperphosphorylates tau to produce pathologic forms [242], while the chaperone HSP70 may suppress α-syn-mediated tau phosphorylation in initial disease stages [243]. In MPTP models, α-syn has been shown to induce GSK-3β-catalyzed tau phosphorylation [244, 245].

Recent postmortem studies showed increased accumulation of tau protein, in particular tau phosphorylated at Ser 262 and 396/404, in the striata of PD patients related to increased GSK-3β activity [149]. Tauopathy in PD striata is restricted to dopaminergic neurons, whereas degeneration in the inferior frontal cortex, associated with increased α-syn deposition because of diminished proteasomal activity in the absence of oxidative stress and pGSK-3β activity, is not associated with tauopathy [149]. Thus, the restricted pattern of tauopathy in PD [246] differs from its generalized affection in AD [247]. Interaction with tubulin suggests that α-syn could be a microtubule-associated protein similar to tau. PD-associated risk factors, for example, environmental toxins and α-syn mutations, may also promote tau phosphorylation, causing microtubule instability, which leads to loss of dopaminergic neurons in PD [248]. Induction of intracellular tau aggregates is promoted by α-syn seeds [249].

There is a strong interaction between α-syn, tau, and β amyloid, particularly in their oligomeric forms, which might synergistically promote their mutual aggregation and vice versa, thereby amplifying neuronal damage [250–252]. Cross-seeding between dissimilar proteins that share β-sheet structures has been described, e.g., for tau and α-syn [253]. Modification of α-syn may induce both Lewy-like and tau pathologies [248], while tau enhances α-syn aggregation and toxicity and disrupts inclusion formation in cellular models [254]. Other links between tau and α-syn are suggested by their co-localization in both neurofibrillary tangles and LBs, especially in neuronal populations vulnerable for both aggregates [178, 235, 239]. LB formation may be triggered, at least in part, by AD pathology and vice versa [255].

Other studies have suggested that β-amyloid is more likely to promote the deposition of α-syn than tau [256], and Aβ is known to initiate hyperphosphorylation of tau [257]. Cortical α-syn load is associated with Aβ plaque burden in a subset of PD patients [258], and α-syn-induced synapse damage is enhanced by Aβ-42 [259]. PD and AD could be linked by progressive accumulation of phospho-tau, GSK-3β, and α-syn, and activation of caspase and caspase-cleft Δ-tau may represent a common way of abnormal intracellular accumulation of both α-syn and tau, promoted by Aβ deposition, thus unifying the pathology of these diseases. Interaction of α-syn, tau, and Aβ may be a molecular mechanism in the overlapping pathology of several proteinopathies, possibly representing a complex continuum characterized by variable amounts of pathologic proteins generated by the same stimulus probably depending upon genetic and environmental factors [260, 261]. Despite documented co-localization of α-syn and tau in LBs and Aβ and phospho-tau in synaptic terminals in AD [262] and in triple transgenic mice [263], the basic mechanisms leading to the intimate association and synergism of these proteins, suggesting a dualism or triad of amyloidogenic neurodegeneration, await further clarification.

Pathophysiology of Clinical Subtypes of Parkinson's Disease

The basal ganglia consist of the caudate, putamen (striatum), and globus pallidus (GP) and are functionally connected to many brain stem nuclei, the basal forebrain, the cortex, and the cerebellum.

Current concepts about the organization of the basal ganglia emphasize the existence of "internal" mechanisms that modulate input/output activity and sustain normal execution of movements. In the normal basal ganglia network, the globus pallidus externus (GPe) emerges as a main regulatory station of output activity (Figs. 4 and 5a). Dopamine not only is an important modulator of basal ganglia function but also may modulate it at sites outside of the striatum, and changes in dopaminergic transmission at these sites may contribute to the symptoms of PD and other disorders [264]. In early stages of PD, overactivation in the basal ganglia is suggested to compensate the dopaminergic deficit in the striatal circuit. In PD, this filtering mechanism is deranged; dopamine depletion shifts the basal ganglia toward inhibiting cortically generated movements by increasing the gain in the GPe-subthalamic nucleus (STN)-GPi network and reducing the activity in "direct" cortico–putaminal–GPi projections (see Fig. 5b). GPi/SNr activity is controlled by the balance between a direct and indirect putaminal–pallidal GABAergic pathway; GPe, in turn, projects via another GABAergic pathway to STN that has a glutamatergic projection to GPi/SNr. Impairment of synaptic plasticity of striatal neurons, in particular medium spiny neurons, may account for the onset and progression of motor symptoms and contribute to the pathogenesis of dyskinesias (see Fig. 5c) [265, 266]. Anatomical connections between the basal ganglia and cerebellum suggest their association in movement disorders [267].

The major clinical subtypes of PD show specific morphological patterns of pathophysiological importance, with different involvement of the striatal and cerebello-thalamic-cortical pathways (Fig. 6) [268].

In the *rigid–akinetic type*, which occurs in about 50 % of all PD patients, the ventrolateral SN projecting to the dorsal putamen shows the brunt of degeneration (see Fig. 5b). There is a gradient loss of TH- and DAT-immunoreactive fibers from the dorsal to the ventral putamen, with prominent involvement of the striosomes projecting to the severely involved ventrolateral SNc. Consequently, nigral cell loss

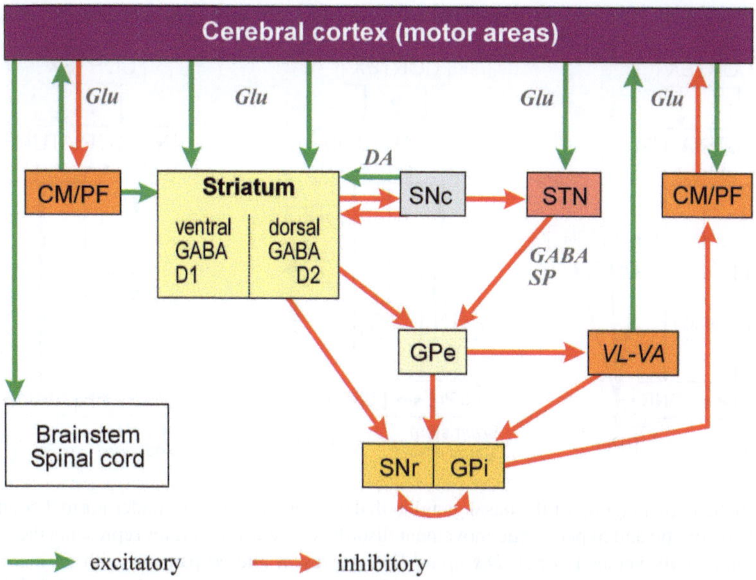

Fig. 4 New model of the basal ganglia. Cortical innervation to the basal ganglia is primarily via corticostriatal and corticosubthalamic projections. The primary basal ganglia projections back to the cortex originate in the GPi (and SNr) and pass through the ventral nuclei of the thalamus (VL-VA). "Internal" or "horizontal" circuits control basal ganglia excitability. These include substantia nigra pars compacta (SNc) dopaminergic projections to the striatum and other basal ganglia, centromedian–parafascicular (CM/Pf) thalamic projections to the striatum and subthalamic nucleus (STN), and reciprocal connections between the external globus pallidus (GPe) and the STN and striatum (Glu, glutamate; DA, dopamine; D1, D2, dopamine receptors; GABA, γ-aminobutyric acid; Enk, enkephalin). Modified with permission from Jellinger KA. Neuropathology of sporadic Parkinson's disease: Evaluation and changes of concepts. Mov Disord 2012; 27: 8–30. Copyright © 2011 Movement Disorder Society

correlates with dopamine loss in the posterior putamen and severity of akinesia–rigidity [65]. Dopamine loss in the GPe and globus pallidus internus (GPi) does not match the more severe dopamine loss in the putamen [56]. Preservation of the calbindin-positive somatostatin-rich matrix, which projects to the GABAergic neurons of the SNr and motor thalamus, suggests that the endings richest in DAT are most sensitive to degeneration. Dopaminergic denervation of the striatum causes severe loss of dendrites on type I medium spiny neurons (MSNs), the principal target of dopaminergic input from the SN [269], and loss of convergent nigrostriatal dopamine and corticostriate glutamate axon integrity. The majority of D1-expressing neurons comprise the "direct" pathway and project to the GPe/SNr, whereas D2-bearing neurons project to the GPe and are part of the "indirect" pathway [270, 271] (see Figs. 4 and 5a).

In early stages of PD, overactivation in the basal ganglia is suggested to compensate for the dopaminergic defect in the striatal motor circuit [272]. The increase in striatal neuronal activity with decreased excitation of D1-bearing

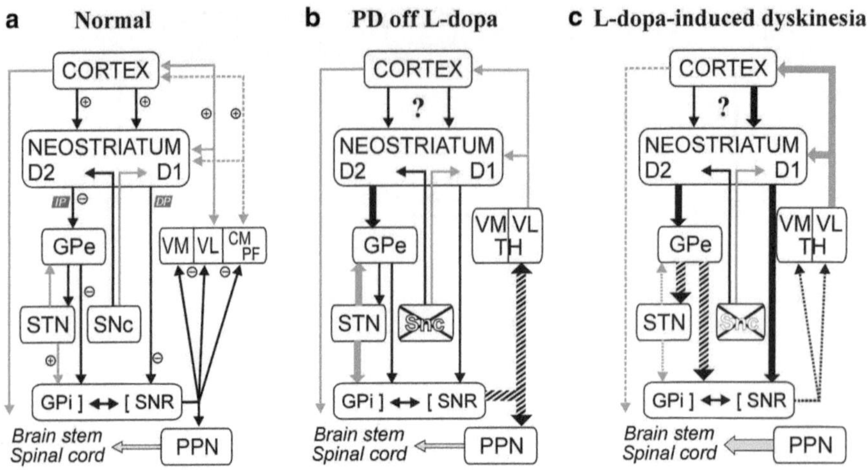

Fig. 5 Schematic diagram of the basal ganglia–thalamocortical circuitry under normal conditions and in hypokinetic and hyperkinetic movement disorders. The *width of lines* represents the relative change in activity versus normal. *Disrupted lines* represent altered patterns with an increase or decrease in neuronal activity. *Dashed arrow*, reduced activity; *solid arrow*, increased activity; D1 and D2, dopamine 1 and 2 receptor subtypes; GPe and GPi, external and internal segment of the globus pallidus; Normal, normal conditions; PPN, pedunculopontine nucleus; PD, Parkinson's disease; PSP, progressive supranuclear palsy; SNc and SNr, substantia nigra pars compacta and reticulata; STN, subthalamic nucleus; TH, thalamus; VM/VL, ventromedial/ventrolateral thalamic nuclei; CM, centromedian nucleus of the thalamus; PF, parafascicular nucleus of the thalamus. Modified with permission from Jellinger KA. Parkinson's disease. In: Dickson DW, Weller RO, editors. Neurodegeneration: The Molecular Pathology of Dementia and Movement Disorders, 2nd ed. Oxford: Blackwell Publishing Ltd.; 2011: pp. 194–223

neurons leads to reduced activity of the "direct" pathway, whereas reduced inhibition of D2-bearing striatal neurons results in decreased activity in striatopallidal (GPe) projections (see Fig. 5b). Later, this filtering mechanism is deranged, and dopamine depletion shifts the basal ganglia toward inhibiting cortically generated movements by increased gain in the indirect GPe–STN–GPi network and reduced activity in the "direct" cortico–putaminal–GPi circuit by dopamine D2 receptors and reduces the inhibition mediated by the direct pathway because of loss of D1 excitation in this pathway [265]. Neuritic changes, α-syn inclusions, and loss of dopaminergic neurons in the neostriatum increase with progression of PD [57, 273]. The essential pathophysiological feature of the rigid–akinetic PD is increased neuronal firing activity in the output nuclei (GPi and SNr) leading to excessive inhibition of thalamocortical and brain stem motor systems [274].

Impairment of synaptic plasticity of striatal MSNs accounts for the onset and progression of motor symptoms and contributes to development dyskinesias [265, 266]. Abundant α-syn pathology in the neostriatum [273, 275], dystrophic neurites in the caudate nucleus, and progressive loss of TH and DAT-immunoreactive nigrostriatal fibers suggest trans-synaptic degeneration as a substrate for the motor deficits and decreased efficacy of dopaminomimetic therapy in late stages of PD [276, 277].

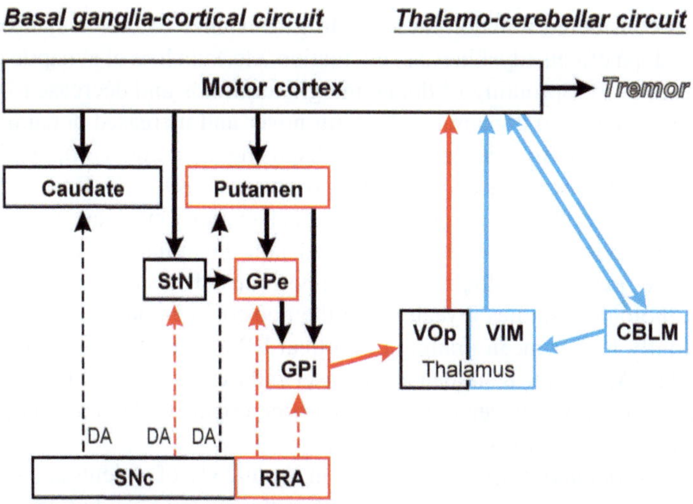

Fig. 6 A model of cerebral mechanisms underlying Parkinson's disease (PD) resting tremor. It emerges from the ventral intermediate nucleus of the thalamus (VIM)–motor cortex (MC)–cerebellum (CBLM) circuit (in *blue*), when triggered by transient pathological signals from the basal ganglia motor loop (in *red*). In tremor-dominant PD, the basal ganglia (globus pallidus internus [GPi], globus pallidus externus [GPe], and putamen) have increased connectivity with the VIM–MC–CBLM circuit through the MC (thick *red line*), and the basal ganglia are activated at critical times in the tremor cycle (onset/offset of tremor episodes). These alterations may be caused by loss of dopaminergic projections from retrorubral area 8 (RRA; in *red*) to the GPi and GPe. These alterations are different from the dopaminergic denervation of the striatum, associated with bradykinesia and rigidity (Vop, thalamic ventralis oralis posterior nucleus; DA, dopamine; SNc, substantia nigra pars compacta; StN, subthalamic nucleus). Reprinted with permission from Jellinger KA. Neuropathology of sporadic Parkinson's disease: Evaluation and changes of concepts. Mov Disord 2012; 27: 8–30. Copyright Â© 2011 Movement Disorder Society

Reduced dopaminergic input to the putamen causes increased activity of the GABAergic indirect efferent loop via SNr and GPi to the ventrolateral thalamus projecting to the cortex. Excessive excitatory glutamatergic drive from the SN and GPi/SNr leads to an akinetic-rigid syndrome through reduced cortical activation (see Fig. 5b). Recent studies suggest that rigidity is associated with widespread changes in the brain, as opposed to a single discrete locus [278].

The increased GABAergic activity is reduced by L-dopa treatment and disappears in the course of the disease, and N-methyl-D-aspartate (NMDA) receptors and glutamatergic synapses may be degenerated, favoring drug resistance and motor complication. Hyperstimulation of dopaminergic receptors may account for the development of motor fluctuations and dyskinesias after L-dopa treatment (see Fig. 5c). Relative preservation of the striatal matrix and its efferents enables restitution of the dopaminergic transmission by L-dopa substitution and maintained the function of the "motor loop," but progressive degeneration with transgression to non-dopaminergic systems in later stages causes loss of postsynaptic D2 and muscarinic cholinergic receptors in the striatum. This uncoupling of receptor systems is considered a major cause of drug resistance of motor symptoms and adverse L-dopa effects (dyskinesias, fluctuation, etc.) via loss of synaptic depotentiation [266, 279]. Sprouting of dopaminergic terminals and decreased DAT may contribute to increased dopamine release/turnover and increased dopamine sensitivity of striatal cholinergic neurons, predisposing to motor complications and L-dopa-induced dyskinesia as the disease progresses [280, 281]. Recent data have shown a differential role of pre- versus postsynaptic mechanisms, dopamine receptor subtypes, glutamate receptors, and non-dopaminergic transmitter systems in the pathophysiology of dopamine-induced dyskinesias [282, 283]. Clinicopathological studies revealed that the non-tremor-dominant subgroup had a significantly higher mean grading of cortical LBs than all other subgroups and more cortical Aβ-plaque load than early-onset and tremor-dominant groups. These data confirm the link between bradykinetic onset, cognitive decline, and LB deposition in the neocortex [37].

The *tremor-dominant type of PD* occurs in about 25 % of patients and shows less severe cell loss (mean 69 %) in the lateral than the medial SNc, but damage to the retrorubral A-8 field, which is usually preserved in rigid–akinetic PD [13, 284]. It projects to the matrix of the dorsolateral striatum and ventrolateral thalamus and influences striatal efflux via the SNc and thalamus to the prefrontal cortex. In contrast to akinetic-rigid PD, dopamine levels in the ventral internal pallidum were normal in PD with predominant tremor, suggesting functional disequilibrium between GABAergic and dopaminergic influences in favor of dopamine in the caudoventral parts of the GPi, which may contribute to rest tremor [56]. Functional neuroimaging in patients with resting tremor suggested increased activity of the ventral intermediate thalamus and dysfunction of cerebellar connections [285]. Morphometric studies demonstrated volume reduction in the cerebellum of these patients, demonstrating involvement of the cerebello-thalamo-cortical circuit [286]. Deficits in cerebellar functions in PD with decreased excitability of the cerebello-thalamo-cortical pathway may be involved in the generation of postural tremor, whereas resting and postural tremors in PD are mediated by different neuronal pathways [287]. Rest tremor is produced by the pathological interaction between the basal ganglia and the cerebellar-thalamo-cortical circuit only in the presence of striatopallidal dopaminergic dysfunction (see Fig. 6) [288, 289], which has been confirmed by recent FDG-PET studies [290]. This has considerable implications for stereotactic treatment of tremor (deep stimulation of the ventral intermediate thalamus) [291, 292].

The current model provides a reasonable explanation for the origin of akinetic features in PD and suggests that rigidity and tremor are generated by basal ganglia downstream mechanisms struggling to compensate for PD akinesia. The stronger association between akinesia and tremor as opposed to the more independent nature of PD tremor indicates that both symptoms are generated by different mechanisms [293]. Recent FR-CIT SPECT studies confirmed the models for a reduced dopaminergic projection to the dorsal putamen in akinetic-rigid PD as well as the lateral putamen and caudate nucleus in tremor-dominant patients in vivo [294].

Neuropathology of Cognitive Changes in Parkinson's Disease

Cognitive deficits are common in PD, but the range of clinical deficits and their structural and molecular/biochemical backgrounds are variable [295]. Cognitive impairment (without dementia) may precede the onset of dementia, with a delay of up to 20 years; it was observed in 19 % of untreated PD patients [296]. PD patients have an increased risk of developing mild cognitive impairment (MCI), the frequency of which is 21–62 %, with a mean of 25.8 % [297, 298], and with a shorter progression to dementia. Its cumulative prevalence is between 48 and 78 %, with a mean of 75 % after survival for more than 10 years [297] and of 83 % after 20 years [299]. Parkinson's disease dementia (PDD) has a 4–6 times increased lifetime incidence rate compared with age-matched controls [298].

The putative brain changes underlying dementia in PD have not yet been explored in sufficient detail to permit a consensus definition. Although some studies indicate LB-type pathology in cortical and limbic structures as the main histological substrate of PDD, it now appears that even widespread α-syn lesions often cannot reliably account for the presence of dementia with frequently encountered concomitant AD-type changes, suggesting a synergism of multiple pathogenic mechanisms [300]. A recent clinicopathologic study confirmed that a combination of Lewy- and Alzheimer-type pathologies is a robust correlate of dementia in PD [301]. A novel classification of LB disorders based upon unbiased statistical methods suggesting pathologic heterogeneity of dementia in PD awaits further validation [302]. In conclusion, the heterogeneity of both motor/nonmotor and neuropsychological symptoms in PD and related LB disorders may emerge from a variety of morphological and neurochemical deficiencies, which need further elucidation and validation.

Mild Cognitive Impairment in Parkinson's Disease

MCI, representing the earliest clinical features of cognitive dysfunction, according to current criteria includes the amnestic and nonamnestic phenotypes (aMCI and naMCI, respectively), which may involve single or multiple domains. Its prevalence ranges from 3.2 to 23.4 %, with an average of 15–18 % for individuals aged 70 years or older. Classification, diagnostic biological markers, outcome, and neuropathology have been reviewed, showing considerable variability among populations [303]. The frequency of MCI in PD (PD-MCI) varies considerably, between 21 and 62 % [304, 305]. Characterization of PD-MCI has been reported recently [306]. Two studies on the neuropathology of PD-MCI showed variable lesions with brain stem, brain stem-limbic, and rare neocortical LB lesions, low Braak AD stages, amyloid but only rare neuritic plaques in the cerebral cortex, and mild CAA, with some cases having an additional mild lacunar state in the basal ganglia or cerebral infarcts

[307, 308]. naMCI cases showed a significantly shorter disease duration than aMCI cases of variable LB stages, lower AD Braak scores (mean 2.1 vs. 2.7), less frequent neuritic cortical plaques but similar cortical amyloid load, as well as similar rare concomitant cerebrovascular lesions. These data in PD-MCI suggest heterogeneous cognitive presentation [309] and heterogeneous neuropathology similar to that found in MCI cases without PD [310, 311]. Recent evidence strengthens the importance of amyloid imaging in vivo as a tool in the diagnosis and prognosis of patients with MCI [312, 313].

Parkinson's Disease and Dementia (PDD)

The morphological substrate of cognitive impairment in LB disorders has been a matter of considerable controversy. The morphologic changes underlying dementia in PD can be classified into three main types: (1) Cognitive impairment may be primarily a result of involvement of subcortical and brain stem structures, (2) an extension of LB pathology into limbic or higher cortical association areas is accepted by others as a plausible substrate for the dementia in LB disorders, and (3) another proposition is that concurrent AD-type pathology underlies the cognitive decline in PD. In general, one of these lesions may not completely explain the development of PDD, whereas at least two or all three conditions may frequently concur [300, 314]. CNS lesions contributing to the cognitive impairment in PD are dysfunctions of the subcorticocortical networks as a result of neuronal loss and atrophy in the amygdala and limbic areas [315], cholinergic deficits in the cortex and thalamus associated with neuronal loss in the NBM (nucleus basalis of Meynert) and decreased striatal dopaminergic function, decreased nicotinic acetylcholine receptors [204, 316], and degeneration of the medial SN and nuclei of other ascending pathways, causing dysfunction of the striato-subfrontal and mesocorticolimbic loops. The cognitive deficits in early PD are associated with impaired nigrostriatal dopaminergic function, which results in abnormal processing in the corticobasal ganglia circuit with reduced prefrontal and parietal metabolism, whereas mesocortical dopaminergic transmission initially appears to be preserved [317]. There is significant subcortical degeneration in PD, with neuronal loss and LBs in the NBM, although this may precede the onset of dementia because of cortical cholinergic denervation [318] and α-syn pathology in the NBM is high in both demented and nondemented PD patients. Severe pathology also involves the noradrenergic LC [319] and the serotonergic dorsal raphe nucleus [318] and the ventral tegmental area [320]. The loss of LC innervation in PD subjects as measured by TH immunoreactivity appears not to lead to LC neuronal loss because TH-IR in AD was robust despite similar loss of LC neurons. These data suggest a differential response of the noradrenergic system in PD compared with AD in response to loss of LC neurons [321].

Dementia with Lewy Bodies and Parkinson's Disease Dementia

DLB and PDD are considered to be parts of an α-syn-associated disease spectrum. DLB, a progressive disorder associated with some core clinical neuropsychiatric features, is considered to be the second most common neurodegenerative dementia syndrome in the elderly [207]. An arbitrary cutoff is used: If dementia develops first or within 1 year of PD diagnosis, then DLB is diagnosed, while if PD develops first and dementia later, this suggests PDD. Distinction between both disorders may be difficult [322]. Their pathological hallmarks are α-syn/Lewy pathology or a variable mixture of Lewy and AD pathologies, which may interact synergistically [301]. Both cortical and subcortical α-syn lesions have been suggested to be predominant [323], whereas for others, AD lesions were more important, the Aβ load being similar to that in AD [173, 174]. Occipital and posterior parietotemporal hypometabolism is a distinguishing feature of DLB that is independent of amyloid pathology [324]. According to revised guidelines, the severity and extent of α-syn are scored semiquantitatively in specific brain regions [207, 325]. Neurofibrillary tangles, being frequent in both DLB and PDD, are often restricted to limbic regions, while extensive tau pathology may be absent. Between 10 and 50 % of PDD cases had enough AD lesions to attain the pathological diagnosis of definite AD. A recent clinicopathologic study identified three subgroups of PDD: (1) predominantly synucleinopathy (Braak LB stages 5–6; 38 %); (2) synucleinopathy with b-amyloid deposition but minimal or no tau pathology (59 %); and (3) synucleinopathy and AD with considerable neocortical tauopathy (Braak tau stages 5–6; 3 %). Patients in group II had significantly shorter survival than those with pure synucleinopathy. Reduced cortical cholinergic innervation in both DLB and PDD is similar and more severe than in AD, while synaptic loss in DLB is similar to that in AD [326]. Elevated APOE ε4 frequency in DLB and PDD cases, in which the overall brain neuritic plaque burden was lower, indicates that ε4 may contribute to neurodegeneration through mechanisms unrelated to amyloid processing [327].

Brains of DLB patients with the first appearance of dementia showed significantly more severe Aβ scores (4–5) than those without apparent dementia, whose scores were lower (0–1), suggesting that Aβ deposits may contribute to the timing of the onset of dementia related to that of parkinsonism in DLB [328]. The presence of Aβ in DLB but not in PD and their great sensitivity to differentiate DLB from PDD with 100 % negative predictive value was confirmed recently [36, 43, 329].

Other differences between PDD and DLB concern neurochemistry findings. Nigrostriatal dopamine changes occur in both disorders, but the severity and distribution of changes differ, with more marked nigral cell loss in PDD. There is postsynaptic dopamine upregulation in PD but not in DLB, which may be related to the increased risk for neuroleptic sensibility reaction in DLB [330]. DLB shows significantly higher frontal 5-HT1A receptor binding compared with PDD [331]. DLB patients with early dementia (less than 10 years after onset of PD) had morphological and neurochemical changes similar to those with DLB, whereas PD patients with later-onset dementia had less cortical pathology (LBs, Aβ plaques, NFTs), but more severe cholinergic deficit in the temporal cortex [161].

Some studies have demonstrated that the number of LBs in the frontal cortex or in the limbic cortex is a better predictor of dementia in PD than is AD pathology [332–335]. Cognitive impairment is often correlated with the density of LNs and neuritic degeneration in the hippocampus and periamygdaloid cortex, which causes disruption of the limbic loop and "disconnection" from key areas, as described in AD [336], and is a major basis for the dementia and visual hallucinations [337]. The density of both limbic LBs and neuritic plaques correlated well with the severity of the dementia, although hippocampal atrophy and cell loss are not necessarily involved in the memory impairment in PD [338]. Increasing cognitive decline with increasing pathologic LB stages secondary to progression of α-syn pathology [123] was not confirmed by others [217, 218, 301, 339–341]. PD patients without dementia may have AD pathology largely restricted to the limbic system (neuritic Braak stage <4), whereas patients with PDD often have severe AD lesions, with or without neocortical atrophy [318]. PDD patients showed significantly more severe AD pathology (neuritic Braak stages, cortical amyloid plaque load, and generalized CAA) than nondemented ones [342] which was in accordance with previous postmortem studies [343, 344] and in vivo neuroimaging studies showing increase amyloid load in human brain [312, 313, 345–347].

The association between cognitive impairment, moderate LB scores, and AD lesions suggests an influence of AD-related pathology on the progression of neurodegeneration and on cognitive decline in PD, whereas it appears to be largely independent of coexisting mild vascular pathology, except in cases with severe CVLs related to CAA and AD pathology [342]. DLB is usually associated with only mild cerebrovascular lesions, showing an inverse relationship with the severity of Lewy pathology [348].

Despite many similarities between DLB and PDD, there are some morphological differences, in particular, higher amyloid plaque load in the striatum, usually absent in nondemented PD [36, 43, 329, 342] and more severe α-syn load in hippocampal CA 2/3 areas [13]. DLB cases had more severe Aβ load than PDD, but no differences in neuritic and α-syn scores, while others reported higher Aβ load in cortical and subcortical areas [301].

Based on available data, both DLB and PDD show heterogeneous pathology and neurochemistry, which depend on the different lesion patterns, supporting the hypothesis that these α-syn-related disorders and AD share a common underlying molecular pathogenesis.

Etiology and Pathogenesis of PD

The etiology of PD is poorly understood, but a molecular interaction between genetic factors and environmental risk factors appears reasonable [349, 350]; multiple etiologies are more likely than a single factor [45, 351]. The impact of various gene mutations, such as α-syn (SNCA), LRRK2, Parkin, PINK 1 and DJ1 on

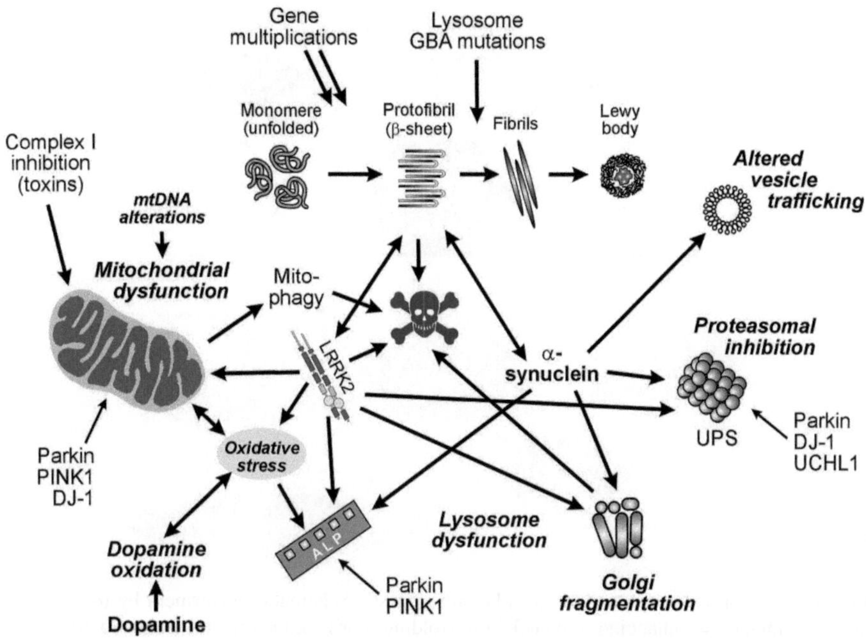

Fig. 7 Simplified scheme of major factors underlying PD pathogenesis. Modified with kind permission from Springer Science+Business Media: Jellinger KA. The role of α-synuclein in neurodegeneration – An update. Translational Neurosci 2012; 3(2)

mitochondrial maintenance, synaptic homeostasis, autophagy, axonal transport, protein regulating systems, oxidative damage, and metabolic functions is well documented (Fig. 7) (see [46, 352]). Genetic susceptibility may be determined in part through impaired metabolism of free radicals or complex I activity, which in turn may be the product of nuclear or mitochondrial genomic deficits [191, 353–355], while environmental interactions include exogenous compounds with uptake and conversion similar to MPTP, cyanide, carbon disulfide, or endogenously generated neurotoxins, such as rotenone or tetrahydroisoquinoline, which are involved in reactive oxidative species and disruption of calcium homeostasis [356]. Recent studies in individuals with POLG mutations showed a selective deficit of the respiratory chain complex I in SNc due to motochondrial DNA deletion, which was or was not associated with clinical parkinsonism [357]. Disturbed calcium homeostasis and abnormal cortical metabolism due to the convergence of multiple deficits have been observed in early stages of PD [190, 358].

A growing body of evidence has been collected regarding the pathogenesis of PD, which has been related to a complex cascade of multiple noxious factors, protein mishandling, in particular misfolded α-syn and its oligomers, perturbation of protein degradation systems, such as the UPS [359], formation of free radicals, oxidative, nitritive, and proteolytic stress [360], production of reactive oxidative species and of advanced glycation products [97], mitochondrial dysfunctions [97, 103, 171, 352, 361–366], impaired bioenergetics [191, 350, 367], lipid peroxidation,

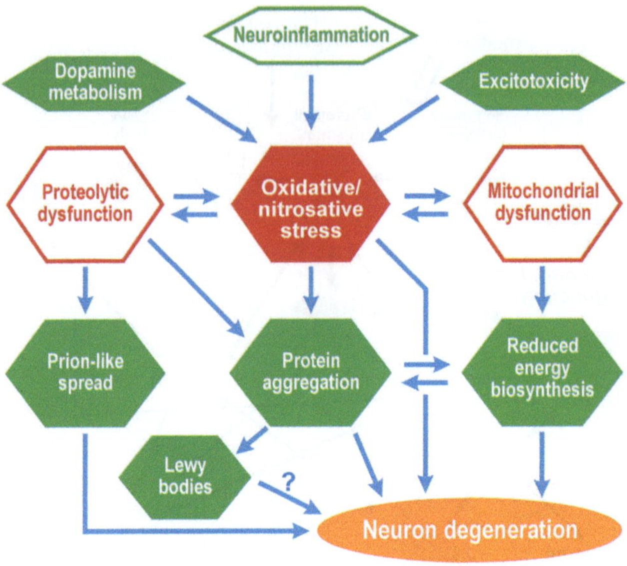

Fig. 8 Common pathways underlying PD pathogenesis. Schematic impairment by α-synuclein and gene mutations enhancing α-synuclein misfolding, fibril formation, and Golgi fractionation; impairing proteasome and mitochondrial functions, altering vesicle traffic and translation. Reprinted from Oxidative and nitrosative stress in Parkinson's disease, 1792/8, Tsang HK, Chung KK, Biochimica et Biophysica Acta (BBA) – Molecular Basis of Disease, 643–650, Copyright 2009, with permission from Elsevier

nuclear RNA deficits, protein–iron and neuromelanin–iron interactions [87, 89, 91, 367, 368], transcriptional α-syn dysregulation [152], disorders of calcium homeostasis, prion-like behavior of misfolded proteins [200, 369, 370], excitotoxicity from increased glutamatergic input, neuroinflammation [45, 79, 133], and interaction between these and other noxious factors (see [46]). The demonstration that α-syn is degraded by both proteasome and autophagy pathways, and the fact that mutated α-syn inhibits the autophagy–lysosome and the autophagy pathways that maintain intracellular proteostasis support its role as the essential trigger for neurodegeneration in PD [104, 359]. Conversely, boosting chaperone-mediated autophagy in vivo mitigates α-syn-induced neurodegeneration [371] (Fig. 8). The complex relationship between autophagy and oxidative stress in PD has been reviewed recently [360, 372], macroautophagy of mitochondria (mitophagy) is thought to be a significant contributor to many different forms of PD [373]. Misfolded α-syn may contribute to oxidative stress through a pathway that induces microglial activation as well as antioxidant responses [81]. Based on the new body of information, the following pathogenic scenario of PD emerges: In dopaminergic neurons, increased calcium conductance and the ensuing greater production of reactive oxygen species lead to higher levels of damaged mitochondria. In normal individuals, Parkin and PINK eliminate damaged mitochondria by macroautophagy allowing neurons to retain a normal pool of healthy mitochondria. In contrast, in PD a loss of Parkin function leads to a progressive buildup of damaged mitochondrial and a defect in Parkin/Pink1 turnover. Thus, over time, the burden caused by mitochondrial dysfunction will reach a pathological threshold, provoking neuronal dysfunction and ultimately cell death [76]. The major components inducing neuronal loss are (1) presynaptic and/or axonal α-syn aggregation, synaptic and axon degeneration, (2) mitochondrial dysfunction, (3) environmental oxidative stress, (4) neuroinflammation, and other noxious factors. Despite speculations as to how aberrant protein activity might lead to neurodegeneration, it is not certain that α-syn aggregation is the primary cause or an epiphenomenon in the pathogenetic process of PD.

To this and other molecular factors, the contribution of other mechanisms must be added, among which complex cell interactions due to a prion-like cell-to-cell spread of α-syn are documented [369, 370, 374, 375]. Worsening of the clinical features over time, the temporal evolution of neuropathology in PD, and postmortem observation of α-syn pathology within embryonic grafted cells in the striata of PD patients implicated that the spread of α-syn (or its toxic truncated forms) from cell to cell is the main mechanism underlying disease progression in PD and other synucleinopathies [133, 376]. This suggests that pathology could spread from one cell to another and that α-syn can be transferred from an affected neuron to a previously healthy neuron by a "prion-like" process [369, 370, 374]. Interestingly, converging preclinical evidence indicates the ability of α-syn to spread throughout the brain through neuronal networks [377]. Extracellular α-syn may also play a role in disease propagation and could further trigger neuroinflammation through microglia activation [378–380]. Recent evidence suggests that a trans-synaptic or transcellular spreading of α-syn may be a more likely explanation for the propagation of the disease than other mechanisms, such as oxidative stress, neuroinflammation, or loss of neurotrophic transport [370]. Cell-to-cell transfer of α-syn can explain the formation of LBs and LNs but may not account for the full spectrum of PD and especially not for the involvement of multiple non-dopaminergic neuronal populations, although a correlation exists between the degree of neuronal degeneration in the dopaminergic SNc and the pedunculopontine nucleus, which sends cholinergic projections directly to nigral dopaminergic neurons. However, the exact mechanisms underlying the prion-like transfer/spread and the relative contributions of soluble and oligomeric species of α-syn or of other pathogenic proteins in the propagation of PD require further elucidation. Of note, recent studies found no evidence to support concerns that proteins underlying PD (or AD) transmit disease to humans.

Animal Models of Parkinson's Disease

Experimental models suggested to shed light on the neuropathobiology of PD come from essentially five sources: pharmacological (e.g., reserpine), toxic (e.g., MPTP [the pyridine toxin 1-methyl-4-phenyl-1,2,3,6-tetrahydropyridine]) [381], rotenone and paraquat [357, 382–384], transgenic [142, 143, 385, 386], and cellular [387]. During recent years, a myriad of different models carrying mutations similar to those found in humans in *Drosophila melanogaster* [388, 389], *Caenorhabditis elegans* [390], rodents [143], and mammalians [391] have been developed to study the pathogenesis of this disease. Although some genetic models reproduced the key features of PD, they did not succeed in reproducing both the pathology and progressive degenerating process in human PD [392–395]. The sole model of DLB reported is an α-syn transgenic mouse [396].

Viral PD models comprising α-syn and LRRK-2-based overexpression or mimicking PARKIN loss of function by overexpression of PARKIN substrates [397], viral-vector-mediated α-syn lesion as a chronic and progressive model [398], and other recent genetic models may provide valuable insights into PD mechanisms in order to contribute to the development of therapeutic targets. The relevance of both pathogenic and etiologic models and their limits for new therapeutic studies have been reviewed recently [393, 399, 400].

Conclusion and Future Directions

Although PD remains as much an enigma as when James Parkinson first described its clinical features, the current knowledge of this devastating disease, its diagnosis, pathogenesis, and development continues to evolve and be challenged by future scientific discovery. Severe damage to the dopaminergic striatonigral system and many non-dopaminergic neuronal systems together with widespread occurrence of α-syn-positive LBs and dystrophic neurites are characteristic pathological findings, Lewy bodies representing its morphological hallmark. However, damage is not restricted to these structures, and PD and other synucleinopathies are now established multiorgan disorders, the etiology and pathogenesis of which are far from being fully elucidated. Recent evidence suggests that the heterogeneous mechanisms leading to sporadic PD are linked and that this progressive disorder is not the result of a single causative factor but is rather multifactorial, integrating the effects of genetic and environmental factors and a complicated cascade of molecular events to work in concert on many cellular systems to induce progressive degeneration in vulnerable neuronal populations. Among the most challenging problems are (1) the mechanisms of selective vulnerability in PD, (2) the factors leading to cell death in the SN and other important neuronal circuits, (3) the pathogenic role of α-syn aggregations and LBs, (4) the interaction of α-syn with other co-deposited proteins, including tau and β-amyloid, (5) the role of inflammation in the pathogenesis of PD, and (6) the better knowledge of the prion-like behavior of proteins and their impact on disease progression. Further research on the dysfunction of protein surveillance identified by the susceptibility genes, the interplay of the degenerative process with α-syn and Lewy pathology, essential pathogenic factors in the development of neurodegeneration, and the nature of triggers that unmask the disease process will be needed to enable the development of reliable biomarkers for early diagnosis, optimal animal models, and disease-modifying treatments of this hitherto incurable movement disorder.

References

1. Wirdefeldt K, Adami HO, Cole P, Trichopoulos D, Mandel J. Epidemiology and etiology of Parkinson's disease: a review of the evidence. Eur J Epidemiol. 2011;26 Suppl 1:S1–58.
2. Bach JP, Ziegler U, Deuschl G, Dodel R, Doblhammer-Reiter G. Projected numbers of people with movement disorders in the years 2030 and 2050. Mov Disord. 2011;26:2286–90.
3. Spillantini MG, Schmidt ML, Lee VM, Trojanowski JQ, Jakes R, Goedert M. Alpha-synuclein in Lewy bodies. Nature. 1997;388:839–40.
4. Jellinger KA. Lewy body disorders. In: Youdim MBH, Riederer P, Mandel SA, Battistin L, Lajtha A, editors. Degenerative diseases of the nervous system. New York: Springer Science; 2007. p. 267–343.
5. Beach TG, Adler CH, Sue LI, Vedders L, Lue L, White Iii CL, et al. Multi-organ distribution of phosphorylated alpha-synuclein histopathology in subjects with Lewy body disorders. Acta Neuropathol. 2010;119:689–702.
6. Braak H, Del Tredici K. Invited article: nervous system pathology in sporadic Parkinson disease. Neurology. 2008;70:1916–25.
7. Fumimura Y, Ikemura M, Saito Y, Sengoku R, Kanemaru K, Sawabe M, et al. Analysis of the adrenal gland is useful for evaluating pathology of the peripheral autonomic nervous system in Lewy body disease. J Neuropathol Exp Neurol. 2007;66:354–62.
8. Ikemura M, Saito Y, Sengoku R, Sakiyama Y, Hatsuta H, Kanemaru K, et al. Lewy body pathology involves cutaneous nerves. J Neuropathol Exp Neurol. 2008;67:945–53.
9. Mu L, Sobotka S, Chen J, Su H, Sanders I, Adler CH, et al. Alpha-synuclein pathology and axonal degeneration of the peripheral motor nerves innervating pharyngeal muscles in Parkinson disease. J Neuropathol Exp Neurol. 2013;72:119–29.
10. Orimo S, Uchihara T, Nakamura A, Mori F, Kakita A, Wakabayashi K, et al. Axonal alpha-synuclein aggregates herald centripetal degeneration of cardiac sympathetic nerve in Parkinson's disease. Brain. 2008;131:642–50.
11. Wakabayashi K, Mori F, Tanji K, Orimo S, Takahashi H. Involvement of the peripheral nervous system in synucleinopathies, tauopathies and other neurodegenerative proteinopathies of the brain. Acta Neuropathol. 2010;120:1–12.
12. Jellinger KA. The role of alpha-synuclein in neurodegeneration – an update. Transl Neurosci. 2012;3:75–122.
13. Jellinger KA. Neuropathology of sporadic Parkinson's disease: evaluation and changes of concepts. Mov Disord. 2012;27:8–30.
14. Wakabayashi K, Tanji K, Odagiri S, Miki Y, Mori F, Takahashi H. The Lewy body in Parkinson's disease and related neurodegenerative disorders. Mol Neurobiol. 2013;47:495–508.
15. Halliday G, McCann H, Shepherd C. Evaluation of the Braak hypothesis: how far can it explain the pathogenesis of Parkinson's disease? Expert Rev Neurother. 2012;12:673–86.
16. DelleDonne A, Klos KJ, Fujishiro H, Ahmed Z, Parisi JE, Josephs KA, et al. Incidental Lewy body disease and preclinical Parkinson disease. Arch Neurol. 2008;65:1074–80.
17. Dickson DW, Fujishiro H, Delledonne A, Menke J, Ahmed Z, Klos KJ, et al. Evidence that incidental Lewy body disease is pre-symptomatic Parkinson's disease. Acta Neuropathol. 2008;115:437–44.
18. Bloch A, Probst A, Bissig H, Adams H, Tolnay M. Alpha-synuclein pathology of the spinal and peripheral autonomic nervous system in neurologically unimpaired elderly subjects. Neuropathol Appl Neurobiol. 2006;32:284–95.
19. Braak H, Sastre M, Bohl JR, de Vos RA, Del Tredici K. Parkinson's disease: lesions in dorsal horn layer I, involvement of parasympathetic and sympathetic pre- and postganglionic neurons. Acta Neuropathol. 2007;113:421–9.
20. Gold A, Turkalp ZT, Munoz DG. Enteric alpha-synuclein expression is increased in Parkinson's disease but not Alzheimer's disease. Mov Disord. 2013;28:237–40.

21. Probst A, Bloch A, Tolnay M. New insights into the pathology of Parkinson's disease: does the peripheral autonomic system become central? Eur J Neurol. 2008;15 Suppl 1:1–4.
22. Lebouvier T, Chaumette T, Paillusson S, Duyckaerts C, Bruley des Varannes S, Neunlist M, et al. The second brain and Parkinson's disease. Eur J Neurosci. 2009;30:735–41.
23. Phillips RJ, Walter GC, Wilder SL, Baronowsky EA, Powley TL. Alpha-synuclein-immunopositive myenteric neurons and vagal preganglionic terminals: autonomic pathway implicated in Parkinson's disease? Neuroscience. 2008;153:733–50.
24. Braak H, Del Tredici K, Rub U, de Vos RA, Jansen Steur EN, Braak E. Staging of brain pathology related to sporadic Parkinson's disease. Neurobiol Aging. 2003;24:197–211.
25. Hawkes CH, Del Tredici K, Braak H. Parkinson's disease: a dual-hit hypothesis. Neuropathol Appl Neurobiol. 2007;33:599–614.
26. Akhtar RS, Stern MB. New concepts in the early and preclinical detection of Parkinson's disease: therapeutic implications. Expert Rev Neurother. 2012;12:1429–38.
27. Chaudhuri KR, Schapira AH. Non-motor symptoms of Parkinson's disease: dopaminergic pathophysiology and treatment. Lancet Neurol. 2009;8:464–74.
28. Lang AE. A critical appraisal of the premotor symptoms of Parkinson's disease: potential usefulness in early diagnosis and design of neuroprotective trials. Mov Disord. 2011;26: 775–83.
29. Massano J, Bhatia KP. Clinical approach to Parkinson's disease: features, diagnosis, and principles of management. Cold Spring Harb Perspect Med. 2012;2:a008870.
30. Pfeiffer RF, Bodis-Wollner I, editors. Parkinson's disease and nonmotor dysfunction. New York: Springer Science + Business Media; 2013.
31. Tolosa E, Santamaria J, Gaig C, Compta Y. Nonmotor aspects of Parkinson's disease. In: Schapira AHV, Lang AET, Fahn S, editors. Movement disorders 4. Philadelphia: Saunders-Elsevier; 2010. p. 229–51.
32. Hely MA, Reid WG, Adena MA, Halliday GM, Morris JG. The Sydney multicenter study of Parkinson's disease: the inevitability of dementia at 20 years. Mov Disord. 2008; 23:837–44.
33. Foltynie T, Brayne C, Barker RA. The heterogeneity of idiopathic Parkinson's disease. J Neurol. 2002;249:138–45.
34. Rajput AH, Voll A, Rajput ML, Robinson CA, Rajput A. Course in Parkinson disease subtypes: A 39-year clinicopathologic study. Neurology. 2009;73:206–12.
35. Stern MB, Lang A, Poewe W. Toward a redefinition of Parkinson's disease. Mov Disord. 2012;27:54–60.
36. Halliday GM, Holton JL, Revesz T, Dickson DW. Neuropathology underlying clinical variability in patients with synucleinopathies. Acta Neuropathol. 2011;122:187–204.
37. Selikhova M, Williams DR, Kempster PA, Holton JL, Revesz T, Lees AJ. A clinicopathological study of subtypes in Parkinson's disease. Brain. 2009;132:2947–57.
38. Hughes AJ, Daniel SE, Ben-Shlomo Y, Lees AJ. The accuracy of diagnosis of Parkinsonian syndromes in a specialist movement disorder service. Brain. 2002;125:861–70.
39. Lees AJ, Hardy J, Revesz T. Parkinson's disease. Lancet. 2009;373:2055–66.
40. Litvan I, Bhatia KP, Burn DJ, Goetz CG, Lang AE, McKeith I, et al. Movement Disorders Society Scientific Issues Committee report: SIC Task Force appraisal of clinical diagnostic criteria for Parkinsonian disorders. Mov Disord. 2003;18:467–86.
41. Dickson DW, Braak H, Duda JE, Duyckaerts C, Gasser T, Halliday GM, et al. Diagnostic criteria for the neuropathological assessment of Parkinson disease: Report of the Neuropathology and Genetics Working Group of the Second International Brainstorming Conference on Parkinson disease. Lancet Neurol. 2009;8:1150–7.
42. Dickson DW. Parkinson's disease and Parkinsonism: neuropathology. Cold Spring Harb Perspect Med. 2012;2:a009258.
43. Halliday G, Lees A, Stern M. Milestones in Parkinson's disease–clinical and pathologic features. Mov Disord. 2011;26:1015–21.
44. Gasser T, Hardy J, Mizuno Y. Milestones in PD genetics. Mov Disord. 2011;26:1042–8.

45. Hirsch EC, Jenner P, Przedborski S. Pathogenesis of Parkinson's disease. Mov Disord. 2013;28:24–30.
46. Jellinger KA. Synuclein and Parkinson's disease: an update. In: Martinez A, Gil C, editors. Emerging drugs and targets for Parkinson's disease. London: The Royal Society of Chemistry; 2013. p. 175–214.
47. Duda JE, Dickson DW. Neuropathology of Parkinson's disease. In: Pfeiffer RF, Wszolek ZK, Ebadi M, editors. Parkinson's disease. 2nd ed. Boca Raton: CRC Press; 2013. p. 492–506.
48. Halliday G, Murphy K. Pathology of Parkinson's disease – an overview. In: Schapira AHV, Lang AET, Fahn S, editors. Movement disorders 4. Philadelphia: Saunders-Elsevier; 2010. p. 132–54.
49. Jellinger KA. Parkinson's disease. In: Dickson DW, Weller RO, editors. Neurodegeneration: the molecular pathology of dementia and movement disorders. 2nd ed. Oxford: Blackwell Publishing Ltd.; 2011. p. 194–223.
50. Houlden H, Singleton AB. The genetics and neuropathology of Parkinson's disease. Acta Neuropathol. 2012;124:325–38.
51. Poulopoulos M, Levy OA, Alcalay RN. The neuropathology of genetic Parkinson's disease. Mov Disord. 2012;27:831–42.
52. Muntane G, Dalfo E, Martinez A, Ferrer I. Phosphorylation of tau and alpha-synuclein in synaptic-enriched fractions of the frontal cortex in Alzheimer's disease, and in Parkinson's disease and related alpha-synucleinopathies. Neuroscience. 2008;152:913–23.
53. Schulz-Schaeffer WJ. The synaptic pathology of alpha-synuclein aggregation in dementia with Lewy bodies, Parkinson's disease and Parkinson's disease dementia. Acta Neuropathol. 2010;120:131–43.
54. Damier P, Hirsch EC, Agid Y, Graybiel AM. The substantia nigra of the human brain. II. Patterns of loss of dopamine-containing neurons in Parkinson's disease. Brain. 1999;122 (Pt 8):1437–48.
55. Kish SJ, Shannak K, Hornykiewicz O. Uneven pattern of dopamine loss in the striatum of patients with idiopathic Parkinson's disease. Pathophysiologic and clinical implications. N Engl J Med. 1988;318:876–80.
56. Rajput AH, Sitte HH, Rajput A, Fenton ME, Pifl C, Hornykiewicz O. Globus pallidus dopamine and Parkinson motor subtypes: clinical and brain biochemical correlation. Neurology. 2008;70:1403–10.
57. Porritt MJ, Kingsbury AE, Hughes AJ, Howells DW. Striatal dopaminergic neurons are lost with Parkinson's disease progression. Mov Disord. 2006;21:2208–11.
58. Tandé D, Hoglinger G, Debeir T, Freundlieb N, Hirsch EC, Francois C. New striatal dopamine neurons in MPTP-treated macaques result from a phenotypic shift and not neurogenesis. Brain. 2006;129:1194–200.
59. Mundinano IC, Caballero MC, Ordonez C, Hernandez M, DiCaudo C, Marcilla I, et al. Increased dopaminergic cells and protein aggregates in the olfactory bulb of patients with neurodegenerative disorders. Acta Neuropathol. 2011;122:61–74.
60. de la Fuente-Fernandez R, Schulzer M, Kuramoto L, Cragg J, Ramachandiran N, Au WL, et al. Age-specific progression of nigrostriatal dysfunction in Parkinson's disease. Ann Neurol. 2011;69:803–10.
61. Lee SH, Kim SS, Tae WS, Lee SY, Choi JW, Koh SB, et al. Regional volume analysis of the Parkinson disease brain in early disease stage: gray matter, white matter, striatum, and thalamus. AJNR Am J Neuroradiol. 2011;32:682–7.
62. Shih MC, Franco de Andrade LA, Amaro Jr E, Felicio AC, Ferraz HB, Wagner J, et al. Higher nigrostriatal dopamine neuron loss in early than late onset Parkinson's disease? – a [99mTc]-TRODAT-1 SPECT study. Mov Disord. 2007;22:863–6.
63. Ma SY, Roytta M, Rinne JO, Collan Y, Rinne UK. Correlation between neuromorphometry in the substantia nigra and clinical features in Parkinson's disease using disector counts. J Neurol Sci. 1997;151:83–7.

64. Pavese N, Rivero-Bosch M, Lewis SJ, Whone AL, Brooks DJ. Progression of monoaminergic dysfunction in Parkinson's disease: a longitudinal (18)F-dopa PET study. Neuroimage. 2011;56:1463–8.
65. Bernheimer H, Birkmayer W, Hornykiewicz O, Jellinger K, Seitelberger F. Brain dopamine and the syndromes of Parkinson and Huntington. Clinical, morphological and neurochemical correlations. J Neurol Sci. 1973;20:415–55.
66. Ziegler DA, Wonderlick JS, Ashourian P, Hansen LA, Young JC, Murphy AJ, et al. Substantia nigra volume loss before basal forebrain degeneration in early Parkinson disease. JAMA Neurol. 2013;70:241–7.
67. Rudow G, O'Brien R, Savonenko AV, Resnick SM, Zonderman AB, Pletnikova O, et al. Morphometry of the human substantia nigra in ageing and Parkinson's disease. Acta Neuropathol. 2008;115:461–70.
68. Djaldetti R, Lorberboym M, Karmon Y, Treves TA, Ziv I, Melamed E. Residual striatal dopaminergic nerve terminals in very long-standing Parkinson's disease: a single photon emission computed tomography imaging study. Mov Disord. 2011;26:327–30.
69. Kovacs GG, Milenkovic IJ, Preusser M, Budka H. Nigral burden of alpha-synuclein correlates with striatal dopamine deficit. Mov Disord. 2008;23:1608–12.
70. Chu Y, Morfini GA, Langhamer LB, He Y, Brady ST, Kordower JH. Alterations in axonal transport motor proteins in sporadic and experimental Parkinson's disease. Brain. 2012;135: 2058–73.
71. Ma SY, Ciliax BJ, Stebbins G, Jaffar S, Joyce JN, Cochran EJ, et al. Dopamine transporter-immunoreactive neurons decrease with age in the human substantia nigra. J Comp Neurol. 1999;409:25–37.
72. Cabello CR, Thune JJ, Pakkenberg H, Pakkenberg B. Ageing of substantia nigra in humans: cell loss may be compensated by hypertrophy. Neuropathol Appl Neurobiol. 2002;28: 283–91.
73. Kingsbury AE, Marsden CD, Foster OJ. The vulnerability of nigral neurons to Parkinson's disease is unrelated to their intrinsic capacity for dopamine synthesis: an in situ hybridization study. Mov Disord. 1999;14:206–18.
74. McGeer PL, McGeer EG. Glial reactions in Parkinson's disease. Mov Disord. 2008;23: 474–83.
75. Dexter DT, Jenner P. Parkinson disease: from pathology to molecular disease mechanisms. Free Radic Biol Med. 2013;62:132–44.
76. Hirsch EC, Hunot S. Neuroinflammation in Parkinson's disease: a target for neuroprotection? Lancet Neurol. 2009;8:382–97.
77. Long-Smith CM, Sullivan AM, Nolan YM. The influence of microglia on the pathogenesis of Parkinson's disease. Prog Neurobiol. 2009;89:277–87.
78. Pradhan S, Andreasson K. Commentary: progressive inflammation as a contributing factor to early development of Parkinson's disease. Exp Neurol. 2013;241:148–55.
79. Tansey MG, Goldberg MS. Neuroinflammation in Parkinson's disease: its role in neuronal death and implications for therapeutic intervention. Neurobiol Dis. 2010;37:510–8.
80. Tufekci KU, Meuwissen R, Genc S, Genc K. Inflammation in Parkinson's disease. Adv Protein Chem Struct Biol. 2012;88:69–132.
81. Alvarez-Erviti L, Couch Y, Richardson J, Cooper JM, Wood MJ. Alpha-synuclein release by neurons activates the inflammatory response in a microglial cell line. Neurosci Res. 2011; 69:337–42.
82. Wakabayashi K, Mori F, Takahashi H. Progression patterns of neuronal loss and Lewy body pathology in the substantia nigra in Parkinson's disease. Parkinsonism Relat Disord. 2006;12(suppl):S92–8.
83. Greffard S, Verny M, Bonnet AM, Seilhean D, Hauw JJ, Duyckaerts C. A stable proportion of Lewy body bearing neurons in the substantia nigra suggests a model in which the Lewy body causes neuronal death. Neurobiol Aging. 2008;31:99–103.
84. Cheng HC, Ulane CM, Burke RE. Clinical progression in Parkinson disease and the neurobiology of axons. Ann Neurol. 2010;67:715–25.

85. Kordower JH, Olanow CW, Dodiya HB, Chu Y, Beach TG, Adler CH, et al. Disease duration and the integrity of the nigrostriatal system in Parkinson's disease. Brain 2013;136: 2419–31.
86. Braak H, Del Tredici K. Neuroanatomy and pathology of sporadic Parkinson's disease. Adv Anat Embryol Cell Biol. 2009;201:1–119.
87. Zhou ZD, Lan YH, Tan EK, Lim TM. Iron species-mediated dopamine oxidation, proteasome inhibition, and dopaminergic cell demise: implications for iron-related dopaminergic neuron degeneration. Free Radic Biol Med. 2010;49:1856–71.
88. Faucheux BA, Martin ME, Beaumont C, Hauw JJ, Agid Y, Hirsch EC. Neuromelanin-associated redox-active iron is increased in the substantia nigra of patients with Parkinson's disease. J Neurochem. 2003;86:1142–8.
89. Lv Z, Jiang H, Xu H, Song N, Xie J. Increased iron levels correlate with the selective nigral dopaminergic neuron degeneration in Parkinson's disease. J Neural Transm. 2011;118: 361–9.
90. Kell DB. Towards a unifying, systems biology understanding of large-scale cellular death and destruction caused by poorly liganded iron: Parkinson's, Huntington's, Alzheimer's, prions, bactericides, chemical toxicology and others as examples. Arch Toxicol. 2010;84:825–89.
91. Sian-Hulsmann J, Mandel S, Youdim MB, Riederer P. The relevance of iron in the pathogenesis of Parkinson's disease. J Neurochem. 2011;118:939–57.
92. Wypijewska A, Galazka-Friedman J, Bauminger ER, Wszolek ZK, Schweitzer KJ, Dickson DW, et al. Iron and reactive oxygen species activity in Parkinsonian substantia nigra. Parkinsonism Relat Disord. 2010;16:329–33.
93. Halliday GM, Ophof A, Broe M, Jensen PH, Kettle E, Fedorow H, et al. Alpha-synuclein redistributes to neuromelanin lipid in the substantia nigra early in Parkinson's disease. Brain. 2005;128:2654–64.
94. Febbraro F, Giorgi M, Caldarola S, Loreni F, Romero-Ramos M. Alpha-Synuclein expression is modulated at the translational level by iron. Neuroreport. 2012;23:576–80.
95. Levin J, Högen T, Hillmer AS, Bader B, Schmidt F, Kamp F, et al. Generation of ferric iron links oxidative stress to alpha-synuclein oligomer formation. J Parkinsons Dis. 2011;1: 205–16.
96. Fasano M, Bergamasco B, Lopiano L. Modifications of the iron-neuromelanin system in Parkinson's disease. J Neurochem. 2006;96:909–16.
97. Guerrero E, Vasudevaraju P, Hegde ML, Britton GB, Rao KS. Recent advances in alpha-synuclein functions, advanced glycation, and toxicity: implications for Parkinson's disease. Mol Neurobiol. 2013;47:525–36.
98. Ruiperez V, Darios F, Davletov B. Alpha-synuclein, lipids and Parkinson's disease. Prog Lipid Res. 2010;49:420–8.
99. Howells DW, Porritt MJ, Wong JY, Batchelor PE, Kalnins R, Hughes AJ, et al. Reduced BDNF mRNA expression in the Parkinson's disease substantia nigra. Exp Neurol. 2000;166: 127–35.
100. Mogi M, Togari A, Kondo T, Mizuno Y, Kogure O, Kuno S, et al. Glial cell line-derived neurotrophic factor in the substantia nigra from control and Parkinsonian brains. Neurosci Lett. 2001;300:179–81.
101. Chauhan NB, Siegel GJ, Lee JM. Depletion of glial cell line-derived neurotrophic factor in substantia nigra neurons of Parkinson's disease brain. J Chem Neuroanat. 2001;21:277–88.
102. Knott C, Stern G, Kingsbury A, Welcher AA, Wilkin GP. Elevated glial brain-derived neurotrophic factor in Parkinson's disease nigra. Parkinsonism Relat Disord. 2002;8:329–41.
103. Gu G, Reyes PE, Golden GT, Woltjer RL, Hulette C, Montine TJ, et al. Mitochondrial DNA deletions/rearrangements in Parkinson disease and related neurodegenerative disorders. J Neuropathol Exp Neurol. 2002;61:634–9.
104. Winslow AR, Rubinsztein DC. The Parkinson disease protein alpha-synuclein inhibits autophagy. Autophagy. 2011;7:429–31.

105. Double KL, Reyes S, Werry EL, Halliday GM. Selective cell death in neurodegeneration: why are some neurons spared in vulnerable regions? Prog Neurobiol. 2010;92:316–29.
106. Fearnley JM, Lees AJ. Ageing and Parkinson's disease: substantia nigra regional selectivity. Brain. 1991;114(Pt 5):2283–301.
107. McRitchie DA, Cartwright HR, Halliday GM. Specific A10 dopaminergic nuclei in the midbrain degenerate in Parkinson's disease. Exp Neurol. 1997;144:202–13.
108. Matzuk MM, Saper CB. Preservation of hypothalamic dopaminergic neurons in Parkinson's disease. Ann Neurol. 1985;18:552–5.
109. Fronczek R, Overeem S, Lee SY, Hegeman IM, van Pelt J, van Duinen SG, et al. Hypocretin (orexin) loss in Parkinson's disease. Brain. 2007;130:1577–85.
110. Thannickal TC, Lai YY, Siegel JM. Hypocretin (orexin) cell loss in Parkinson's disease. Brain. 2007;130:1586–95.
111. Saxena S, Caroni P. Selective neuronal vulnerability in neurodegenerative diseases: from stressor thresholds to degeneration. Neuron. 2011;71:35–48.
112. Uchikado H, Lin WL, DeLucia MW, Dickson DW. Alzheimer disease with amygdala Lewy bodies: a distinct form of alpha-synucleinopathy. J Neuropathol Exp Neurol. 2006;65: 685–97.
113. Jellinger KA. Pathology of Parkinson's disease. Changes other than the nigrostriatal pathway. Mol Chem Neuropathol. 1991;14:153–97.
114. Benarroch EE, Schmeichel AM, Low PA, Boeve BF, Sandroni P, Parisi JE. Involvement of medullary regions controlling sympathetic output in Lewy body disease. Brain. 2005;128: 338–44.
115. Benarroch EE, Schmeichel AM, Low PA, Parisi JE. Depletion of putative chemosensitive respiratory neurons in the ventral medullary surface in multiple system atrophy. Brain. 2007;130:469–75.
116. Grinberg LT, Rueb U, Alho AT, Heinsen H. Brainstem pathology and non-motor symptoms in PD. J Neurol Sci. 2010;289:81–8.
117. Dickson DW, Fujishiro H, Orr C, DelleDonne A, Josephs KA, Frigerio R, et al. Neuropathology of non-motor features of Parkinson disease. Parkinsonism Relat Disord. 2009;15 Suppl 3:S1–5.
118. Silveira-Moriyama L, Holton JL, Kingsbury A, Ayling H, Petrie A, Sterlacci W, et al. Regional differences in the severity of Lewy body pathology across the olfactory cortex. Neurosci Lett. 2009;453:77–80.
119. Tamura T, Yoshida M, Hashizume Y, Sobue G. Lewy body-related alpha-synucleinopathy in the spinal cord of cases with incidental Lewy body disease. Neuropathology. 2012;32: 13–22.
120. Del Tredici K, Braak H. Spinal cord lesions in sporadic Parkinson's disease. Acta Neuropathol. 2012;124:643–64.
121. Djaldetti R, Lev N, Melamed E. Lesions outside the CNS in Parkinson's disease. Mov Disord. 2009;24:793–800.
122. Duda JE. Olfactory system pathology as a model of Lewy neurodegenerative disease. J Neurol Sci. 2010;289:49–54.
123. Braak H, Rub U, Jansen Steur EN, Del Tredici K, de Vos RA. Cognitive status correlates with neuropathologic stage in Parkinson disease. Neurology. 2005;64:1404–10.
124. Amino T, Orimo S, Itoh Y, Takahashi A, Uchihara T, Mizusawa H. Profound cardiac sympathetic denervation occurs in Parkinson disease. Brain Pathol. 2005;15:29–34.
125. Ghebremedhin E, Del Tredici K, Langston JW, Braak H. Diminished tyrosine hydroxylase immunoreactivity in the cardiac conduction system and myocardium in Parkinson's disease: an anatomical study. Acta Neuropathol. 2009;118:777–84.
126. Orimo S, Takahashi A, Uchihara T, Mori F, Kakita A, Wakabayashi K, et al. Degeneration of cardiac sympathetic nerve begins in the early disease process of Parkinson's disease. Brain Pathol. 2007;17:24–30.
127. Orimo S, Kanazawa T, Nakamura A, Uchihara T, Mori F, Kakita A, et al. Degeneration of cardiac sympathetic nerve can occur in multiple system atrophy. Acta Neuropathol. 2007; 113:81–6.

128. Archibald NK, Clarke MP, Mosimann UP, Burn DJ. The retina in Parkinson's disease. Brain. 2009;132:1128–45.
129. Beach TG, Adler CH, Lue L, Sue LI, Bachalakuri J, Henry-Watson J, et al. Unified staging system for Lewy body disorders: correlation with nigrostriatal degeneration, cognitive impairment and motor dysfunction. Acta Neuropathol. 2009;117:613–34.
130. Annerino DM, Arshad S, Taylor GM, Adler CH, Beach TG, Greene JG. Parkinson's disease is not associated with gastrointestinal myenteric ganglion neuron loss. Acta Neuropathol. 2012;124:665–80.
131. Beach TG, Adler CH, Sue LI, Peirce JB, Bachalakuri J, Dalsing-Hernandez JE, et al. Reduced striatal tyrosine hydroxylase in incidental Lewy body disease. Acta Neuropathol. 2008;115:445–51.
132. Frigerio R, Fujishiro H, Ahn TB, Josephs KA, Maraganore DM, DelleDonne A, et al. Incidental Lewy body disease: do some cases represent a preclinical stage of dementia with Lewy bodies? Neurobiol Aging. 2011;32:857–63.
132a. Doppler K, Ebert s, Üçeyler N, Trenkwalder C, Ebentheuer J, Volkmann J, et al. Cutaneous neuropathy in Parkinson's disease: a window into brain pathology. Acta Neuropathol 2014; 128:99–109.
133. Lema Tomé CM, Tyson T, Rey NL, Grathwohl S, Britschgi M, Brundin P. Inflammation and alpha-synuclein's prion-like behavior in Parkinson's disease–is there a link? Mol Neurobiol. 2013;47:561–74.
134. Freundt EC, Maynard N, Clancy EK, Roy S, Bousset L, Sourigues Y, et al. Neuron-to-neuron transmission of alpha-synuclein fibrils through axonal transport. Ann Neurol. 2012;72:517–24.
135. Lue L-F, Walker DG, Adler CH, Shill H, Tran H, Akiyama H, et al. Biochemical increase in phosphorylated a-synuclein precedes histopathology of Lewy-type synucleinopathies. Brain Pathol. 2012;22:745–56.
136. Minguez-Castellanos A, Chamorro CE, Escamilla-Sevilla F, Ortega-Moreno A, Rebollo AC, Gomez-Rio M, et al. Do alpha-synuclein aggregates in autonomic plexuses predate Lewy body disorders?: a cohort study. Neurology. 2007;68:2012–8.
137. Burke RE, Dauer WT, Vonsattel JP. A critical evaluation of the Braak staging scheme for Parkinson's disease. Ann Neurol. 2008;64:485–91.
138. Kanazawa T, Adachi E, Orimo S, Nakamura A, Mizusawa H, Uchihara T. Pale neurites, premature alpha-synuclein aggregates with centripetal extension from axon collaterals. Brain Pathol. 2012;22:67–78.
139. Dale GE, Probst A, Luthert P, Martin J, Anderton BH, Leigh PN. Relationships between Lewy bodies and pale bodies in Parkinson's disease. Acta Neuropathol. 1992;83:525–9.
140. Katsuse O, Iseki E, Marui W, Kosaka K. Developmental stages of cortical Lewy bodies and their relation to axonal transport blockage in brains of patients with dementia with Lewy bodies. J Neurol Sci. 2003;211:29–35.
141. Lundblad M, Decressac M, Mattsson B, Bjorklund A. Impaired neurotransmission caused by overexpression of alpha-synuclein in nigral dopamine neurons. Proc Natl Acad Sci U S A. 2012;109:3213–9.
141a. Garcia-Reitböck P, Anichtchik O, Bellucci A, Iovino M, Ballini C, Fineberg E, et al. SNARE protein redistribution and synaptic failure in a transgenic mouse model of Parkinson's disease. Brain 2010;133:2032–44.
142. Li Y, Liu W, Oo TF, Wang L, Tang Y, Jackson-Lewis V, et al. Mutant LRRK2(R1441G) BAC transgenic mice recapitulate cardinal features of Parkinson's disease. Nat Neurosci. 2009;12:826–8.
143. Stoica G, Lungu G, Bjorklund NL, Taglialatela G, Zhang X, Chiu V, et al. Potential role of alpha-synuclein in neurodegeneration: studies in a rat animal model. J Neurochem. 2012; 122:812–22.
143a. Nakata Y, Yasuda T, Fukaya M, Yamamori S, Itakura M, Nihira T, et al. Accumulation of alpha-synuclein triggered by presynaptic dysfunction. J Neurosci 2012;32:17186–96.

144. Milber JM, Noorigian JV, Morley JF, Petrovitch H, White L, Ross GW, et al. Lewy pathology is not the first sign of degeneration in vulnerable neurons in Parkinson disease. Neurology. 2012;79:2307–14.
145. Bellucci A, Zaltieri M, Navarria L, Grigoletto J, Missale C, Spano P. From alpha-synuclein to synaptic dysfunctions: new insights into the pathophysiology of Parkinson's disease. Brain Res. 2012;1476:183–202.
146. Mori F, Nishie M, Kakita A, Yoshimoto M, Takahashi H, Wakabayashi K. Relationship among alpha-synuclein accumulation, dopamine synthesis, and neurodegeneration in Parkinson disease substantia nigra. J Neuropathol Exp Neurol. 2006;65:808–15.
147. Sidhu A, Wersinger C, Vernier P. Does alpha-synuclein modulate dopaminergic synaptic content and tone at the synapse? FASEB J. 2004;18:637–47.
148. Tong J, Wong H, Guttman M, Ang LC, Forno LS, Shimadzu M, et al. Brain alpha-synuclein accumulation in multiple system atrophy, Parkinson's disease and progressive supranuclear palsy: a comparative investigation. Brain. 2010;133:172–88.
149. Wills J, Jones J, Haggerty T, Duka V, Joyce JN, Sidhu A. Elevated tauopathy and alpha-synuclein pathology in postmortem Parkinson's disease brains with and without dementia. Exp Neurol. 2010;225:210–8.
150. Quinn JG, Coulson DT, Brockbank S, Beyer N, Ravid R, Hellemans J, et al. Alpha-synuclein mRNA and soluble alpha-synuclein protein levels in post-mortem brain from patients with Parkinson's disease, dementia with Lewy bodies, and Alzheimer's disease. Brain Res. 2012;1459:71–80.
151. Fujiwara H, Hasegawa M, Dohmae N, Kawashima A, Masliah E, Goldberg MS, et al. Alpha-synuclein is phosphorylated in synucleinopathy lesions. Nat Cell Biol. 2002; 4:160–4.
152. Beyer K, Ariza A. Alpha-synuclein posttranslational modification and alternative splicing as a trigger for neurodegeneration. Mol Neurobiol. 2013;47:509–24.
153. Kuusisto E, Parkkinen L, Alafuzoff I. Morphogenesis of Lewy bodies: dissimilar incorporation of alpha-synuclein, ubiquitin, and p62. J Neuropathol Exp Neurol. 2003;62:1241–53.
153a. Walker DG, Lue LF, Adler CH, Shill HA, Caviness JN, Sabbagh MN, et al. Changes in properties of serine 129 phosphorylated alpha-synuclein with progression of Lewy-type histopathology in human brains. Exp Neurol 2013;240:190–204.
154. Wilhelmus MM, Verhaar R, Andringa G, Bol JG, Cras P, Shan L, et al. Presence of tissue transglutaminase in granular endoplasmic reticulum is characteristic of melanized neurons in Parkinson's disease brain. Brain Pathol. 2011;21:130–9.
155. Nath S, Goodwin J, Engelborghs Y, Pountney DL. Raised calcium promotes alpha-synuclein aggregate formation. Mol Cell Neurosci. 2011;46:516–26.
156. Izumi Y, Kume T, Akaike A. Regulation of dopaminergic neuronal death by endogenous dopamine and proteasome activity. Yakugaku Zasshi. 2011;131:21–7.
157. Halliday G, Hely M, Reid W, Morris J. The progression of pathology in longitudinally followed patients with Parkinson's disease. Acta Neuropathol. 2008;115:409–15.
158. Sugeno N, Takeda A, Hasegawa T, Kobayashi M, Kikuchi A, Mori F, et al. Serine 129 phosphorylation of alpha-synuclein induces unfolded protein response-mediated cell death. J Biol Chem. 2008;283:23179–88.
159. Greffard S, Verny M, Bonnet AM, Beinis JY, Gallinari C, Meaume S, et al. Motor score of the Unified Parkinson Disease Rating Scale as a good predictor of Lewy body-associated neuronal loss in the substantia nigra. Arch Neurol. 2006;63:584–8.
160. Sossi V, de la Fuente-Fernandez R, Schulzer M, Troiano AR, Ruth TJ, Stoessl AJ. Dopamine transporter relation to dopamine turnover in Parkinson's disease: a positron emission tomography study. Ann Neurol. 2007;62:468–74.
161. Ballard C, Ziabreva I, Perry R, Larsen JP, O'Brien J, McKeith I, et al. Differences in neuropathologic characteristics across the Lewy body dementia spectrum. Neurology. 2006;67: 1931–4.
162. Halliday GM, McCann H. The progression of pathology in Parkinson's disease. Ann N Y Acad Sci. 2010;1184:188–95.

163. Kempster PA, Williams DR, Selikhova M, Holton J, Revesz T, Lees AJ. Patterns of levodopa response in Parkinson's disease: a clinico-pathological study. Brain. 2007;130:2123–8.
164. Chu Y, Kordower JH. Age-associated increases of alpha-synuclein in monkeys and humans are associated with nigrostriatal dopamine depletion: Is this the target for Parkinson's disease? Neurobiol Dis. 2007;25:134–49.
165. Forno LS. Neuropathology of Parkinson's disease. J Neuropathol Exp Neurol. 1996;55: 259–72.
166. Ishiyama M, Yagishita S, Hasegawa K, Yokoyama T. Ultrastructural study (tEM and sEM) of cortical Lewy bodies. Neuropathol. 2006;26:A58.
167. Walker DG, Lue LF, Adler CH, Shill HA, Caviness JN, Sabbagh MN, et al. Changes in properties of serine 129 phosphorylated alpha-synuclein with progression of Lewy-type histopathology in human brains. Exp Neurol. 2013;240:190–204.
168. Ince PG, Clark B, Holton JL, Revesz T, Wharton SB. Disorders of movement and system degeneration. In: Love S, Louis DN, Ellison DW, editors. Greenfield's neuropathology. 8th ed. London: Hodder Arnold; 2008. p. 889–1030.
169. Waxman EA, Duda JE, Giasson BI. Characterization of antibodies that selectively detect alpha-synuclein in pathological inclusions. Acta Neuropathol. 2008;116:37–46.
170. Sharma N, Hewett J, Ozelius LJ, Ramesh V, McLean PJ, Breakefield XO, et al. A close association of torsinA and alpha-synuclein in Lewy bodies: a fluorescence resonance energy transfer study. Am J Pathol. 2001;159:339–44.
171. Banerjee R, Starkov AA, Beal MF, Thomas B. Mitochondrial dysfunction in the limelight of Parkinson's disease pathogenesis. Biochim Biophys Acta. 2009;1792:651–63.
172. Dugger BN, Dickson DW. Cell type specific sequestration of choline acetyltransferase and tyrosine hydroxylase within Lewy bodies. Acta Neuropathol. 2010;120:633–9.
173. Dugger BN, Murray ME, Boeve BF, Parisi JE, Benarroch EE, Ferman TJ, et al. Neuropathological analysis of brainstem cholinergic and catecholaminergic nuclei in relation to rapid eye movement (REM) sleep behaviour disorder. Neuropathol Appl Neurobiol. 2012;38:142–52.
174. Dugger BN, Serrano GE, Sue LI, Walker DG, Adler CH, Shill HA, et al. Presence of striatal amyloid plaques in Parkinson's disease dementia predicts concomitant Alzheimer's disease: usefulness for amyloid imaging. J Parkinsons Dis. 2012;2:57–65.
175. Odagiri S, Tanji K, Mori F, Kakita A, Takahashi H, Wakabayashi K. Autophagic adapter protein NBR1 is localized in Lewy bodies and glial cytoplasmic inclusions and is involved in aggregate formation in alpha-synucleinopathy. Acta Neuropathol. 2012;124:173–86.
176. Schlossmacher MG, Frosch MP, Gai WP, Medina M, Sharma N, Forno L, et al. Parkin localizes to the Lewy bodies of Parkinson disease and dementia with Lewy bodies. Am J Pathol. 2002;160:1655–67.
177. Sulzer D. Clues to how alpha-synuclein damages neurons in Parkinson's disease. Mov Disord. 2010;25 Suppl 1:S27–31.
178. Leverenz JB, Umar I, Wang Q, Montine TJ, McMillan PJ, Tsuang DW, et al. Proteomic identification of novel proteins in cortical Lewy bodies. Brain Pathol. 2007;17:139–45.
179. Proteomic analysis of the substantia nigra in patients with Parkinson's disease. In: Abstracts of the movement disorder society's thirteenth international congress of Parkinson's disease and movement disorders. June 8–10, 2009. Mov Disord 2009; 24 Suppl 1: S39.
180. van Dijk KD, Berendse HW, Drukarch B, Fratantoni SA, Pham TV, Piersma SR, et al. The proteome of the locus ceruleus in Parkinson's disease: relevance to pathogenesis. Brain Pathol. 2012;22:485–98.
181. Kovacs GG, Wagner U, Dumont B, Pikkarainen M, Osman AA, Streichenberger N, et al. An antibody with high reactivity for disease-associated alpha-synuclein reveals extensive brain pathology. Acta Neuropathol. 2012;124:37–50.
182. Power JH, Blumbergs PC. Cellular glutathione peroxidase in human brain: cellular distribution, and its potential role in the degradation of Lewy bodies in Parkinson's disease and dementia with Lewy bodies. Acta Neuropathol. 2009;117:63–73.

183. Kanazawa T, Uchihara T, Takahashi A, Nakamura A, Orimo S, Mizusawa H. Three-layered structure shared between Lewy bodies and Lewy neurites – three-dimensional reconstruction of triple-labeled sections. Brain Pathol. 2008;18:415–22.
184. Ugrumov MV. Non-dopaminergic neurons partly expressing dopaminergic phenotype: distribution in the brain, development and functional significance. J Chem Neuroanat. 2009;38: 241–56.
185. Halliday GM, Stevens CH. Glia: initiators and progressors of pathology in Parkinson's disease. Mov Disord. 2011;26:6–17.
186. Hishikawa N, Hashizume Y, Yoshida M, Sobue G. Widespread occurrence of argyrophilic glial inclusions in Parkinson's disease. Neuropathol Appl Neurobiol. 2001;27:362–72.
187. Beach TG, Walker DG, Sue LI, Newell A, Adler CC, Joyce JN. Substantia nigra Marinesco bodies are associated with decreased striatal expression of dopaminergic markers. J Neuropathol Exp Neurol. 2004;63:329–37.
188. Jellinger KA. Basic mechanisms of neurodegeneration: a critical update. J Cell Mol Med. 2010;14:457–87.
189. Devi L, Raghavendran V, Prabhu BM, Avadhani NG, Anandatheerthavarada HK. Mitochondrial import and accumulation of alpha-synuclein impair complex I in human dopaminergic neuronal cultures and Parkinson disease brain. J Biol Chem. 2008;283: 9089–100.
190. Ferrer I. Early involvement of the cerebral cortex in Parkinson's disease: convergence of multiple metabolic defects. Prog Neurobiol. 2009;88:89–103.
191. Mullin S, Schapira A. Alpha-synuclein and mitochondrial dysfunction in Parkinson's disease. Mol Neurobiol. 2013;47:587–97.
192. Breydo L, Wu JW, Uversky VN. Alpha-synuclein misfolding and Parkinson's disease. Biochim Biophys Acta. 1822;2012:261–85.
193. Stefanis L. Alpha-synuclein in Parkinson's disease. Cold Spring Harb Perspect Med. 2012;2:a009399.
194. Wan OW, Chung KK. The role of alpha-synuclein oligomerization and aggregation in cellular and animal models of Parkinson's disease. PLoS One. 2012;7:e38545.
195. Colla E, Coune P, Liu Y, Pletnikova O, Troncoso JC, Iwatsubo T, et al. Endoplasmic reticulum stress is important for the manifestations of alpha-synucleinopathy in vivo. J Neurosci. 2012;32:3306–20.
196. Winner B, Jappelli R, Maji SK, Desplats PA, Boyer L, Aigner S, et al. In vivo demonstration that alpha-synuclein oligomers are toxic. Proc Natl Acad Sci U S A. 2011;108:4194–9.
197. Gadad BS, Britton GB, Rao KS. Targeting oligomers in neurodegenerative disorders: lessons from alpha-synuclein, tau, and amyloid-beta peptide. J Alzheimers Dis. 2011;24 Suppl 2:223–32.
198. Kalia LV, Kalia SK, McLean PJ, Lozano AM, Lang AE. Alpha-synuclein oligomers and clinical implications for Parkinson disease. Ann Neurol. 2013;73:155–69.
199. Tashiro M, Kojima M, Kihara H, Kasai K, Kamiyoshihara T, Uéda K, et al. Characterization of fibrillation process of alpha-synuclein at the initial stage. Biochem Biophys Res Commun. 2008;369:910–4.
200. Dimant H, Kalia SK, Kalia LV, Zhu LN, Kibuuka L, Ebrahimi-Fakhari D, et al. Direct detection of alpha synuclein oligomers in vivo. Acta Neuropathol Commun. 2013;1:1. doi:10.1186/2051-5960-1-6.
201. Yasuda T, Nakata Y, Mochizuki H. Alpha-synuclein and neuronal cell death. Mol Neurobiol. 2013;47:466–83.
202. Johansen T, Lamark T. Selective autophagy mediated by autophagic adapter proteins. Autophagy. 2011;7:279–96.
203. Xilouri M, Brekk OR, Stefanis L. Alpha-synuclein and protein degradation systems: a reciprocal relationship. Mol Neurobiol. 2013;47:537–51.
204. Fujita Y, Ohama E, Takatama M, Al-Sarraj S, Okamoto K. Fragmentation of Golgi apparatus of nigral neurons with alpha-synuclein-positive inclusions in patients with Parkinson's disease. Acta Neuropathol (Berl). 2006;112:261–5.

205. Muller SK, Bender A, Laub C, Högen T, Schlaudraff F, Liss B, et al. Lewy body pathology is associated with mitochondrial DNA damage in Parkinson's disease. Neurobiol Aging. 2013;34:2231–3.
206. Braak H, Bohl JR, Muller CM, Rub U, de Vos RA, Del Tredici K. Stanley Fahn Lecture 2005: the staging procedure for the inclusion body pathology associated with sporadic Parkinson's disease reconsidered. Mov Disord. 2006;21:2042–51.
207. McKeith IG, Dickson DW, Lowe J, Emre M, O'Brien JT, Feldman H, et al. Diagnosis and management of dementia with Lewy bodies: third report of the DLB consortium. Neurology. 2005;65:1863–72.
208. Zaccai J, Brayne C, McKeith I, Matthews F, Ince PG. Patterns and stages of alpha-synucleinopathy: relevance in a population-based cohort. Neurology. 2008;70:1042–8.
209. Braak H, Ghebremedhin E, Rub U, Bratzke H, Del Tredici K. Stages in the development of Parkinson's disease-related pathology. Cell Tissue Res. 2004;318:121–34.
210. Doty RL. Olfactory dysfunction in Parkinson disease. Nat Rev Neurol. 2012;8:329–39.
211. Ferrer I, Martinez A, Blanco R, Dalfo E, Carmona M. Neuropathology of sporadic Parkinson disease before the appearance of parkinsonism: preclinical Parkinson disease. J Neural Transm. 2011;118:821–39.
212. Kosaka K, Tsuchiya K, Yoshimura M. Lewy body disease with and without dementia: a clinicopathological study of 35 cases. Clin Neuropathol. 1988;7:299–305.
213. Dickson DW, Uchikado H, Fujishiro H, Tsuboi Y. Evidence in favor of Braak staging of Parkinson's disease. Mov Disord. 2010;25 Suppl 1:S78–82.
214. Halliday GM, Del Tredici K, Braak H. Critical appraisal of brain pathology staging related to presymptomatic and symptomatic cases of sporadic Parkinson's disease. J Neural Transm Suppl. 2006;70:99–103.
215. Kempster PA, O'Sullivan SS, Holton JL, Revesz T, Lees AJ. Relationships between age and late progression of Parkinson's disease: a clinico-pathological study. Brain. 2010;133:1755–62.
216. Muller CM, de Vos RA, Maurage CA, Thal DR, Tolnay M, Braak H. Staging of sporadic Parkinson disease-related alpha-synuclein pathology: inter- and intra-rater reliability. J Neuropathol Exp Neurol. 2005;64:623–8.
217. Jellinger KA. A critical evaluation of current staging of alpha-synuclein pathology in Lewy body disorders. Biochim Biophys Acta. 2009;1792:730–40.
218. Kalaitzakis ME, Graeber MB, Gentleman SM, Pearce RK. Controversies over the staging of alpha-synuclein pathology in Parkinson's disease. Acta Neuropathol. 2008;116:125–8. author reply 129–31.
219. Kalaitzakis ME, Graeber MB, Gentleman SM, Pearce RK. The dorsal motor nucleus of the vagus is not an obligatory trigger site of Parkinson's disease: a critical analysis of alpha-synuclein staging. Neuropathol Appl Neurobiol. 2008;34:284–95.
220. Parkkinen L, Pirttila T, Alafuzoff I. Applicability of current staging/categorization of alpha-synuclein pathology and their clinical relevance. Acta Neuropathol. 2008;115:399–407.
221. Leverenz JB, Hamilton R, Tsuang DW, Schantz A, Vavrek D, Larson EB, et al. Empiric refinement of the pathologic assessment of Lewy-related pathology in the dementia patient. Brain Pathol. 2008;18:220–4.
222. Mikolaenko I, Pletnikova O, Kawas CH, O'Brien R, Resnick SM, Crain B, et al. Alpha-synuclein lesions in normal aging, Parkinson disease, and Alzheimer disease: evidence from the Baltimore Longitudinal Study of Aging (BLSA). J Neuropathol Exp Neurol. 2005;64:156–62.
223. Marui W, Iseki E, Kato M, Akatsu H, Kosaka K. Pathological entity of dementia with Lewy bodies and its differentiation from Alzheimer's disease. Acta Neuropathol. 2004;108:121–8.
224. Boeve BF, Dickson DW, Olson EJ, Shepard JW, Silber MH, Ferman TJ, et al. Insights into REM sleep behavior disorder pathophysiology in brainstem-predominant Lewy body disease. Sleep Med. 2007;8:60–4.

225. Frigerio R, Fujishiro H, Ahn TB, Josephs KA, Maraganore DM, Delledonne A, et al. Incidental Lewy body disease: Do some cases represent a preclinical stage of dementia with Lewy bodies? Neurobiol Aging 2011;32:857–63.
226. Claassen DO, Josephs KA, Ahlskog JE, Silber MH, Tippmann-Peikert M, Boeve BF. REM sleep behavior disorder preceding other aspects of synucleinopathies by up to half a century. Neurology. 2010;75:494–9.
227. Postuma RB, Gagnon JF, Vendette M, Desjardins C, Montplaisir JY. Olfaction and color vision identify impending neurodegeneration in rapid eye movement sleep behavior disorder. Ann Neurol. 2011;69:811–8.
228. Jellinger KA. Lewy body-related alpha-synucleinopathy in the aged human brain. J Neural Transm. 2004;111:1219–35.
229. Aho L, Parkkinen L, Pirttila T, Alafuzoff I. Systematic appraisal using immunohistochemistry of brain pathology in aged and demented subjects. Dement Geriatr Cogn Disord. 2008; 25:423–32.
230. Markesbery WR, Jicha GA, Liu H, Schmitt FA. Lewy body pathology in normal elderly subjects. J Neuropathol Exp Neurol. 2009;68:816–22.
231. Parkkinen L, Soininen H, Alafuzoff I. Regional distribution of alpha-synuclein pathology in unimpaired aging and Alzheimer disease. J Neuropathol Exp Neurol. 2003;62:363–7.
232. Saito Y, Ruberu NN, Sawabe M, Arai T, Kazama H, Hosoi T, et al. Lewy body-related alpha-synucleinopathy in aging. J Neuropathol Exp Neurol. 2004;63:742–9.
233. Wakisaka Y, Furuta A, Tanizaki Y, Kiyohara Y, Iida M, Iwaki T. Age-associated prevalence and risk factors of Lewy body pathology in a general population: the Hisayama study. Acta Neuropathol. 2003;106:374–82.
234. Ding ZT, Wang Y, Jiang YP, Hashizume Y, Yoshida M, Mimuro M, et al. Characteristics of alpha-synucleinopathy in centenarians. Acta Neuropathol. 2006;111:450–8.
235. Fujishiro H, Tsuboi Y, Lin WL, Uchikado H, Dickson DW. Co-localization of tau and alpha-synuclein in the olfactory bulb in Alzheimer's disease with amygdala Lewy bodies. Acta Neuropathol. 2008;116:17–24.
236. Parkkinen L, Pirttila T, Tervahauta M, Alafuzoff I. Widespread and abundant alpha-synuclein pathology in a neurologically unimpaired subject. Neuropathology. 2005;25:304–14.
237. Jellinger KA. Interaction between alpha-synuclein and tau in Parkinson's disease comment on Wills et al.: elevated tauopathy and alpha-synuclein pathology in postmortem Parkinson's disease brains with and without dementia. Exp Neurol 2010; 225: 210–218. Exp Neurol. 2011;227:13–8.
238. Kovacs GG, Botond G, Budka H. Protein coding of neurodegenerative dementias: the neuropathological basis of biomarker diagnostics. Acta Neuropathol. 2010;119:389–408.
239. Arai Y, Yamazaki M, Mori O, Muramatsu H, Asano G, Katayama Y. Alpha-synuclein-positive structures in cases with sporadic Alzheimer's disease: morphology and its relationship to tau aggregation. Brain Res. 2001;888:287–96.
240. Iseki E, Togo T, Suzuki K, Katsuse O, Marui W, de Silva R, et al. Dementia with Lewy bodies from the perspective of tauopathy. Acta Neuropathol (Berl). 2003;105:265–70.
241. Maries E, Dass B, Collier TJ, Kordower JH, Steece-Collier K. The role of alpha-synuclein in Parkinson's disease: insights from animal models. Nat Rev Neurosci. 2003;4:727–38.
242. Baum L, Seger R, Woodgett JR, Kawabata S, Maruyama K, Koyama M, et al. Overexpressed tau protein in cultured cells is phosphorylated without formation of PHF: implication of phosphoprotein phosphatase involvement. Brain Res Mol Brain Res. 1995;34:1–17.
243. Kawakami F, Suzuki M, Shimada N, Kagiya G, Ohta E, Tamura K, et al. Stimulatory effect of alpha-synuclein on the tau-phosphorylation by GSK-3beta. FEBS J. 2011; 278:4895–904.
244. Duka T, Duka V, Joyce JN, Sidhu A. Alpha-synuclein contributes to GSK-3beta-catalyzed tau phosphorylation in Parkinson's disease models. FASEB J. 2009;23:2820–30.
245. Kozikowski AP, Gaisina IN, Petukhov PA, Sridhar J, King LT, Blond SY, et al. Highly potent and specific GSK-3beta inhibitors that block tau phosphorylation and decrease alpha-

synuclein protein expression in a cellular model of Parkinson's disease. ChemMedChem. 2006;1:256–66.
246. Kaul T, Credle J, Haggerty T, Oaks AW, Masliah E, Sidhu A. Region-specific tauopathy and synucleinopathy in brain of the alpha-synuclein overexpressing mouse model of Parkinson's disease. BMC Neurosci. 2011;12:79.
247. Wills J, Credle J, Haggerty T, Lee JH, Oaks AW, Sidhu A. Tauopathic changes in the striatum of A53T alpha-synuclein mutant mouse model of Parkinson's disease. PLoS One. 2011; 6:e17953.
248. Qureshi HY, Paudel HK. Parkinsonian neurotoxin 1-methyl-4-phenyl-1,2,3,6-tetrahydropyridine (MPTP) and alpha-synuclein mutations promote tau protein phosphorylation at ser262 and destabilize microtubule cytoskeleton in vitro. J Biol Chem. 2011;286: 5055–68.
249. Waxman EA, Giasson BI. Induction of intracellular tau aggregation is promoted by alpha-synuclein seeds and provides novel insights into the hyperphosphorylation of tau. J Neurosci. 2011;31:7604–18.
250. Badiola N, de Oliveira RM, Herrera F, Guardia-Laguarta C, Gonçalves SA, Pera M, et al. Tau enhances a-synuclein aggregation and toxicity in cellular models of synucleinopathy. PLoS One. 2011;6:e26609. doi:10.1371/journal.pone.0026609.
251. Giasson BI, Forman MS, Higuchi M, Golbe LI, Graves CL, Kotzbauer PT, et al. Initiation and synergistic fibrillization of tau and alpha-synuclein. Science. 2003;300:636–40.
252. Lei P, Ayton S, Finkelstein DI, Adlard PA, Masters CL, Bush AI. Tau protein: relevance to Parkinson's disease. Int J Biochem Cell Biol. 2010;42:1775–8.
253. Kotzbauer PT, Giasson BI, Kravitz AV, Golbe LI, Mark MH, Trojanowski JQ, et al. Fibrillization of alpha-synuclein and tau in familial Parkinson's disease caused by the A53T alpha-synuclein mutation. Exp Neurol. 2004;187:279–88.
254. Emmer KL, Waxman EA, Covy JP, Giasson BI. E46K human alpha-synuclein transgenic mice develop Lewy-like and tau pathology associated with age-dependent detrimental motor impairments. J Biol Chem. 2011;286:35104–18.
255. Toledo JB, Korff A, Shaw LM, Trojanowski JQ, Zhang J. Alpha-Synuclein improves diagnostic and prognostic performance of tau and A-beta in Alzheimer's disease. Acta Neuropathol. 2013. doi:10.1007/s00401-013-1148-z.
256. Pletnikova O, West N, Lee MK, Rudow GL, Skolasky RL, Dawson TM, et al. Abeta deposition is associated with enhanced cortical alpha-synuclein lesions in Lewy body diseases. Neurobiol Aging. 2005;26:1183–92.
257. Huang HC, Jiang ZF. Accumulated amyloid-beta peptide and hyperphosphorylated tau protein: relationship and links in Alzheimer's disease. J Alzheimers Dis. 2009;16:15–27.
258. Lashley T, Holton JL, Gray E, Kirkham K, O'Sullivan SS, Hilbig A, et al. Cortical alpha-synuclein load is associated with amyloid-beta plaque burden in a subset of Parkinson's disease patients. Acta Neuropathol. 2008;115:417–25.
259. Bate C, Gentleman S, Williams A. Alpha-synuclein induced synapse damage is enhanced by amyloid-beta1-42. Mol Neurodegener. 2010;5:55.
260. Obi K, Akiyama H, Kondo H, Shimomura Y, Hasegawa M, Iwatsubo T, et al. Relationship of phosphorylated alpha-synuclein and tau accumulation to Abeta deposition in the cerebral cortex of dementia with Lewy bodies. Exp Neurol. 2008;210:409–20.
261. Mandal PK, Pettegrew JW, Masliah E, Hamilton RL, Mandal R. Interaction between Abeta peptide and alpha synuclein: molecular mechanisms in overlapping pathology of Alzheimer's and Parkinson's in dementia with Lewy body disease. Neurochem Res. 2006;31:1153–62.
262. Takahashi RH, Capetillo-Zarate E, Lin MT, Milner TA, Gouras GK. Co-occurrence of Alzheimer's disease ss-amyloid and tau pathologies at synapses. Neurobiol Aging 2010; 31:1145–52.
263. Rhein V, Song X, Wiesner A, Ittner LM, Baysang G, Meier F, et al. Amyloid-beta and tau synergistically impair the oxidative phosphorylation system in triple transgenic Alzheimer's disease mice. Proc Natl Acad Sci U S A. 2009;106:20057–62.
264. Obeso JA, Lanciego JL. Past, present, and future of the pathophysiological model of the Basal Ganglia. Front Neuroanat 2011;5:39.

265. Calabresi P, Mercuri NB, Di Filippo M. Synaptic plasticity, dopamine and Parkinson's disease: one step ahead. Brain. 2009;132:285–7.
266. Bagetta V, Ghiglieri V, Sgobio C, Calabresi P, Picconi B. Synaptic dysfunction in Parkinson's disease. Biochem Soc Trans. 2010;38:493–7.
267. Wu T, Hallett M. The cerebellum in Parkinson's disease. Brain. 2013;136:696–709.
268. Jellinger KA. Post mortem studies in Parkinson's disease – is it possible to detect brain areas for specific symptoms? J Neural Transm Suppl. 1999;56:1–29.
269. Zaja-Milatovic S, Milatovic D, Schantz AM, Zhang J, Montine KS, Samii A, et al. Dendritic degeneration in neostriatal medium spiny neurons in Parkinson disease. Neurology. 2005; 64:545–7.
270. Lee FJ, Wang YT, Liu F. Direct receptor cross-talk can mediate the modulation of excitatory and inhibitory neurotransmission by dopamine. J Mol Neurosci. 2005;26:245–52.
271. West AR, Grace AA. Opposite influences of endogenous dopamine D1 and D2 receptor activation on activity states and electrophysiological properties of striatal neurons: studies combining in vivo intracellular recordings and reverse microdialysis. J Neurosci. 2002;22: 294–304.
272. Reetz K, Gaser C, Klein C, Hagenah J, Büchel C, Gottschalk S, et al. Structural findings in the basal ganglia in genetically determined and idiopathic Parkinson's disease. Mov Disord. 2009;24:99–103.
273. Mori F, Tanji K, Zhang H, Kakita A, Takahashi H, Wakabayashi K. Alpha-synuclein pathology in the neostriatum in Parkinson's disease. Acta Neuropathol. 2008;115:453–9.
274. Wichmann T, DeLong MR, Guridi J, Obeso JA. Milestones in research on the pathophysiology of Parkinson's disease. Mov Disord. 2011;26:1032–41.
275. Duda JE, Giasson BI, Mabon ME, Lee VM, Trojanowski JQ. Novel antibodies to synuclein show abundant striatal pathology in Lewy body diseases. Ann Neurol. 2002;52:205–10.
276. Deutch AY, Colbran RJ, Winder DJ. Striatal plasticity and medium spiny neuron dendritic remodeling in parkinsonism. Parkinsonism Relat Disord. 2007;13 Suppl 3:S251–8.
277. Ito H, Kusaka H, Matsumoto S, Imai T. Striatal efferent involvement and its correlation to levodopa efficacy in patients with multiple system atrophy. Neurology. 1996;47:1291–9.
278. Baradaran N, Tan SN, Liu A, Ashoori A, Palmer SJ, Wang ZJ, et al. Parkinson's disease rigidity: relation to brain connectivity and motor performance. Front Neurol. 2013;4:67.
279. Picconi B, Paille V, Ghiglieri V, Bagetta V, Barone I, Lindgren HS, et al. L-DOPA dosage is critically involved in dyskinesia via loss of synaptic depotentiation. Neurobiol Dis. 2008; 29:327–35.
280. Ding Y, Won L, Britt JP, Lim SA, McGehee DS, Kang UJ. Enhanced striatal cholinergic neuronal activity mediates L-DOPA-induced dyskinesia in Parkinsonian mice. Proc Natl Acad Sci U S A. 2011;108:840–5.
281. Lee J, Zhu WM, Stanic D, Finkelstein DI, Horne MH, Henderson J, et al. Sprouting of dopamine terminals and altered dopamine release and uptake in Parkinsonian dyskinaesia. Brain. 2008;131:1574–87.
282. Ahmed I, Bose SK, Pavese N, Ramlackhansingh A, Turkheimer F, Hotton G, et al. Glutamate NMDA receptor dysregulation in Parkinson's disease with dyskinesias. Brain. 2011;134: 979–86.
283. Calabresi P, Di Filippo M, Ghiglieri V, Tambasco N, Picconi B. Levodopa-induced dyskinesias in patients with Parkinson's disease: filling the bench-to-bedside gap. Lancet Neurol. 2010;9:1106–17.
284. Paulus W, Jellinger K. The neuropathologic basis of different clinical subgroups of Parkinson's disease. J Neuropathol Exp Neurol. 1991;50:743–55.
285. Elias S, Israel Z, Bergman H. Physiology of Parkinson's disease. In: Hallett M, Poewe W, editors. Therapeutics of Parkinson's disease and other movement disorders. Chichester: Wiley-Blackwell; 2008. p. 25–36.
286. Benninger DH, Thees S, Kollias SS, Bassetti CL, Waldvogel D. Morphological differences in Parkinson's disease with and without rest tremor. J Neurol. 2009;256:256–63.

287. Ni Z, Pinto AD, Lang AE, Chen R. Involvement of the cerebellothalamocortical pathway in Parkinson disease. Ann Neurol. 2010;68:816–24.
288. Helmich RC, Janssen MJ, Oyen WJ, Bloem BR, Toni I. Pallidal dysfunction drives a cerebellothalamic circuit into Parkinson tremor. Ann Neurol. 2011;69:269–81.
289. Helmich RC, Hallett M, Deuschl G, Toni I, Bloem BR. Cerebral causes and consequences of Parkinsonian resting tremor: a tale of two circuits? Brain. 2012;135:3206–26.
290. Mure H, Hirano S, Tang CC, Isaias IU, Antonini A, Ma Y, et al. Parkinson's disease tremor-related metabolic network: characterization, progression, and treatment effects. Neuroimage. 2011;54:1244–53.
291. Volkmann J. Surgery Parkinson's disease. In: Hallett M, Poewe W, editors. Therapeutics of Parkinson's disease and other movement disorders. Oxford: Wiley-Blackwell; 2008. p. 120–43.
292. Desouza RM, Moro E, Lang AE, Schapira AH. Timing of deep brain stimulation in Parkinson disease: a need for reappraisal? Ann Neurol. 2013;73:565–75.
293. Hallett M, Deuschl G. Are we making progress in the understanding of tremor in Parkinson's disease? Ann Neurol. 2010;68:780–1.
294. Eggers C, Kahraman D, Fink GR, Schmidt M, Timmermann L. Akinetic-rigid and tremor-dominant Parkinson's disease patients show different patterns of FP-CIT SPECT. Basal Ganglia. 2011;1:34.
295. Kehagia AA, Barker RA, Robbins TW. Neuropsychological and clinical heterogeneity of cognitive impairment and dementia in patients with Parkinson's disease. Lancet Neurol. 2010;9:1200–13.
296. Aarsland D, Bronnick K, Larsen JP, Tysnes OB, Alves G. Cognitive impairment in incident, untreated Parkinson disease: the Norwegian ParkWest study. Neurology. 2009;72:1121–6.
297. Aarsland D, Bronnick K, Williams-Gray C, Weintraub D, Marder K, Kulisevsky J, et al. Mild cognitive impairment in Parkinson disease: a multicenter pooled analysis. Neurology. 2010;75:1062–9.
298. Aarsland D, Kurz MW. The epidemiology of dementia associated with Parkinson's disease. Brain Pathol. 2010;20:633–9.
299. Hely MA, Morris JG, Reid WG, Trafficante R. Sydney Multicenter Study of Parkinson's disease: non-L-dopa-responsive problems dominate at 15 years. Mov Disord. 2005;20:190–9.
300. Kalaitzakis ME, Pearce RK. The morbid anatomy of dementia in Parkinson's disease. Acta Neuropathol. 2009;118:587–98.
301. Compta Y, Parkkinen L, O'Sullivan SS, Vandrovcova J, Holton JL, Collins C, et al. Lewy- and Alzheimer-type pathologies in Parkinson's disease dementia: which is more important? Brain. 2011;134:1493–505.
302. Dickson D, Orr C, Murray M, Pahwa R, Lyons K, Goldman S, et al. Hierarchical cluster analysis of cortical pathology suggests pathologic heterogeneity of dementia in Parkinson's disease (abs). J Neuropathol Exp Neurol. 2011;70:505.
303. Petersen RC, Roberts RO, Knopman DS, Boeve BF, Geda YE, Ivnik RJ, et al. Mild cognitive impairment: ten years later. Arch Neurol. 2009;66:1447–55.
304. Caviness JN, Driver-Dunckley E, Connor DJ, Sabbagh MN, Hentz JG, Noble B, et al. Defining mild cognitive impairment in Parkinson's disease. Mov Disord. 2007;22:1272–7.
305. Williams-Gray CH, Foltynie T, Brayne CE, Robbins TW, Barker RA. Evolution of cognitive dysfunction in an incident Parkinson's disease cohort. Brain. 2007;130:1787–98.
306. Dalrymple-Alford JC, Livingston L, MacAskill MR, Graham C, Melzer TR, Porter RJ, et al. Characterizing mild cognitive impairment in Parkinson's disease. Mov Disord. 2011;26:629–36.
307. Adler CH, Caviness JN, Sabbagh MN, Shill HA, Connor DJ, Sue L, et al. Heterogeneous neuropathological findings in Parkinson's disease with mild cognitive impairment. Acta Neuropathol. 2010;120:827–8.
308. Jellinger KA. Neuropathology in Parkinson's disease with mild cognitive impairment. Acta Neuropathol. 2010;120:829–30.

309. McKinlay A, Grace RC, Dalrymple-Alford JC, Roger D. Cognitive characteristics associated with mild cognitive impairment in Parkinson's disease. Dement Geriatr Cogn Disord. 2009;28:121–9.
310. Petersen RC, Parisi JE, Dickson DW, Johnson KA, Knopman DS, Boeve BF, et al. Neuropathologic features of amnestic mild cognitive impairment. Arch Neurol. 2006;63: 665–72.
311. Markesbery WR. Neuropathologic alterations in mild cognitive impairment: a review. J Alzheimers Dis. 2010;19:221–8.
312. Silbert LC, Kaye J. Neuroimaging and cognition in Parkinson's disease dementia. Brain Pathol. 2010;20:646–53.
313. Burack MA, Hartlein J, Flores HP, Taylor-Reinwald L, Perlmutter JS, Cairns NJ. In vivo amyloid imaging in autopsy-confirmed Parkinson disease with dementia. Neurology. 2010; 74:77–84.
314. Evans JR, Revesz T, Barker RA. Lesions associated with cognitive impairment and dementia. In: Halliday G, Barker RA, Rowe DB, editors. Non-dopamine lesions in Parkinson's disease. Oxford: Oxford University Press; 2011. p. 261–87.
315. Bouchard TP, Malykhin N, Martin WR, Hanstock CC, Emery DJ, Fisher NJ, et al. Age and dementia-associated atrophy predominates in the hippocampal head and amygdala in Parkinson's disease. Neurobiol Aging. 2008;29:1027–39.
316. Fujita M, Ichise M, Zoghbi SS, Liow JS, Ghose S, Vines DC, et al. Widespread decrease of nicotinic acetylcholine receptors in Parkinson's disease. Ann Neurol. 2006;59:174–7.
317. Huang C, Mattis P, Perrine K, Brown N, Dhawan V, Eidelberg D. Metabolic abnormalities associated with mild cognitive impairment in Parkinson disease. Neurology. 2008;70: 1470–7.
318. Jellinger KA. Morphological substrates of dementia in parkinsonism. A critical update. J Neural Transm Suppl. 1997;51:57–82.
319. Del Tredici K, Braak H. Dysfunction of the locus coeruleus-norepinephrine system and related circuitry in Parkinson's disease-related dementia. J Neurol Neurosurg Psychiatry. 2013;84:774–83.
320. Zweig RM, Cardillo JE, Cohen M, Giere S, Hedreen JC. The locus ceruleus and dementia in Parkinson's disease. Neurology. 1993;43:986–91.
321. McMillan PJ, White SS, Franklin A, Greenup JL, Leverenz JB, Raskind MA, et al. Differential response of the central noradrenergic nervous system to the loss of locus coeruleus neurons in Parkinson's disease and Alzheimer's disease. Brain Res. 2011;1373:240–52.
322. Aarsland D, Londos E, Ballard C. Parkinson's disease dementia and dementia with Lewy bodies: different aspects of one entity. Int Psychogeriatr. 2009;21:216–9.
323. Kraybill ML, Larson EB, Tsuang DW, Teri L, McCormick WC, Bowen JD, et al. Cognitive differences in dementia patients with autopsy-verified AD, Lewy body pathology, or both. Neurology. 2005;64:2069–73.
324. Kantarci K, Lowe VJ, Boeve BF, Weigand SD, Senjem ML, Przybelski SA, et al. Multimodality imaging characteristics of dementia with Lewy bodies. Neurobiol Aging. 2012;33:2091–105.
325. Alafuzoff I, Ince PG, Arzberger T, Al-Sarraj S, Bell J, Bodi I, et al. Staging/typing of Lewy body related alpha-synuclein pathology: a study of the BrainNet Europe Consortium. Acta Neuropathol. 2009;117:635–52.
326. Kotzbauer PT, Cairns NJ, Campbell MC, Willis AW, Racette BA, Tabbal SD, et al. Pathologic accumulation of alpha-synuclein and A-beta in Parkinson disease patients with dementia. Arch Neurol. 2012;69:1326–31.
327. Tsuang D, Leverenz JB, Lopez OL, Hamilton RL, Bennett DA, Schneider JA, et al. APOE epsilon4 increases risk for dementia in pure synucleinopathies. JAMA Neurol. 2013;70: 223–8.

328. Fujishiro H, Iseki E, Higashi S, Kasanuki K, Murayama N, Togo T, et al. Distribution of cerebral amyloid deposition and its relevance to clinical phenotype in Lewy body dementia. Neurosci Lett. 2010;486:19–23.
329. Halliday GM, Song YJ, Harding AJ. Striatal beta-amyloid in dementia with Lewy bodies but not Parkinson's disease. J Neural Transm. 2011;118:713.
330. Piggott MA, Perry EK, Marshall EF, McKeith IG, Johnson M, Melrose HL, et al. Nigrostriatal dopaminergic activities in dementia with Lewy bodies in relation to neuroleptic sensitivity: comparisons with Parkinson's disease. Biol Psychiatry. 1998;44:765–74.
331. Francis PT, Perry EK. Cholinergic and other neurotransmitter mechanisms in Parkinson's disease, Parkinson's disease dementia, and dementia with Lewy bodies. Mov Disord. 2007;22 Suppl 17:S351–7.
332. Hurtig HI, Trojanowski JQ, Galvin J, Ewbank D, Schmidt ML, Lee VM, et al. Alpha-synuclein cortical Lewy bodies correlate with dementia in Parkinson's disease. Neurology. 2000;54:1916–21.
333. Apaydin H, Ahlskog JE, Parisi JE, Boeve BF, Dickson DW. Parkinson disease neuropathology: later-developing dementia and loss of the levodopa response. Arch Neurol. 2002; 59:102–12.
334. Kovari E, Gold G, Herrmann FR, Canuto A, Hof PR, Bouras C, et al. Lewy body densities in the entorhinal and anterior cingulate cortex predict cognitive deficits in Parkinson's disease. Acta Neuropathol (Berl). 2003;106:83–8.
335. Mattila PM, Rinne JO, Helenius H, Dickson DW, Roytta M. Alpha-Synuclein-immunoreactive cortical Lewy bodies are associated with cognitive impairment in Parkinson's disease. Acta Neuropathol. 2000;100:285–90.
336. Mattila PM, Rinne JO, Helenius H, Roytta M. Neuritic degeneration in the hippocampus and amygdala in Parkinson's disease in relation to Alzheimer pathology. Acta Neuropathol (Berl). 1999;98:157–64.
337. Harding AJ, Halliday GM. Simplified neuropathological diagnosis of dementia with Lewy bodies. Neuropathol Appl Neurobiol. 1998;24:195–201.
338. Joelving FC, Billeskov R, Christensen JR, West M, Pakkenberg B. Hippocampal neuron and glial cell numbers in Parkinson's disease – a stereological study. Hippocampus. 2006; 16:826–33.
339. Colosimo C, Hughes AJ, Kilford L, Lees AJ. Lewy body cortical involvement may not always predict dementia in Parkinson's disease. J Neurol Neurosurg Psychiatry. 2003;74: 852–6.
340. Libow LS, Frisina PG, Haroutunian V, Perl DP, Purohit DP. Parkinson's disease dementia: a diminished role for the Lewy body. Parkinsonism Relat Disord. 2009;15:572–5.
341. Weisman D, Cho M, Taylor C, Adame A, Thal LJ, Hansen LA. In dementia with Lewy bodies, Braak stage determines phenotype, not Lewy body distribution. Neurology. 2007;69: 356–9.
342. Jellinger KA, Attems J. Prevalence and impact of vascular and Alzheimer pathologies in Lewy body disease. Acta Neuropathol. 2008;115:127–36.
343. Jendroska K, Lees AJ, Poewe W, Daniel SE. Amyloid beta-peptide and the dementia of Parkinson's disease. Mov Disord. 1996;11:647–53.
344. Mastaglia FL, Johnsen RD, Byrnes ML, Kakulas BA. Prevalence of amyloid-beta deposition in the cerebral cortex in Parkinson's disease. Mov Disord. 2003;18:81–6.
345. Edison P, Rowe CC, Rinne JO, Ng S, Ahmed I, Kemppainen N, et al. Amyloid load in Parkinson's disease dementia and Lewy body dementia measured with [11C]PIB positron emission tomography. J Neurol Neurosurg Psychiatry. 2008;79:1331–8.
346. Gomperts SN, Rentz DM, Moran E, Becker JA, Locascio JJ, Klunk WE, et al. Imaging amyloid deposition in Lewy body diseases. Neurology. 2008;71:903–10.
347. Maetzler W, Reimold M, Liepelt I, Solbach C, Leyhe T, Schweitzer K, et al. [11C]PIB binding in Parkinson's disease dementia. Neuroimage. 2008;39:1027–33.

348. Ghebremedhin E, Rosenberger A, Rub U, Vuksic M, Berhe T, Bickeböller H, et al. Inverse relationship between cerebrovascular lesions and severity of Lewy body pathology in patients with Lewy body diseases. J Neuropathol Exp Neurol. 2010;69:442–8.
349. Devine MJ, Gwinn K, Singleton A, Hardy J. Parkinson's disease and alpha-synuclein expression. Mov Disord. 2011;26:2160–8.
350. Pilsl A, Winklhofer KF. Parkin, PINK1 and mitochondrial integrity: emerging concepts of mitochondrial dysfunction in Parkinson's disease. Acta Neuropathol. 2012;123:173–88.
351. Sulzer D, Surmeier DJ. Neuronal vulnerability, pathogenesis, and Parkinson's disease. Mov Disord. 2013;28:41–50.
352. Schapira AH, Gegg M. Mitochondrial contribution to Parkinson's disease pathogenesis. Parkinsons Dis. 2011;2011:159160.
353. Reynolds NP, Soragni A, Rabe M, Verdes D, Liverani E, Handschin S, et al. Mechanism of membrane interaction and disruption by alpha-synuclein. J Am Chem Soc. 2011;133: 19366–75.
354. Piccoli G, Condliffe SB, Bauer M, Giesert F, Boldt K, De Astis S, et al. LRRK2 controls synaptic vesicle storage and mobilization within the recycling pool. J Neurosci. 2011; 31:2225–37.
355. Wang X, Winter D, Ashrafi G, Schlehe J, Wong YL, Selkoe D, et al. PINK1 and Parkin target Miro for phosphorylation and degradation to arrest mitochondrial motility. Cell. 2011;147:893–906.
356. Cook C, Stetler C, Petrucelli L. Disruption of protein quality control in Parkinson's disease. Cold Spring Harb Perspect Med. 2012;2:a009423.
357. Tzoulis C, Tran GT, Schwarzlmuller T, Specht K, Haugarvoll K, Balafkan N et al. Severe nigrostriatal degeneration without clinical parkinsonism in patients with polymerase gamma mutations. Brain 2013;136:2393–404.
358. Hurley MJ, Brandon B, Gentleman SM, Dexter DT. Parkinson's disease is associated with altered expression of CaV1 channels and calcium-binding proteins. Brain. 2013;136: 2077–97.
359. Pan T, Kondo S, Le W, Jankovic J. The role of autophagy–lysosome pathway in neurodegeneration associated with Parkinson's disease. Brain. 2008;131:1969–78.
360. Janda E, Isidoro C, Carresi C, Mollace V. Defective autophagy in Parkinson's disease: role of oxidative stress. Mol Neurobiol. 2012;46:639–61.
361. Exner N, Lutz AK, Haass C, Winklhofer KF. Mitochondrial dysfunction in Parkinson's disease: molecular mechanisms and pathophysiological consequences. EMBO J. 2012;31: 3038–62.
362. Bueler H. Mitochondrial dynamics, cell death and the pathogenesis of Parkinson's disease. Apoptosis. 2010;15:1336–53.
363. Schon EA, Przedborski S. Mitochondria: the next (neurode)generation. Neuron. 2011;70: 1033–53.
364. Coskun P, Wyrembak J, Schriner SE, Chen HW, Marciniack C, Laferla F, et al. A mitochondrial etiology of Alzheimer and Parkinson disease. Biochim Biophys Acta. 2012;1820: 553–64.
365. Karbowski M, Neutzner A. Neurodegeneration as a consequence of failed mitochondrial maintenance. Acta Neuropathol. 2012;123:157–71.
366. McCoy MK, Cookson MR. Mitochondrial quality control and dynamics in Parkinson's disease. Antioxid Redox Signal. 2012;16:869–82.
367. Schapira AH, Jenner P. Etiology and pathogenesis of Parkinson's disease. Mov Disord. 2011;26:1049–55.
368. Altamura S, Muckenthaler MU. Iron toxicity in diseases of aging: Alzheimer's disease, Parkinson's disease and atherosclerosis. J Alzheimers Dis. 2009;16:879–95.
369. Angot E, Steiner JA, Lema Tome CM, Ekström P, Mattsson B, Björklund A, et al. Alpha-synuclein cell-to-cell transfer and seeding in grafted dopaminergic neurons in vivo. PLoS One. 2012;7:e39465.

370. Brundin P, Melki R, Kopito R. Prion-like transmission of protein aggregates in neurodegenerative diseases. Nat Rev Mol Cell Biol. 2010;11:301–7.
371. Xilouri M, Brekk OR, Landeck N, Pitychoutis PM, Papasilekas T, Papadopoulou-Daifoti Z, et al. Boosting chaperone-mediated autophagy in vivo mitigates alpha-synuclein-induced neurodegeneration. Brain. 2013;136:2130–46.
372. Tsang AH, Chung KK. Oxidative and nitrosative stress in Parkinson's disease. Biochim Biophys Acta. 2009;1792:643–50.
373. Huang Y, Chegini F, Chua G, Murphy K, Gai W, Halliday GM. Macroautophagy in sporadic and the genetic form of Parkinson's disease with the A53T a-synuclein mutation. Translat Neurodeg. 2012;1:2. doi:10.1186/2047-9158-1-2.
374. Visanji NP, Brooks PL, Hazrati L-N, Lang AE. The prion hypothesis in Parkinson's disease: Braak to the future. Acta Neuropathol Commun. 2013;1:2. doi:10.1186/2051-5960-1-2.
375. Olanow CW, McNaught K. Parkinson's disease, proteins, and prions: milestones. Mov Disord. 2011;26:1056–71.
376. Danzer KM, Kranich LR, Ruf WP, Cagsal-Getkin O, Winslow AR, Zhu L, et al. Exosomal cell-to-cell transmission of alpha synuclein oligomers. Mol Neurodegener. 2012;7:42.
377. Marques O, Outeiro TF. Alpha-synuclein: from secretion to dysfunction and death. Cell Death Dis. 2012;3:e350.
378. Fellner L, Jellinger KA, Wenning GK, Stefanova N. Glial dysfunction in the pathogenesis of alpha-synucleinopathies: emerging concepts. Acta Neuropathol. 2011;121:675–93.
379. Martin ZS, Neugebauer V, Dineley KT, Kayed R, Zhang W, Reese LC, et al. Alpha-synuclein oligomers oppose long-term potentiation and impair memory through a calcineurin-dependent mechanism: relevance to human synucleopathic diseases. J Neurochem. 2012;120:440–52.
380. Vekrellis K, Xilouri M, Emmanouilidou E, Rideout HJ, Stefanis L. Pathological roles of alpha-synuclein in neurological disorders. Lancet Neurol. 2011;10:1015–25.
381. Bove J, Perier C. Neurotoxin-based models of Parkinson's disease. Neuroscience. 2012; 211:51–76.
382. Cannon JR, Greenamyre JT. Neurotoxic in vivo models of Parkinson's disease recent advances. Prog Brain Res. 2010;184:17–33.
383. Tanner CM, Kamel F, Ross GW, Hoppin JA, Goldman SM, Korell M, et al. Rotenone, paraquat, and Parkinson's disease. Environ Health Perspect. 2011;119:866–72.
384. Nistico R, Mehdawy B, Piccirilli S, Mercuri N. Paraquat- and rotenone-induced models of Parkinson's disease. Int J Immunopathol Pharmacol. 2011;24:313–22.
385. Dawson TM, Ko HS, Dawson VL. Genetic animal models of Parkinson's disease. Neuron. 2010;66:646–61.
386. Welchko RM, Leveque XT, Dunbar GL. Genetic rat models of Parkinson's disease. Parkinsons Dis. 2012;2012:128356.
387. Alberio T, Lopiano L, Fasano M. Cellular models to investigate biochemical pathways in Parkinson's disease. FEBS J. 2012;279:1146–55.
388. Mizuno H, Fujikake N, Wada K, Nagai Y. Alpha-synuclein transgenic drosophila as a model of Parkinson's disease and related synucleinopathies. Parkinsons Dis. 2010;2011:212706.
389. Whitworth AJ. Drosophila models of Parkinson's disease. Adv Genet. 2011;73:1–50.
390. Yao C, El Khoury R, Wang W, Byrd TA, Pehek EA, Thacker C, et al. LRRK2-mediated neurodegeneration and dysfunction of dopaminergic neurons in a Caenorhabditis elegans model of Parkinson's disease. Neurobiol Dis. 2010;40:73–81.
391. Antony PM, Diederich NJ, Balling R. Parkinson's disease mouse models in translational research. Mamm Genome. 2011;22:401–19.
392. Bezard E, Przedborski S. A tale on animal models of Parkinson's disease. Mov Disord. 2011;26:993–1002.
393. Bezard E, Yue Z, Kirik D, Spillantini MG. Animal models of Parkinson's disease: limits and relevance to neuroprotection studies. Mov Disord. 2013;28:61–70. doi:10.1002/mds.25108.
394. Blesa J, Phani S, Jackson-Lewis V, Przedborski S. Classic and new animal models of Parkinson's disease. J Biomed Biotechnol. 2012;2012:845618. doi:10.1155/2012/845618.

395. Chesselet MF, Richter F. Modelling of Parkinson's disease in mice. Lancet Neurol. 2011;10:1108–18.
396. Lim Y, Kehm VM, Lee EB, Soper JH, Li C, Trojanowski JQ, et al. alpha-Syn suppression reverses synaptic and memory defects in a mouse model of dementia with Lewy bodies. J Neurosci. 2011;31:10076–87.
397. Low K, Aebischer P. Use of viral vectors to create animal models for Parkinson's disease. Neurobiol Dis. 2012;48:189–201.
398. Ulusoy A, Bjorklund T, Buck K, Kirik D. Dysregulated dopamine storage increases the vulnerability to alpha-synuclein in nigral neurons. Neurobiol Dis. 2012;47:367–77.
399. Eschbach J, Danzer KM. α-Synuclein in Parkinson's Disease: Pathogenic Function and Translation into Animal Models. Neurodegener Dis 2014;14:1–17.
400. Blandini F, Armentero MT. Animal models of Parkinson's disease. FEBS J. 2012;279: 1156–66.

Role of the Innate and Adaptive Immune System in the Pathogenesis of PD

George T. Kannarkat and Malú G. Tansey

Introduction

In our current understanding of PD, there is a dearth of disease-modifying therapies, comprehension of disease pathogenesis, and relevant biomarkers [1]. Inflammation has been increasingly recognized as an important process in disease pathogenesis. The role of inflammation needs to be clarified, particularly in relation to etiology and disease progression. Immunomodulatory therapeutics may be able to delay or attenuate disease, while functional profiling of peripheral immune cells could provide insight into biologic markers of disease [2]. The vast majority of research in PD has focused on neuronal and glial dysfunction independent of contribution of immune-related factors. In this chapter, we review the latest evidence for the role of inflammation and immunity in promoting disease susceptibility and progression.

Immune-Relevant Parkinson's Disease Pathology

Chronic neuroinflammation, Lewy body inclusions, and loss of dopamine-producing (DA) neurons in the substantia nigra parts compacta (SNpc) of the midbrain characterize PD pathology [3, 4]. The clinical diagnosis of PD and other Lewy-body diseases is confirmed postmortem by the histologic presence of Lewy bodies [4]. Intraneuronal aggregates of various proteins such as α-synuclein, tau, and ubiquitin make up Lewy bodies. The Braak hypothesis puts forth a comprehensive pattern for the spread of Lewy body pathology in PD. This hypothesis proposes that Lewy bodies initially form in the olfactory bulb or the gastrointestinal tract (areas that are constantly exposed to the environment). With disease progression, it is proposed that pathological hallmarks then appear in the vagus or olfactory nerve and

G.T. Kannarkat, M.D., Ph.D. (✉) • M.G. Tansey, Ph.D.
Department of Physiology, Emory University School of Medicine, Atlanta, GA, USA

M. Thomas (ed.), *Inflammation in Parkinson's Disease: Scientific and Clinical Aspects*,
DOI 10.1007/978-3-319-08046-8_3,

subsequently in the brainstem. Neurodegeneration of greater than 70 % of DA neurons occurs before onset of clinical symptoms. In addition, significant Lewy body pathology and neuroinflammation is present in that region. Pathology also occurs in the forebrain and cortical regions in the final stages of the disease [5]. This hypothesis is attractive for two reasons. First, it can explain the presence and timing of both nonmotor and motor symptoms. Second, it takes into account the multisystemic nature of the disease. Inflammation and the immune system would fit well into this hypothesis as a mediator of the spread of disease pathology.

One of the foremost challenges in the field is to identify the at-risk population for PD in order to understand early pathologic changes. Screening protocols using nonmotor symptom-based mechanisms are underway at various centers to identify people at risk for PD. Prospective study of such at-risk individuals can lead to further understanding the Braak hypothesis [5]. Furthermore, assessment of the inflammatory status of at-risk patients could serve to pinpoint the critical period in which immunomodulation could alter disease onset and progression. Understanding the neuroinflammatory changes that occur early in the progression of PD will also clarify the immune system's contribution to disease. The chronic neuroinflammatory hallmarks of PD such as microglial activation and immune cell infiltration will be discussed in detail later in the chapter.

Potential Inflammatory Etiology of Sporadic Parkinson's Disease

At clinical presentation, over 70 % of DA neurons in the SNpc have undergone degeneration. The severity of pathology at the time of presentation has precluded researchers from identifying the precise etiology of PD [6]. Despite this hurdle, there is general agreement in the field that both genetic and environmental factors contribute. Genome-wide association studies (GWAS) have identified multiple genetic polymorphisms that are associated with increased risk for sporadic PD. These identified genetic loci are thought to contribute to disease susceptibility. Examples of such loci include genes for α-synuclein, glucocerebrosidase, and tau. These polymorphisms could contribute to risk for disease in the context of disease-promoting environmental factors. Thus, specific environmental exposures combined with genetic background could promote pathologic process underlying PD.

Epidemiological studies and case reports have helped identify environmental exposures that promote the development of PD. In this way, we now understand that environmental exposures also modify the risk for PD. Indeed, the identification of 1-methyl-4-phenyl-1,2,3,6-tetrahydropyridine (MPTP) was critical in recognizing a link between environmental exposures and the hallmark of PD pathology, the loss of DA neurons in the SNpc [7]. Before this discovery, no mechanisms were known that would selectively destroy cells of the nigrostriatal pathway. MPTP is metabolized into the cytotoxic MPP+ in DA neurons leading to neuronal death [7, 8]. MPTP has become routinely used in animal models of PD. The contribution of the immune system to these models will be discussed later in the chapter.

Unlike MPTP, the mechanisms through which other environmental exposures modulate risk of PD are unclear. The risk for PD is increased by pesticide/organophosphate exposure and head trauma while it is decreased by moderate amounts of cigarette use and caffeine consumption [9–11]. In terms of inflammation-related exposures, positive associations of PD with influenza, toxoplasmosis, and autoimmunity have been reported, while non-steroidal anti-inflammatory drugs decrease risk for PD [12–20]. In summary, genetic factors, as well as environmental factors, clearly contribute to the development of PD; however, neither is believed to be independently sufficient to cause sporadic disease. Thus, the complex interplay between genetic and environmental factors predisposes people to the development of sporadic PD. Determining the relative contributions from genes and environment and the pathologic processes such as inflammation which link them is important for understanding PD etiology. The immune system may be the nexus between genetics and environment.

The immune system interacts constantly with our environment. It must tolerate certain exposures or antigens while it responds to and eliminates others. Similar to other biological systems, abnormal immune function can lead to disease. An inadequate response to an infection leads to microbial invasion of the bloodstream, while hyper-reactivity to a harmless antigen can cause allergy or autoimmunity. The immune system is composed of both innate and adaptive immune cells. Innate immune cells respond to general patterns of antigens in the environment. These innate cells become activated in response to recognizing these antigen patterns, after which they recruit and activate cells of the adaptive immune system. The adaptive immune system actually develops a specific, tailored response to the antigens that activated the innate immune cells. Adaptive immune cells are uniquely suited to modulate inflammation in the context of certain environmental exposures and neuronal dysfunction. These adaptive immune cells can be activated by specific environmental exposures that cause these cells to become toxic to specific neuronal populations. The Braak hypothesis suggests that mucosal sites (nasal and intestinal) may be the initial focus of PD pathology. Furthermore, many complex immunoregulatory processes occur at mucosal surfaces that are constantly exposed to antigens. Thus, the immune system is uniquely poised to determine the body's response to various environmental exposures in predisposing to or protecting against PD. The immune system's capacity to play a role in propagating neuronal dysfunction and pathology within the central nervous system (CNS) could explain the systemic, progressive nature of PD. The contributions from genetic background, neuronal dysfunction, environmental exposure, and immunologic memory to immune function and risk for PD will make it difficult to contextualize its role in pathology. A survey of our current knowledge of the role of the immune system in PD is presented below.

Evidence for Inflammation in PD

There is a complex interplay between inflammation and neuronal dysfunction. Inflammation can induce neuronal death and neuronal death can induce inflammation. Mechanisms of neuronal dysfunction such as proteasome-mediated protein degradation, mitochondrial dysfunction, and oxidative stress have been implicated in PD pathogenesis [21]. The mechanisms by which neuronal dysfunction is caused by inflammation have also been well established. Specifically in PD, midbrain DA neurons are very sensitive to cytokines such as TNF and IFN-γ [22–25]. Often, these cytokines are produced by microglia, CNS-resident immune cells. The SN's enhanced sensitivity to inflammatory stimuli is likely explained by the high density of microglia in this region [26]. Lipopolysaccharide (LPS), a bacterial endotoxin, is an activating ligand for TLR4 receptors on microglia. Because it can trigger the production of pro-inflammatory factors, a number of different LPS regimens have been used to model inflammatory signaling and its relationship to PD [27].

Abundant evidence in humans also demonstrates a role of chronic neuroinflammation in PD. CSF and postmortem nigrostriatal brain regions of individuals with PD relative have been reported to have elevated levels of cytokines (including IL-1β, TGF-β, IFN-γ, and IL-6) relative to those in age-matched healthy controls [24, 28–30] as well as complement proteins in extraneuronal Lewy bodies [31]. Interestingly, several studies have reported elevated levels of cytokines in the peripheral blood of PD patients relative to healthy controls, and these often correlate to Hoehn and Yahr staging [32] or nonmotor symptoms like depression [33]. Taken together, this evidence indicates that an active inflammatory process is ongoing in the CNS of PD patients that may also be reflected in the peripheral circulation.

An important challenge facing the field is the need for early diagnosis because this limitation impacts not only our ability to intervene with disease-modifying therapies in a timely manner but also our ability to definitely establish whether inflammation is a cause or consequence of the pathophysiology of PD. Nevertheless, thanks to cutting-edge neuroimaging technology, neuroinflammation is now recognized to be definitively present in the PD brain and has also been reproducibly detected in most animal models of PD [34]. LPS models are useful to test the extent to which inflammation alone can initiate neuronal dysfunction and nigral cell death. On the other hand, direct toxin models may better reflect how neuronal death induces inflammation, which then propagates further neuronal injury [35]. In many of these PD models, inflammation is often present before detectable neuronal dysfunction or death occurs, and in neurotoxin animal models such as MPTP and 6-hydroxydopamine (6-OHDA), anti-inflammatory immunosuppressive drugs like dexamethasone can attenuate DA neuron loss [36]. Viral overexpression of human α-synuclein in the rat or mouse SN induces inflammation and microglial activation that is followed months later by progressive death of TH+neurons [37, 38]. Importantly, inflammation is also observed in various transgenic mouse models of α-synuclein overexpression. Multiple models of transgenic mutant and wild-type human α-synuclein overexpression display chronic microgliosis [39–42]. Transgenic overexpression of wild-type human α-synuclein under the direction of the Thy1 promoter results in microglial activation and striatal TNF expression at 1 month of age, progressing to the SN at 5–6 months of age and persisting up to 14 months of age [43].

In summary, neurotoxin models (MPTP, 6-OHDA) directly damage DA neurons thereby initiating an inflammatory response, whereas in LPS and α-synuclein overexpression models, inflammatory responses appear to precipitate neuronal dysfunction and death. It has yet to be determined which of these two pathogenic processes predominates in PD since, at the present time, we are only able to diagnose the disease upon clinical presentation of motor symptoms in an already advanced stage. Investigation of inflammation in the context of multiple animal models remains extremely important because it will allow investigators to clarify the relationship between neuronal dysfunction, neuroinflammation, and the contribution of the peripheral immune system in disease risk and progression.

Peripheral inflammation is typically accompanied by elevated levels of pro-inflammatory cytokines that can alter the permeability of the BBB allowing increased influx of innate and adaptive immune cells from the periphery. These can in turn promote inflammation and propagate a feed-forward cycle to accelerate dopamine neuron loss and acceleration of PD motor symptoms [25]. PET imaging has enabled researchers to visualize inflammation in vivo, and evidence for increased blood brain permeability has been revealed through uptake by the molecular efflux pump P-glycoprotein and increased albumin in the CSF of PD patients [44, 45]. Possible mechanisms for this increased BBB permeability include cerebral capillary basement membrane thickening and collagen accumulation [46], as well as increased proliferation of blood vessels or endothelial cells [47]. Upregulation of ICAM-1, an important adhesion molecule for immune cell diapedesis or entry into brain parenchyma, has been reported in MPTP-induced rodent and nonhuman primate PD models [48, 49] and in blood vessels near the SN in postmortem brain tissue from PD patients [49]. Functionally, inflammatory responses that enhance BBB permeability may create permissive conditions for greater influx of peripheral immune cells that further propagate inflammation and efflux of an immunogen from the CNS to lymphoid organs where adaptive immunity can be engaged and maintained. In fact, the selective loss of specific neuronal populations while others are spared suggests a role for adaptive immunity in this process. Understanding how adaptive immune cells are exposed to neuronal antigens and are then recruited to the CNS in PD will be important for developing a coherent model of PD pathogenesis and will aid in the development of therapeutic approaches to promote neuroprotective immune responses.

Overall, because DA neurons are especially susceptible to damage from inflammatory stimuli, the role of neuroinflammation as a key pathogenic process in PD has become more than a curiosity and is now at center-stage. However, it is important to recognize that until earlier diagnosis or biomarkers are established, it will be rather difficult to unequivocally establish whether inflammation precedes neuronal injury by a significant extent and has a causal role in the process. Nevertheless, because the brains of PD patients with motor symptoms display chronic neuroinflammation, it may be possible to target inflammatory mediators that can be shown to actively contribute to disease progression and achieve disease modification.

Microglial Activation and MHC in PD

Some of the earliest evidence for inflammation in PD is from identification of chronic microglial activation in postmortem brains [50, 51]. Microglia are CNS-resident immune cells that play an important role in immune surveillance and tissue repair [52–54]. They are critical for recruitment of peripheral immune cells and thus amplify inflammatory signals in the CNS. The inflammatory signals that activate microglia originate from normal cross-talk between neurons and glia, neuronal dysfunction, or external insults (including trauma, pathogens, toxicants, etc.). Among the confirmed signals that activate microglia are bacterial and viral products, α-synuclein, complement proteins, antibodies, and cytokines [55–58]. Neuronal death may trigger microglial activation through loss of inhibitory CD200:CD200R signaling, ligation of microglial receptors that recognize factors released during apoptosis, release of α-synuclein, and/or through binding of complement or antibodies bound to neurons [56, 58]. In response to these stimuli, microglia produce cytokines [58–60], reactive oxygen species [61, 62], prostanoids that have immunomodulatory functions [63], and chemokines that recruit peripheral immune cells [64, 65]. While it has become increasingly clear that cytokines such as TNF have important roles in modulating synaptic plasticity [66], neuronal death can occur in response to cytokines through ligation of receptors with "death domains" such as TNFRs and Fas, reactive oxygen species, and phagocytosis of opsonized neurons [58, 64]. Activated microglia and other cells with antigen-presentation functions (B lymphocytes, macrophages, monocytes, dendritic cells) will express Major Histocompatibility Class II (MHC-II) molecules that present endocytosed or lysosomal peptides to CD4+ T lymphocytes. MHC-II genes are commonly known for their use in tissue typing for organ donation. MHC-II molecules are α/β heterodimers that require binding of a peptide approximately 8–10 amino acids in length to be stably expressed on the surface of activated antigen-presenting cells. The majority of these peptides are derived from the processing of endocytosed proteins or from the typical protein constituents of endolysosomes. Recognition of a specific peptide:MHC-II complex by a cognate CD4+ T cell through its unique receptor will activate the T cell and allow it to perform its effector functions: proliferation, cytokine secretion, assisting B cells to differentiate into plasma cells that produce higher affinity antibodies (through a process called hyperaffinity maturation), and allow for proper activation and maintenance of cytotoxic CD8+ T cells [67–70].

Microglial expression of MHC-II molecules has been reported in the states of chronic neuroinflammation, including neurodegenerative diseases [71]. In the healthy CNS, microglial MHC-II expression is difficult to detect. In PD brains, HLA-DR+microglia are found throughout the nigrostriatal tract and other parts of the CNS, including the hippocampus, entorhinal cortex, and cingulated cortex [50, 51, 72]. Positive correlations between disease duration and the microglial/macrophage activation marker CD68 and between MHC-II expression and amount of α-synuclein deposition in the SN of postmortem human brain sections have been observed [34, 55]. These activated microglia are associated with damaged neurons and Lewy body pathology [72]. In vivo PET imaging of PD patients reveals that while the SN region of the midbrain has the highest level of microglia activation, other brain regions including cortical areas also display increased inflammatory signal. Interestingly, microglial activation does not increase linearly with the number of years after diagnosis, suggesting that neuroinflammation may start early in the disease and is maintained throughout the duration of the disease [73]. PET studies have also correlated microglial activation in the human midbrain with increased motor score as measured by the Unified Parkinson's Disease Rating Scale (UPDRS) [74]. After accidental exposure to MPTP in a synthetic heroine generated with faulty chemistry, microglia activation in the brains of drug addicts persisted for decades after initial exposure [75]. Similar observations have been made in nonhuman primates exposed to acute or chronic MPTP dosing [76–78]. In summary, microglial activation is prevalent in PD and MPTP-induced parkinsonism and occurs early in the degenerative process, raising the interesting possibility that some inflammatory processes and microglial effector functions may play a prominent role in promoting degeneration and neuronal loss. Microglial effector functions are likely to engage adaptive immunity in this context and together accelerate the progressive neurodegenerative process.

Particularly relevant for adaptive immunity, common single nucleotide polymorphisms (SNPs) in the MHC-II locus have been associated with increased risk for late-onset PD. Specifically, people homozygous for a risk-conferring SNP at rs3129882 in the first intron of HLA-DRA have a 1.7-fold higher risk for PD than in individuals homozygous for the non-risk-conferring allele [79, 80]. Other SNPs in the MHC-II locus associated with PD have also been reported in the HLA-DRB1 and -DRB5 genes. Another study has shown an association with the HLA-DQB1*06 allele in a German cohort [81–85]. The upregulation of MHC-II mRNA (HLA-DRA, HLA-DPA1, HLA-DQA1) and increased expression of HLA-DR on monocytes in cerebrospinal fluid (CSF) has been reported [86, 87]. Additional studies will be needed to assess whether any of these SNPs have functional consequences on MHC-II expression. Nevertheless, associations between late-onset PD and common variants in the MHC-II locus suggest that certain antigens or patterns of MHC-II expression may increase the risk for development of PD perhaps in response to some environmental trigger or pathogen. The quality of the interaction between CD4+ T cell receptors and peptide:MHC-II impacts CD4+ T cell expansion and differentiation [68, 69]. Thus, MHC-II expression in immune cells in the brain could modulate the overall quality of the neuroinflammatory response. Individuals with a certain MHC-II expression pattern or haplotype could more readily propagate inflammation initiated by neuronal dysfunction or death and in turn, such a mechanism may act to promote and/or exacerbate PD progression [88]. The evidence for involvement of T cells, B cells, and antibodies in promoting inflammation in PD is discussed below.

Given that gene–environment interactions are strongly suspected to underlie the etiology of late-onset PD, certain antigens or environmental exposures could synergize with a person's MHC-II genome to put them at risk for developing PD. In this manner, it could be said that the immune system plays a role in pathogenesis. Peptides presented on MHC-II would then activate T cells to influence neuronal function through secretion of cytokines with known cytotoxic effects on vulnerable neuronal populations. This idea is supported by the association between PD and autoimmune diseases, such as bullous pemphigoid, systemic lupus erythematosus, and Sjögren's syndrome [12, 13, 15, 16]. In addition, gut inflammation is hypothesized to play a role in the development of sporadic PD. Given the extensive neuronal network of the GI tract, its constant interaction with the environment, and its extensive, unique immunological repertoire, the GI tract represents a potential initiation site of PD pathogenesis. Overrepresentation of *CARD15* mutations associated with Crohn's disease and *Helicobacter pylori* seropositivity before age 75 in people with sporadic PD supports this hypothesis [89, 90]. Additionally, a GWAS study identified associations between polymorphisms in the *LRRK2* gene (which encodes a MAP kinase kinase) and Crohn's disease, a type of inflammatory bowel disease. Interestingly, several mutations in the *LRRK2* gene give rise to an autosomal dominant form of PD (see below).

Also implicated in PD are immune responses to infections such as influenza, toxoplasmosis, and Epstein-Barr virus (EBV) [14, 17, 91]. In support of the idea that immune responses to certain viruses may predispose an individual to PD are the numerous cases of post-encephalitic parkinsonism after the 1918 Spanish Flu pandemic and a cross-reactive antibody between EBV and α-synuclein. Japanese encephalitis virus (JEV) has also induced a post-encephalitic parkinsonism with similar neuropathologic features and locomotor dysfunction as seen in people with sporadic PD [92]. JEV infection in rats results in hypokinesia attributable to depletion of catecholamines in the CNS [93]. Lastly, intranasal infection of mice with the H5N1 influenza A/VN/1203/04 strain induced α-synuclein phosphorylation and aggregation in the enteric nervous system [94] and resulted in viral replication in the gut, microglial activation, and increased proinflammatory cytokine and chemokine expression in the CNS lasting 90 days after viral clearance [95]; a transient decrease in tyrosine hydroxylase (TH) expression in the SN was also observed, suggesting that dopaminergic neurons displayed transient neurotoxicity and dysfunction. Because this specific strain of H5N1 was not detected in the brain, these studies provide compelling evidence that an immune response initiated solely by inflammation can induce PD-related neurologic dysfunction. In these examples, MHC expression would play a critical role in determining which antigens are presented to the adaptive immune system. Activated adaptive immune cells would then propagate the inflammatory reaction. The use of animal models of PD such as the human α-synuclein-overexpressing adenoassociated virus (AAV-Syn) model [38] that more directly engages adaptive immunity could help address the validity of these associations. Other neurotoxin models employing MPTP or 6-hydroxydopamine (6-OHDA) may be less likely to engage adaptive immune mechanisms because they are mainly driven by neuronal toxicity; but the role of adaptive immune cells in these neurotoxin models has also been investigated [48]. Clarifying whether the immune system acts as an etiologic factor in PD or simply propagates inflammation initiated by neuronal dysfunction will be an important part of determining PD pathogenesis and disease progression. A more clear and in-depth understanding of the immune system's role in PD and other neurodegenerative disorders will certainly help accelerate development of immunomodulatory strategies to delay or attenuate this progressive disease.

T Lymphocytes in PD

Naïve and memory T cells perform homeostatic surveillance in the CNS [96, 97], and as such these lymphocytes may be involved in both initiating and propagating steps of PD pathogenesis. In both PD patients and animal models, infiltration of T cells into the SN has been demonstrated [48, 50, 51]. In conjunction with HLA-DR expression on microglia, T-cell infiltration has been shown in postmortem brain sections of PD patients [48]. This evidence suggests potential direct interaction with antigen-presenting functions of microglia [50, 51]. Furthermore, levels of B2 microglobulin, a protein required for stability of MHC-I molecules, are increased in the striatum of PD patients [28]. MHC-I molecules activate CD8+ T cells by presenting cytosolic peptides processed through the proteasome pathway. Unlike MHC-II, MHC-I molecules are ubiquitously expressed on all cells (including neurons) except erythrocytes. Upon engagement of peptide:MHC-I, CD8+ T cells can directly kill cells by engagement of death receptors via Fas or TNF or by direct lysis through release of granzymes and perforin [98]. In addition to CD4+ T-cell-mediated toxicity, direct neuronal injury may be caused by CD8+ T cells that are reactive against neuronal antigens presented on MHC-I molecules [99]. Thus, T-cell-mediated neurotoxicity may be driven by direct cell lysis, engagement of cell death receptors, and cytokine secretion through recognition of peptide:MHC molecules.

Several studies have analyzed the composition of T-cell subsets in the peripheral blood of PD patients and have shed light on how adaptive immune responses are altered in this disease. PD patients are reported to have decreased overall numbers of lymphocytes without a change in frequency [100, 101]. Compared to people with other neurologic diseases, individuals with PD have increased memory T cells but decreased naïve T cells [86]. Memory T cells respond faster and with greater magnitude than activated naïve T cells [102]. A more activated, cytotoxic T-cell response is suggested by decreased CD4+:CD8+ ratios and a shift to more IFNγ− versus IL-4-producing T cells in PD patients [100, 101, 103]. Within the CD4+ T cell compartment, PD patients have been reported to have an increase in CD45RO+T cells, which signal an activated and/or memory T-cell population [104]. CD45RO+expression also positively correlates with UPDRS motor score [104]. Naïve CD4+ T cells have increased Fas expression, which may explain why their frequency is decreased [100]. Fas expression is normally upregulated after T-cell activation and ligation by FasL induces apoptosis. This process enables T lymphocytes to maintain immune privilege or initiate contraction after an immune response [105]. Increased memory and activated CD4+ T cells in conjunction with a relative increase in CD8+ T cells could suggest an active inflammatory process. Conflicting reports of changes in relative frequencies of CD4+CD25+ T cells in the peripheral blood of PD patients exist, but without further characterization of this subpopulation, the functional significance of this is unclear [100, 101, 103, 106]. CD25 is increased on activated or memory T cells, as well as regulatory T (T_{reg}) cells. CD4+CD25+CD127- regulatory T cells from PD patients have been reported to have less suppressive capacity compared to cells from healthy controls [104]. The relative number of effector to regulatory T-cell responses is thought to regulate immune responses [107]. Decreased effectiveness of regulatory T cells could promote a chronic neuroinflammatory state or allow for breaking of tolerance to neuronal antigens that would lead to abnormal immune responses against CNS proteins. A more clear understanding of why these regulatory T cells have reduced suppressive capacity could also provide insight into PD pathogenesis and disease progression.

Although some information about the changes in relative frequency of T-cell subsets in patients with PD relative to age-matched healthy controls is emerging, nothing is known about the identity of CNS antigens to which activated and memory T cells are responding in people with PD. One study looked at whether specific T-cell receptor genes are preferentially expressed in PD patients and reported that CD8+ T cells have a lower frequency of Vβ8 expressing cells [108]. The use of deep sequencing techniques to identify patterns of T-cell receptor usage in PD patients could provide evidence for response to specific antigens and aid in identification of those antigens whose patterns could also be potentially useful biomarkers of disease risk or progression. T-cell biomarkers have been investigated and some candidate proteins have been identified within these cells such as β-fibrinogen and transaldolase [109]. The pathogenic relevance of these changes remains to be established.

Other overall pathogenic changes in peripheral blood lymphocytes from PD patients have been reported. Lymphocytes from PD patients display an increased incidence of micronuclei, single-strand DNA breaks, and oxidized purine bases [110]. Interestingly, levodopa treatment seems to reduce this DNA damage in peripheral blood lymphocytes [111]. Markers of apoptosis, caspase-3 activation, and Cu/Zn superoxide dismutase activity are increased in lymphocytes from individuals with PD [112]. This DNA damage and increased level of apoptosis could be representative of a systemic, pathogenic process involving oxidative stress, specific immune responses, and/or intrinsic genetic factors. The use of animal models to assess the contribution of lymphocytes will inform how these in vivo changes in immune cell subsets may contribute to the disease etiology and progression in humans.

The contribution of T cells to PD-like pathology in animal models has been assessed but mainly in neurotoxin models. CD8+ T cells are detectable in greater numbers compared to CD4+ T cells in the acute MPTP neurotoxin model. In this model, these lymphocytes have increased expression of LFA-1, an integrin that binds endothelial adhesion molecules to allow for diapedesis across the BBB [113]. DA neuron loss and behavioral deficits caused by both chronic and acute MPTP administration are attenuated in RAG2 knockout mice that lack both T and B cells [48, 114]. Mice in which there is a global loss of αβ-T cells through knockout of the T cell receptor β-chain, as well as mice lacking CD4 T cells (*CD4−/−*), are also protected in the MPTP model [48]. The loss of CD8 T cells was not protective. Reconstitution of *Rag1−/−* mice with FasL-mutant splenocytes attenuated DA neuron cell death, while reconstitution with *IFNγ−/−* splenocytes did not. These findings suggest that Fas–FasL interactions involving CD4+ T cells play an important role in promoting MPTP-induced neurodegeneration. As discussed above, cytotoxic T cells use FasL to induce apoptosis in target cells but Fas receptor is also important in T-cell homeostasis and contraction. Impaired FasL–Fas interactions result in unchecked T-cell activation and proliferation. An extreme example manifests itself in autoimmune lymphoproliferative syndrome caused by unchecked T-cell proliferation [115]. Dysregulation of this pathway may also leave chronically activated macrophages or microglia unchecked allowing for propagation of the inflammatory response. Fas–FasL signaling may also indirectly contribute to neuronal damage by inducing Fas-induced apoptosis-resistant astrocytes to produce proinflammatory cytokines that damage neurons [116]. In the intranigral AAV-human-α-synuclein overexpression mouse model, B- and T-lymphocyte infiltration in the SN persists after peak of microglial activation, suggesting that microglia in the SN engage adaptive immune cells to propagate inflammation in this model of PD [38].

Nitrated α-synuclein draining from the CNS into cervical lymph nodes may represent one molecular mechanism by which adaptive immune engagement occurs after MPTP-induced neuronal damage. Robust T-cell responses were initiated when mice were immunized with the C-terminus of the nitrated α-synuclein. Transfer of T cells from immunized mice into MPTP-treated mice enhanced neuroinflammation to a slight but significant degree [117]. T cells from mice immunized with nitrated α-synuclein produced mostly IL-17 and TNF after ex vivo restimulation. Adoptive transfer of Th17-polarized T cells from nitrated α-synuclein-immunized mice into wild-type mice greatly exacerbated MPTP-induced neurodegeneration. Unexpectedly, neurodegeneration was not exacerbated by adoptive transfer of T cells polarized to Th1 (IFNγ-producing) or Th2 (IL-4-producing) phenotypes. Yet, adoptive transfer of ex vivo differentiated regulatory T cells into MPTP-induced mice attenuated neurodegeneration [65]. The novelty of this study is that it demonstrates that modulation of the adaptive immune response can indeed determine the outcome of neurodegeneration in a model of PD.

Together, this evidence supports a model in which T-cell responses to modified α-synuclein or other modified antigens from DA neurons initiate an adaptive immune response that further propagates neuronal death. These responses would differ based on the context of antigen presentation. Various etiologies could allow for the adaptive immune system to be exposed to modified α-synuclein (i.e., toxins) or increased escape of CNS antigen (i.e., head trauma). These mechanisms would break normal tolerance mechanisms by presenting self-antigens that are cross-reactive with cognate peptide:MHC of existing memory T cells. These antigens could also activate naive T cells by presenting self-antigens for which T cells are not normally negatively selected or tolerized against in the context of an inflammatory response. Additional studies to identify specific antigens to which T cells respond in animal models of PD and in humans with PD will be critical to our understanding of the role of the adaptive immune system in pathogenesis and progression of PD.

Antibodies and B Lymphocytes in PD

B lymphocytes are the key mediators of humoral immunity in that their secreted immunoglobulins can have effects at sites far from the actual site of secretion [118]. Unique antibodies, as well as increased antibody levels against CNS proteins, are present in people with PD [119, 120]. However, infiltration of antibody-producing B lymphocytes into the CNS is not a common histopathological postmortem finding in brains of PD patients [48, 50, 51]. While infiltration of B lymphocytes is present under some inflammatory conditions, the aggregation of antibodies at a specific site is enough to promote inflammation without the presence of actual B cells. Antibodies can precipitate inflammatory reactions through activation of the complement system or effector cells through surface immunoglobulin receptors [118]. A decrease in the number of peripheral blood B cells in PD patients has been reported but the functional significance of this finding needs to be contextualized [100, 101]. For instance, reduced peripheral blood B cell counts in other autoimmune or inflammatory diseases are due to decreased circulating memory B cells. Thus, the reduction in B cell number may be related to active inflammation and cellular activation [121–123]. Additional research is needed to understand the role for B cells in PD beyond their antibody-secreting functions which are discussed below.

Antibodies against DA neurons that are not present in healthy people have been reported in PD patients [119, 120, 124, 125]. At present, the lack of a universal antibody or "PD"-specific antigen refutes an etiologic role for B cells and antibodies but does not rule out a pathogenic or protective role in modulating inflammation in PD. Alternatively, it is entirely possible that a universal antibody or antigen in PD will not be found because no single antigen is required for disease induction. On the other hand, it may not be possible to identify such an antigen because antibody production is typically assessed during the late stages of disease. In neurohistological evaluation of postmortem PD brains, immunoglobulins have been reported to colocalize with pigmented DA neurons in close proximity to FcγR-positive microglia [126]. The number of IgG-immunoreactive neurons positively correlated with the number of MHC-II-positive microglia, suggesting a link between antibody-mediated destruction of neurons and antigen presentation. Further supporting this link, these microglia contained intracellular pigmented granules, suggesting their participation in antibody-mediated phagocytosis of pigmented DA neurons. A pathogenic role for anti-neuronal antibodies in PD is further supported by studies in which immunoglobulins from PD patients induced neurotoxicity in a rat model when injected into the SN resulting in a loss of TH+neurons while sparing acetylcholinesterase-positive neurons in the medial septal region [127]. The injected immunoglobulins induced perivascular inflammation, microgliosis, and loss of TH+neurons in the SN in an Fcγ receptor-dependent fashion [128]. Similarly, Fcγ receptor knockout mice are resistant to chronic but not acute MPTP administration [114]. One caveat to these results is that the deletion of Fcγ receptors in mouse models impacts numerous cell types (monocytes, microglia, neutrophils, basophils, mast cells, NK cells) and reduces the ability to respond to cellular-bound IgG through multiple mechanisms. These mice are also resistant to neurodegeneration and microglial activation induced by AAV-induced intranigral expression of human wild-type α-synuclein [129]. The AAV-α-synuclein model also leads to significant IgG deposition, suggesting that humoral immunity and/or breakdown of the BBB is playing a role in the degenerative process [38]. Together, these findings strongly suggest that the humoral arm of the immune system can play a role in chronic neuroinflammation and demise of DA neurons.

Given the chronic inflammatory nature of PD, humoral immunity could play an important role in the progression of PD while T-cell immunity may be more important for disease onset. Intuitively, this idea makes rational sense because CD4+ T-cell activation is essential for potent engagement of humoral immunity. In contrast, antibodies may also play a protective role. The use of a mouse antibody against α-synuclein demonstrates that microglia can take up antibody-bound α-synuclein in vivo and prevent neuron-to-astrocyte transmission of α-synuclein [130]. It is unknown whether this phenomenon can happen in the PD brain, but it raises the distinct possibility that certain sets of antibodies could play a pathogenic versus a protective role. Lastly, pathogenic antibodies could promote inflammatory reactions or propagate α-synuclein spread through uptake by Fc receptor-expressing cells, while other antibodies may be protective by aiding in clearance of α-synuclein aggregates.

A handful of studies have investigated the extent to which antibodies could be used as biomarkers for PD. One study found decreased levels of anti-α-synuclein antibodies in PD patients but not in controls or patients with other neurodegenerative conditions with sensitivity and specificity of 85 and 25 %, respectively. These antibodies did not correlate with age, duration of disease, or Hoehn and Yahr staging [119]. It should be noted that while the presence of α-synuclein antibodies may hint at pathologic mechanisms, it is unclear whether they could be used alone for diagnostic purposes. Another study demonstrated the ability to use ten autoantibody biomarkers to differentiate PD from normal aging, Alzheimer's disease, breast cancer, and multiple sclerosis with accuracies of over 85 % [120]. Yet other studies reported negative findings in that the frequency of anti-α-synuclein antibodies in patients with sporadic PD is not significantly different from those in healthy controls [125]. However, around 90 % of people with familial PD have these antibodies. The authors suggest that the antibodies in familial PD may represent more pathogenic epitopes rather than incidental ones resulting from secondary tissue damage. Additional research aimed at detecting antibodies at earlier stages of disease will likely provide more insight into the role of antibodies in PD pathogenesis. Antibodies generated in the earliest stages of PD are more likely to be related to pathogenic epitopes and less likely to be incidental (i.e., from the release of CNS antigens) as inflammation becomes exacerbated during the progressive neuronal damage in the disease.

Genetic Mutations that Cause PD and Adaptive Immunity

Many of the genetic causes of familial PD have been identified [131, 132]. Hereditary forms of PD, caused by specific gene mutations, only comprise 5–10 % of PD cases [4, 133]. These genetic forms of PD typically have an earlier age of onset and provide insight into the potential role of ubiquitously expressed proteins in neuronal and immune dysfunction in sporadic PD [133]. Yet, it is generally believed that genetic and sporadic forms of the disease are likely to share common mechanisms. Therefore, the study of these genetic mutations has provided insight into how perturbation of certain pathways may contribute to the development of sporadic PD. Despite the fact that most of these PD-linked genes have been shown to be expressed in immune cells and may contribute to nonautonomous cell death of neurons, the majority of research efforts to date have investigated the pathogenic roles of these mutations in neurons only. Yet, it is important to recognize that dysfunction of these proteins in both neurons and immune cells would allow for synergy of inflammatory and neuronal death mechanisms that promote the development and/or progression of PD.

The *SNCA* gene, which encodes α-synuclein, was the first mutation linked to a familial form of PD [134]. Since then, a gene triplication in SNCA has also been linked to a familial form of PD [134], and polymorphisms in the promoter region of SNCA that drive increased expression of α-synuclein have also been identified as genetic risk loci [135]. But while α-synuclein was once believed to be primarily expressed in neurons, it should be noted that the *SNCA* gene and therefore the α-synuclein protein are also expressed in a wide variety of immune cells including T cells, B cells, NK cells, microglia, and monocytes [136–139] as are most of the genes implicated in familial forms of PD including parkin and DJ-1. In microglia, α-synuclein has been shown to have a homeostatic role. Microglia from mice lacking *SNCA* have a more activated phenotype in terms of morphology and cytokine secretion in addition to decreased phagocytic ability [139, 140]. Consistent with the idea that it may have some regulatory role in inflammatory responses, the level of α-synuclein protein increases after LPS stimulation of monocytes and lymphocytes [141]. Autophagy plays a critical role in maintenance, activation, and proliferation of T cells [142], and individuals with the autoimmune disorder systemic lupus erythematosus CD4+ T cells express five times higher levels of α-synuclein that correlate with higher basal levels of autophagy [143]. Therefore, changes in immune cell levels of α-synuclein could modulate cellular function via mechanisms such as altered autophagy. This last point may be especially relevant as altered number or frequency of T and B cells have been reported in PD patients. In mice expressing human wild-type α-synuclein on the Thy1 promoter, frequencies of CD4 and CD8 T cells are increased in the peripheral blood [43]. α-Synuclein is also overexpressed in the T cells of these mice; thus the role of this protein in immune cells versus neurons will need to be evaluated in greater depth. It is unknown whether the inflammatory phenotype is attributed to primary deficits in immune cells overexpressing α-synuclein versus to secondary activation of immune cells as a result of overexpression of α-synuclein in neurons and neuronal dysfunction. The critical point here is that the functional significance of mutations or polymorphisms in α-synuclein in immune cells has been understudied. In addition, perturbations in the levels of α-synuclein by various stimuli, such as LPS, in the context of genetic polymorphisms inherent in immune gene loci could lead to immune dysfunction in those individuals that may synergize with and exacerbate neuronal dysfunction. Consistent with these observations, signs of synergy between inflammation and α-synuclein-induced degeneration have been observed in numerous cell culture and animal model studies as discussed previously. This synergy is likely to have important consequences in the brains of humans affected with PD.

Mutations in *LRRK2* (*PARK8*), a gene encoding a protein kinase with an MAPK-kinase–kinase, GTPase, and ankyrin domains, cause an autosomal dominant form of PD with a clinical presentation and age of onset similar to sporadic PD [144]. The incomplete penetrance (estimated at 33–67 %) of these mutations also suggests a strong environmental and/or immune component that modifies disease onset [145, 146]. Genetic variants in this gene have also been associated with increased susceptibility for sporadic PD [83, 147]. Early studies analyzing LRRK2 function and expression in neurons demonstrated that its expression is low in the SN and greater in areas of the brain that receive dopamine signals [148–151]. *LRRK2–/–* mice are more susceptible to dextran sodium sulfate-induced colitis [152]. In vitro and targeted in vivo overexpression of mutant LRRK2 induces neurotoxicity in a kinase- and GTPase-dependent manner [153–157]. However, germ-line mutant LRRK2 transgenic mice do not completely replicate PD-like phenotypes or show spontaneous DA neuron degeneration [158–161]. However, these mouse models do show behavioral alterations and impaired dopamine release in the nigrostriatal system. Indeed, perturbations in LRRK2 function alone may not be sufficient to induce PD-like pathology, but may require a second insult such as inflammation.

Interestingly, LRRK2 expression occurs in many immune cells: dendritic cells, monocytes, microglia, B cells, and T cells [162, 163]; yet the role of LRRK2 in various immune cell populations has not received much attention in recent years. The level of expression in many immune cell subsets is significantly greater than in neuronal populations [164]. Mouse bone marrow-derived macrophages (BMDMs) significantly upregulate LRRK2 mRNA expression after stimulation with LPS and lentiviral particles. BMDMs from R144C-LRRK2 mutant mice have reduced LC3-II expression, a marker of autophagy [162]. LRRK2 expression is consistently upregulated in immune cells after IFNγ stimulation and activation of the NF-κB, a key pathway important for production of microbicidal reactive oxygen species during phagocytosis of pathogens during intracellular infection [164]. In microglia, LRRK2 expression can be detected upon in vivo activation with LPS and is upregulated by ex vivo LPS treatment [165]. Furthermore, LRRK2 inhibition or knockdown in microglia attenuated LPS-induced inflammatory signaling as measured by cytokine secretion, microglial chemotaxis, and morphologic remodeling. Specific LRRK2 SNPs have been shown to associate with leprosy and Crohn's disease [166, 167]. In fact, increased LRRK2 expression is found in the epithelium of Crohn's disease patients in many cell types including macrophages, dendritic cells, and B lymphocytes [164]. Of direct relevance to adaptive immunity, LRRK2 inhibits the nuclear translocation of NFAT, a master regulator of transcriptional activation in T cells [152]. Overall, it is clear that LRRK2 is likely to be involved in regulating the activation status and effector functions in multiple kinds of immune cells. Therefore, the role of pathogenic *LRRK2* mutations in specific LRRK2 domains is worthy of investigation within the context of the immune system and its role in predisposing an individual for age-related degeneration.

The *Parkin* gene encodes a multidomain protein that contains E3 ubiquitin ligase activity that plays a role in the regulation of numerous cellular activities including proteasomal degradation and ubiquitin-mediated signaling; and loss of function mutations and deletions in the *Parkin* (*PARK2*) gene cause autosomal recessive forms of juvenile PD [168]. Although the physiologic substrates of parkin are unknown [169], the potential roles for this protein include a role in preventing protein aggregation and/or promoting mitophagy [170–172]. Parkin has also been suggested to function as a transcription factor that regulates p53 expression [173] independent of its ligase activity. Parkin knockout animals do not have loss of DA neurons in the SN and do not have increased vulnerability to MPTP, yet they do show nonmotor behavioral changes related to changes in the nigrostriatal pathway [174, 175]. This phenotype suggests compensatory changes in the global Parkin knockout animal that prevent death of DA neurons or that a second insult is required in conjunction with lack of Parkin expression. Consistent with this idea, Parkin knockout mice display increased vulnerability to inflammation-related degeneration. Specifically, chronic peripheral low-dose intraperitoneal injections of LPS in Parkin knockout mice trigger fine-motor deficits and loss of DA neurons in the SN [176]. In addition, in microglia, neurons, and peripheral macrophages, LPS and TNF dose-dependently reduce *Parkin* expression due to the presence of an NF-κB response element in the *Parkin* promoter [177]. Therefore, chronic inflammation may downregulate Parkin and phenocopy loss of function *Parkin* mutations. Interestingly, Parkin has also been implicated as a susceptibility locus for leprosy and typhoid fever [178, 179] and more recently was demonstrated to be critical for host defense against *Mycobacterium tuberculosis* [180]. In summary, current evidence implicates a protective role for *Parkin* in inflammation-induced degeneration, and inflammatory pathways negatively regulate Parkin expression. Therefore, the role of Parkin in inflammation and immune cells merits a more thorough evaluation as it may represent an important point of convergence for the functional consequences of inflammatory stress and its effects on PD pathogenesis and progression.

Identification of the normal physiological role of proteins wherein pathogenic mutations cause genetic forms of PD will be critical for a clear mechanistic understanding of PD pathogenesis. It is clear that in the last decade, most of the research focus on the role of these proteins has been neuron-centric despite the fact that most PD-linked genes are expressed in many other cell types. Immune cells in particular are poised to interact with the environment and respond in a coordinated manner. In genetic forms of PD, dysfunction of these proteins may render neurons more vulnerable and promote their dysfunction. In sporadic PD, environmental exposures may alter the expression of these genes in immune cells which could then indirectly modify neuronal function and promote the development of PD. Therefore, further research of this normal and pathogenic role of these proteins in immune cells is well-justified and is expected to advance our understanding of nonautonomous cell processes that contribute to degeneration in PD.

Immunomodulatory Therapies

Given the chronic, progressive nature of PD and the large amount of neurodegeneration that has already occurred before clinical presentation of motor symptoms, it is highly unlikely that immunomodulatory therapies will have a significant impact in altering the course of PD. Therefore, efforts to enable early diagnosis in premotor stages and timely treatment will be necessary to significantly impact disease. Nevertheless, because intense investigation into biomarkers of early disease is in progress, it is critical that we continue identifying immunomodulatory therapies that could be translated to the clinic. To this end, we will review a handful of therapies that have targeted immune pathways in animal models of PD and shown some therapeutic benefit.

Modulation of the T-cell repertoire to suppress T effector and boost regulatory T-cell function is one such example. Copaxone, also known as glatiramer acetate, is a random polymer of amino acids from myelin basic protein used in the treatment of multiple sclerosis. This mixture is thought to mimic the antigenic properties of myelin basic protein but alters the T-cell response to a more anti-inflammatory phenotype [181]. Adoptive transfer of T cells from a copaxone-immunized animal afforded protection against neurodegeneration in an MPTP mouse model of PD [182], suggesting that T-cell skewing to dampen the adaptive immune response could potentially have a disease-modifying effect. The adoptively transferred T cells accumulate in the SN, suppress microglial activation, and are correlated with an increase in neurotrophic factors [183]. Consistent with this mechanism, adoptive transfer of T_{regs} also attenuated neurodegeneration in an MPTP mouse model of PD [65]. Decreased effectiveness of regulatory T cells in their suppressive capacities and changes in the T-cell compartment suggest that correcting phenotypic T-cell changes in PD patients may provide a beneficial disease-modifying effect [104]. To this end, Gendelman and colleagues are initiating a clinical trial to assess the efficacy of Sargramostim, a granulocyte–monocyte colony-stimulating factor analog thought to promote the development of T_{regs}, in the treatment of PD. If successful, this trial could demonstrate the usefulness of immunomodulatory therapies in slowing down progression of PD.

The use of a dominant-negative inhibitor of TNF (DN-TNF) in PD animal models suggests that anti-TNF biological agents may also be of clinical value to delay or attenuate nigral DA neuron degeneration if administered in a timely fashion. Specifically, administration of soluble DN-TNF peptides whose mechanism of action renders them selective for the soluble form of TNF [184] via osmotic pump or lentiviral overexpression in the SN shows protection in 6-OHDA models [185, 186]. Even delayed lentiviral overexpression of DN-TNF in the SN can be protective against progressive DA neuron loss [187]. Therefore, if the idea is to dampen overall levels of peripheral or central inflammation, anti-TNF biologics may be of therapeutic value in PD.

Passive immunization in animal models with anti-α-synuclein antibodies have also been investigated as a potential mechanism for clearing accumulations of α-synuclein. In mice expressing human α-synuclein under the platelet-derived growth factor β promoter, administration of an anti-α-synuclein antibody improved behavioral performance and promoted degradation of accumulated α-synuclein [188, 189]. Clearance of α-synuclein is thought to occur via uptake through Fc-receptor-expressing cells such as microglia. These observations will need to be replicated using other human α-synuclein overexpression models independently to confirm the promising potential of synuclein immunotherapy. While it is unclear if removal or prevention of α-synuclein-containing Lewy body formation is required to ameliorate PD progression, it is an important question that requires investigation in order to determine whether such therapies should be translated to the clinic.

Lastly, in light of the possibility that adaptive immune cells may contribute to the pathogenesis and/or progression of PD as highlighted in this review, several other strategies to modulate T-cell function may merit investigation in preclinical animal models of PD. Specifically, immunosuppressive therapies that block T-cell proliferation may be useful in modifying progression or onset of PD. Such therapeutics could include corticosteroids, colchicine, or peripheral T-cell-depleting antibodies such as muromonab-CD3. Colchicine blocks mitosis and thereby prevents proliferation of rapidly dividing cells such as activated immune cells; although medicinal chemistry to modify this drug may be needed as is has significant gastrointestinal side effects. In a rat model of the pesticide rotenone wherein microglial activation is believed to be critical for nigral degeneration [190], colchicine showed benefit in preventing neurodegeneration [191]. Muromonab initially activates CD3+ T cells but then these activated cells die; this antibody is currently used to prevent transplant rejection [192].

A second avenue for immunomodulation is the use of drugs that block T-cell activation or recruitment. Abatacept and belatacept block the interaction between CD28 on T cells and CD80/CD86 molecules on antigen-presenting cells [192, 193]. These drugs have been used in transplant rejection and rheumatoid arthritis with great success [193, 194]. Given the documented changes in activated and memory T-cell subsets in people with PD, these drugs could have therapeutic success in limiting such T-cell populations. The antibody against the α4 integrin, natalizumab, has been successful in the treatment of multiple sclerosis because it blocks the recruitment of T cells to sites of inflammation [195]. Therefore, it may be possible to dampen neuroinflammation and lessen degeneration in PD by blocking activation and recruitment of T cells to sites where vulnerable neuronal populations reside.

Ex vivo modification of autologous T cells to make them produce anti-inflammatory molecules or have them target effector T cells that are pathogenic in PD might also be another useful therapeutic approach. This approach would require identification of pathogenic T-cell populations or the relevant antigens to which pathogenic T cells are responding in PD. Such technologies are currently being explored in harnessing immune responses against cancer [196].

Therapies to target humoral immunity do exist and have shown effectiveness in autoimmune diseases where antibodies are known to play a pathogenic role. Rituximab is an example of a B-cell depleting antibody that has shown some effectiveness in SLE [197]. Intravenous immunoglobulin (IVIG) has been effective in treating diseases that are mediated by pathogenic antibody responses such as erythroblastosis fetalis, autoimmune thrombocytopenia, and chronic inflammatory demyelinating polyneuropathy. IVIG is thought to block proinflammatory antibody-mediated responses through many pathways including modulating Fc-receptor expression, expansion of T_{regs}, and blocking activating Fc receptors [198]. IVIG is generally well tolerated with less than 5 % of people experiencing headache, fever, or nausea. In a recent Phase III trial by Baxter, IVIG did not show efficacy in the treatment of mild to moderate Alzheimer's disease; however, since the underlying pathogenic mechanisms in PD are different, the lack of success in AD may not reflect on its potential in PD. It should be noted that this study demonstrated that IVIG was safe in elderly persons with a neurodegenerative disease. Thus, IVIG could be a safe immunomodulatory therapy potentially useful in PD.

As with any immunomodulatory therapy, immunosuppression or off-target effects are of great concern, especially in an elderly population that is at increased susceptibility to infections. But as learned in the transplant field, timing of these and any other therapeutic intervention is also critical [192]. The use of these therapeutics at the time when inflammation is beginning or is primed could have significant positive impact on the course of disease while having minimal effects much later in the course of the disease. Additional research in preclinical models of disease should enhance our understanding of the role of the adaptive immune system in PD pathogenesis and progression and will inform which immunomodulatory therapies are most suitable for advancing to clinical trials in PD.

Conclusion

The adaptive immune system normally responds to specific pathogens or antigens and has various effector mechanisms to clear them, i.e., direct cytotoxicity, cytokine production, and antibody production. The adaptive immune system must receive the appropriate signals from innate immune cells to be activated in order to respond to specific antigens recognized by uniquely specific receptors. T cells recognize peptides presented on MHC molecules while B cells recognize antigens through their cell surface receptors. Abundant evidence exists for the role of inflammation in human PD as well as in animal models of the disease. Environmental and genetic factors synergize to create susceptibility to PD. It remains to be seen whether these factors create susceptibility primarily through inducing neuronal dysfunction or through direct activation of the immune system that then propagates neuronal dysfunction. Regardless, engagement of the adaptive immune system can further precipitate neuronal dysfunction in a specific manner, i.e., from antigens derived from DA neurons. Modification of these antigens by inflammation and environmental factors may allow for an adaptive immune response in bypassing normal tolerance mechanisms. Nitrated α-synuclein is one potential antigen in this case. From the initiation site of this inflammation, a chronic adaptive immune reaction could spread neuronal damage and dysfunction to other CNS pathways implicated in sporadic PD. The adaptive immune system may prove to be the missing link between environment, genetics, and the spread of pathology put forth by the Braak hypothesis. Further investigations aimed at delineating the role of the adaptive immune system in PD pathogenesis and progression and the specific peptides that are being presented to T cells is prerequisite for development of suitable immunomodulatory therapies that can delay onset or modify the course of the disease.

In this review, the evidence for activation of the adaptive immune system in human PD has been presented, as well as our present understanding of how the effector functions of adaptive immune cells damage DA neurons in animal models of PD. Immune cell expression and functions of proteins encoded by genes wherein mutations give rise to familial forms of PD have also been presented. Taken together, exciting clues for a newly recognized role of the adaptive immune system exist but much work remains to be done in this area. Closer and more in-depth examination of this important topic may provide a better understanding of PD as well as an opportunity to engage in paradigm-shifting research to identify immune-related biomarkers of PD and disease-modifying therapies to prevent, arrest, or at least delay the onset of this debilitating disease.

References

1. Chen JJ. Parkinson's disease: health-related quality of life, economic cost, and implications of early treatment. Am J Manag Care. 2010;16:S87–93.
2. Henchcliffe C, Severt WL. Disease modification in Parkinson's disease. Drugs Aging. 2011;28:605–15.
3. Gelb DJ, Oliver E, Gilman S. Diagnostic criteria for Parkinson disease. Arch Neurol. 1999;56: 33–9.
4. Samii A, Nutt JG, Ransom BR. Parkinson's disease. Lancet. 2004;363:1783–93.
5. Hawkes CH, Del Tredici K, Braak H. A timeline for Parkinson's disease. Parkinsonism Relat Disord. 2010;16:79–84.
6. Brooks DJ. The early diagnosis of Parkinson's disease. Ann Neurol. 1998;44(3 Suppl 1) :S10–8.
7. Ballard PA, Tetrud JW, Langston JW. Permanent human parkinsonism due to 1-methyl-4-phenyl-1,2,3,6-tetrahydropyridine (MPTP): seven cases. Neurology. 1985;35:949–56.
8. Davis GC, Williams AC, Markey SP, Ebert MH, Caine ED, Reichert CM, et al. Chronic Parkinsonism secondary to intravenous injection of meperidine analogues. Psychiatry Res. 1979;1:249–54.
9. Bower JH, Maraganore DM, Peterson BJ, McDonnell SK, Ahlskog JE, Rocca WA. Head trauma preceding PD: a case–control study. Neurology. 2003;60:1610–5.
10. Hernan MA, Takkouche B, Caamano-Isorna F, Gestal-Otero JJ. A meta-analysis of coffee drinking, cigarette smoking, and the risk of Parkinson's disease. Ann Neurol. 2002;52: 276–84.
11. Chen H, Huang X, Guo X, Mailman RB, Park Y, Kamel F, et al. Smoking duration, intensity, and risk of Parkinson disease. Neurology. 2010;74:878–84.
12. Chemaly RE, Moussalli AS. Parkinsonian syndrome as a complication of systemic lupus erythematosus. Report of a case and review of the literature. J Med Liban. 2012;60:103–5.
13. Walker RH, Spiera H, Brin MF, Olanow CW. Parkinsonism associated with Sjögren's syndrome: three cases and a review of the literature. Mov Disord. 1999;14:262–8.
14. Ravenholt RT, Foege WH. 1918 influenza, encephalitis lethargica, parkinsonism. Lancet. 1982;2:860–4.
15. Li X, Sundquist J, Sundquist K. Subsequent risks of Parkinson disease in patients with autoimmune and related disorders: a nationwide epidemiological study from Sweden. Neurodgener Dis. 2012;10:277–84.
16. Langan SM, Groves RW, West J. The relationship between neurological disease and bullous pemphigoid: a population-based case–control study. J Invest Dermatol. 2011;131:631–6.

17. Miman O, Kusbeci OY, Aktepe OC, Cetinkaya Z. The probable relation between Toxoplasma gondii and Parkinson's disease. Neurosci Lett. 2010;475:129–31.
18. Rugbjerg K, Friis S, Ritz B, Schernhammer ES, Korbo L, Olsen JH. Autoimmune disease and risk for Parkinson disease: a population-based case–control study. Neurology. 2009;73: 1462–8.
19. Samii A, Etminan M, Wiens MO, Jafari S. NSAID use and the risk of Parkinson's disease: systematic review and meta-analysis of observational studies. Drugs Aging. 2009;26:769–79.
20. Chen H, Zhang SM, Hernan MA, Schwarzschild MA, Willett WC, Colditz GA, et al. Nonsteroidal anti-inflammatory drugs and the risk of Parkinson disease. Arch Neurol. 2003;60:1059–64.
21. Dauer W, Przedborski S. Parkinson's disease: mechanisms and models. Neuron. 2003; 39:889–909.
22. McGuire SO, Ling ZD, Lipton JW, Sortwell CE, Collier TJ, Carvey PM. Tumor necrosis factor alpha is toxic to embryonic mesencephalic dopamine neurons. Exp Neurol. 2001;169: 219–30.
23. Block ML, Zecca L, Hong JS. Microglia-mediated neurotoxicity: uncovering the molecular mechanisms. Nat Rev Neurosci. 2007;8:57–69.
24. Mount MP, Lira A, Grimes D, Smith PD, Faucher S, Slack R, et al. Involvement of interferon-gamma in microglial-mediated loss of dopaminergic neurons. J Neurosci. 2007;27: 3328–37.
25. Tansey MG, Goldberg MS. Neuroinflammation in Parkinson's disease: its role in neuronal death and implications for therapeutic intervention. Neurobiol Dis. 2010;37:510–8.
26. Lawson LJ, Perry VH, Dri P, Gordon S. Heterogeneity in the distribution and morphology of microglia in the normal adult mouse brain. Neuroscience. 1990;39:151–70.
27. Barnum CJ, Tansey MG. Modeling neuroinflammatory pathogenesis of Parkinson's disease. Prog Brain Res. 2010;184:113–32.
28. Mogi M, Harada M, Kondo T, Riederer P, Nagatsu T. Brain beta 2-microglobulin levels are elevated in the striatum in Parkinson's disease. J Neural Transm Park Dis Dement Sect. 1995;9:87–92.
29. Mogi M, Harada M, Kondo T, Riederer P, Inagaki H, Minami M, et al. Interleukin-1 beta, interleukin-6, epidermal growth factor and transforming growth factor-alpha are elevated in the brain from Parkinsonian patients. Neurosci Lett. 1994;180:147–50.
30. Blum-Degen D, Müller T, Kuhn W, Gerlach M, Przuntek H, Riederer P. Interleukin-1 beta and interleukin-6 are elevated in the cerebrospinal fluid of Alzheimer's and de novo Parkinson's disease patients. Neurosci Lett. 1995;202:17–20.
31. Yamada T, McGeer PL, McGeer EG. Lewy bodies in Parkinson's disease are recognized by antibodies to complement proteins. Acta Neuropathol. 1992;84:100–4.
32. Koziorowski D, Tomasiuk R, Szlufik S, Friedman A. Inflammatory cytokines and NT-proCNP in Parkinson's disease patients. Cytokine. 2012;60:762–6.
33. Petit GH, Berkovich E, Hickery M, Kallunki P, Fog K, Fitzer-Attas C, et al. Rasagiline ameliorates olfactory deficits in an alpha-synuclein mouse model of Parkinson's disease. PLoS One. 2013;8:e60691.
34. Sanchez-Guajardo V, Barnum CJ, Tansey MG, Romero-Ramos M. Neuroimmunological processes in Parkinson's disease and their relation to alpha-synuclein: microglia as the referee between neuronal processes and peripheral immunity. ASN Neuro. 2013;5:113–39.
35. Herrera AJ, Castano A, Venero JL, Cano J, Machado A. The single intranigral injection of LPS as a new model for studying the selective effects of inflammatory reactions on dopaminergic system. Neurobiol Dis. 2000;7:429–47.
36. Mogi M, Togari A, Tanaka K, Ogawa N, Ichinose H, Nagatsu T. Increase in level of tumor necrosis factor-alpha in 6-hydroxydopamine-lesioned striatum in rats is suppressed by immunosuppressant FK506. Neurosci Lett. 2000;289:165–8.
37. McFarland NR, Lee JS, Hyman BT, McLean PJ. Comparison of transduction efficiency of recombinant AAV serotypes 1, 2, 5, and 8 in the rat nigrostriatal system. J Neurochem. 2009;109:838–45.

38. Theodore S, Cao S, McLean PJ, Standaert DG. Targeted overexpression of human alpha-synuclein triggers microglial activation and an adaptive immune response in a mouse model of Parkinson disease. J Neuropathol Exp Neurol. 2008;67:1149–58.
39. Tofaris GK, Garcia Reitbock P, Humby T, Lambourne SL, O'Connell M, Ghetti B, et al. Pathological changes in dopaminergic nerve cells of the substantia nigra and olfactory bulb in mice transgenic for truncated human alpha-synuclein (1–120): implications for Lewy body disorders. J Neurosci. 2006;26:3942–50.
40. Emmer KL, Waxman EA, Covy JP, Giasson BI. E46K human alpha-synuclein transgenic mice develop Lewy-like and tau pathology associated with age-dependent, detrimental motor impairment. J Biol Chem. 2011;286:35104–18.
41. Lee MK, Stirling W, Xu Y, Xu X, Qui D, Mandir AS, et al. Human alpha-synuclein-harboring familial Parkinson's disease-linked Ala-53 Thr mutation causes neurodegenerative disease with alpha-synuclein aggregation in transgenic mice. Proc Natl Acad Sci U S A. 2002; 99:8968–73.
42. Miller RM, Kiser GL, Kaysser-Kranich T, Casaceli C, Colla E, Lee MK, et al. Wild-type and mutant alpha-synuclein induce a multi-component gene expression profile consistent with shared pathophysiology in different transgenic mouse models of PD. Exp Neurol. 2007; 204:421–32.
43. Watson MB, Richter F, Lee SK, Gabby L, Wu J, Masliah E, et al. Regionally-specific microglial activation in young mice over-expressing human wildtype alpha-synuclein. Exp Neurol. 2012;237:318–34.
44. Pisani V, Stefani A, Pierantozzi M, Natoli S, Stanzione P, Franciotta D, et al. Increased blood-cerebrospinal fluid transfer of albumin in advanced Parkinson's disease. J Neuroinflammation. 2012;9:188.
45. Kortekaas R, Leenders KL, van Oostrom JC, Vaalburg W, Bart J, Willemsen AT, et al. Blood–brain barrier dysfunction in Parkinsonian midbrain in vivo. Ann Neurol. 2005;57: 176–9.
46. Farkas E, De Jong GI, de Vos RA, Jansen Steur EN, Luiten PG. Pathological features of cerebral cortical capillaries are doubled in Alzheimer's disease and Parkinson's disease. Acta Neuropathol. 2000;100:395–402.
47. Faucheux BA, Bonnet A-M, Agid Y, Hirsch EC. Blood vessels change in the mesencephalon of patients with Parkinson's disease. Lancet. 1999;353:981–2.
48. Brochard V, Combadiere B, Prigent A, Laouar Y, Perrin A, Beray-Berthat V, et al. Infiltration of CD4+ lymphocytes into the brain contributes to neurodegeneration in a mouse model of Parkinson disease. J Clin Invest. 2009;119:182–92.
49. Miklossy J, Doudet DD, Schwab C, Yu S, McGeer EG, McGeer PL. Role of ICAM-1 in persisting inflammation in Parkinson disease and MPTP monkeys. Exp Neurol. 2006;197: 275–83.
50. McGeer PL, Itagaki S, Boyes BE, McGeer EG. Reactive microglia are positive for HLA-DR in the substantia nigra of Parkinson's and Alzheimer's disease brains. Neurology. 1988;38: 1285–91.
51. McGeer PL, Itagaki S, McGeer EG. Expression of the histocompatibility glycoprotein HLA-DR in neurological disease. Acta Neuropathol. 1988;76:550–7.
52. Carson MJ, Bilousova TV, Puntambekar SS, Melchior B, Doose JM, Ethell IM. A rose by any other name? The potential consequences of microglial heterogeneity during CNS health and disease. Neurotherapeutics. 2007;4:571–9.
53. Ransohoff RM, Brown MA. Innate immunity in the central nervous system. J Clin Invest. 2012;122:1164–71.
54. Colton CA. Heterogeneity of microglial activation in the innate immune response in the brain. J Neuroimmune Pharmacol. 2009;4:399–418.
55. Croisier E, Moran LB, Dexter DT, Pearce RK, Graeber MB. Microglial inflammation in the Parkinsonian substantia nigra: relationship to alpha-synuclein deposition. J Neuroinflammation. 2005;2:14.

56. Kim SU, de Vellis J. Microglia in health and disease. J Neurosci Res. 2005;81:302–13.
57. Klegeris A, Pelech S, Giasson BI, Maguire J, Zhang H, McGeer EG, et al. Alpha-synuclein activates stress signaling protein kinases in THP-1 cells and microglia. Neurobiol Aging. 2008;29:739–52.
58. Aloisi F. Immune function of microglia. Glia. 2001;36:165–79.
59. Su X, Maguire-Zeiss KA, Giuliano R, Prifti L, Venkatesh K, Federoff HJ. Synuclein activates microglia in a model of Parkinson's disease. Neurobiol Aging. 2008;29:1690–701.
60. Su X, Federoff HJ, Maguire-Zeiss KA. Mutant alpha-synuclein overexpression mediates early proinflammatory activity. Neurotoxicity Res. 2009;16:238–54.
61. Wilms H, Rosenstiel P, Romero-Ramos M, Arlt A, Schäfer H, Seegert D, et al. Suppression of MAP kinases inhibits microglial activation and attenuates neuronal cell death induced by alpha-synuclein protofibrils. Int J Immunopathol Pharmacol. 2009;22:897–909.
62. Lee EJ, Woo MS, Moon PG, Baek MC, Choi IY, Kim WK, et al. Alpha-synuclein activates microglia by inducing the expressions of matrix metalloproteinases and the subsequent activation of protease-activated receptor-1. J Immunol. 2010;185:615–23.
63. Couch Y, Alvarez-Erviti L, Sibson NR, Wood MJ, Anthony DC. The acute inflammatory response to intranigral alpha-synuclein differs significantly from intranigral lipopolysaccharide and is exacerbated by peripheral inflammation. J Neuroinflammation. 2011;8:166.
64. Marin-Teva JL, Cuadros MA, Martin-Oliva D, Navascues J. Microglia and neuronal cell death. Neuron Glia Biol. 2011;7:25–40.
65. Reynolds AD, Stone DK, Hutter JA, Benner EJ, Mosley RL, Gendelman HE. Regulatory T cells attenuate Th17 cell-mediated nigrostriatal dopaminergic neurodegeneration in a model of Parkinson's disease. J Immunol. 2010;184:2261–71.
66. Stellwagen D, Malenka RC. Synaptic scaling mediated by glial TNF-alpha. Nature. 2006; 440:1054–9.
67. Waldburger JM, Masternak K, Muhlethaler-Mottet A, Villard J, Peretti M, Landmann S, et al. Lessons from the bare lymphocyte syndrome: molecular mechanisms regulating MHC class II expression. Immunol Rev. 2000;178:148–65.
68. Luckheeram RV, Zhou R, Verma AD, Xia B. CD4(+)T cells: differentiation and functions. Clin Dev Immunol. 2012;2012:925135.
69. Yamane H, Paul WE. Cytokines of the gamma(c) family control CD4+ T cell differentiation and function. Nat Immunol. 2012;13:1037–44.
70. Marsh SG, System WHONCfFotH. Nomenclature for factors of the HLA system, update December 2012. Tissue Antigens. 2013;81:253–7.
71. Getts MT, Miller SD. 99th Dahlem conference on infection, inflammation and chronic inflammatory disorders: triggering of autoimmune diseases by infections. Clin Exp Immunol. 2010;160:15–21.
72. Imamura K, Hishikawa N, Sawada M, Nagatsu T, Yoshida M, Hashizume Y. Distribution of major histocompatibility complex class II-positive microglia and cytokine profile of Parkinson's disease brains. Acta Neuropathol. 2003;106:518–26.
73. Gerhard A, Pavese N, Hotton G, Turkheimer F, Es M, Hammers A, et al. In vivo imaging of microglial activation with [11C](R)-PK11195 PET in idiopathic Parkinson's disease. Neurobiol Dis. 2006;21:404–12.
74. Ouchi Y, Yoshikawa E, Sekine Y, Futatsubashi M, Kanno T, Ogusu T, et al. Microglial activation and dopamine terminal loss in early Parkinson's disease. Ann Neurol. 2005;57:168–75.
75. Langston JW, Forno LS, Tetrud J, Reeves AG, Kaplan JA, Karluk D. Evidence of active nerve cell degeneration in the substantia nigra of humans years after 1-methyl-4-phenyl-1,2,3,6-tetrahydropyridine exposure. Ann Neurol. 1999;46:598–605.
76. McGeer PL, Schwab C, Parent A, Doudet D. Presence of reactive microglia in monkey substantia nigra years after 1-methyl-4-phenyl-1,2,3,6-tetrahydropyridine administration. Ann Neurol. 2003;54:599–604.
77. Barcia C, Sanchez Bahillo A, Fernandez-Villalba E, Bautista V, Poza YPM, Fernandez-Barreiro A, et al. Evidence of active microglia in substantia nigra pars compacta of Parkinsonian monkeys 1 year after MPTP exposure. Glia. 2004;46:402–9.

78. Vázquez-Claverie M, Garrido-Gil P, San Sebastián W, Izal-Azcárate A, Belzunegui S, Marcilla I, et al. Acute and chronic 1-methyl-4-phenyl-1,2,3,6-tetrahydropyridine administrations elicit similar microglial activation in the substantia nigra of monkeys. J Neuropathol Exp Neurol. 2009;68:977–84.
79. Hamza TH, Zabetian CP, Tenesa A, Laederach A, Montimurro J, Yearout D, et al. Common genetic variation in the HLA region is associated with late-onset sporadic Parkinson's disease. Nat Genet. 2010;42:781–5.
80. Guo Y, Deng X, Zheng W, Xu H, Song Z, Liang H, et al. HLA rs3129882 variant in Chinese Han patients with late-onset sporadic Parkinson disease. Neurosci Lett. 2011;501:185–7.
81. Ahmed I, Tamouza R, Delord M, Krishnamoorthy R, Tzourio C, Mulot C, et al. Association between Parkinson's disease and the HLA-DRB1 locus. Mov Disord. 2012;27:1104–10.
82. Hill-Burns EM, Factor SA, Zabetian CP, Thomson G, Payami H. Evidence for more than one Parkinson's disease-associated variant within the HLA region. PLoS One. 2011;6:e27109.
83. Satake W, Nakabayashi Y, Mizuta I, Hirota Y, Ito C, Kubo M, et al. Genome-wide association study identifies common variants at four loci as genetic risk factors for Parkinson's disease. Nat Genet. 2009;41:1303–7.
84. International Parkinson Disease Genomics C, Nalls MA, Plagnol V, Hernandez DG, Sharma M, Sheerin UM, et al. Imputation of sequence variants for identification of genetic risks for Parkinson's disease: a meta-analysis of genome-wide association studies. Lancet. 2011;377: 641–9.
85. Sun C, Wei L, Luo F, Li Y, Li J, Zhu F, et al. HLA-DRB1 alleles are associated with the susceptibility to sporadic Parkinson's disease in Chinese Han population. PLoS One. 2012;7: e48594.
86. Fiszer U, Mix E, Fredrikson S, Kostulas V, Link H. Parkinson's disease and immunological abnormalities: increase of HLA-DR expression on monocytes in cerebrospinal fluid and of CD45RO+T cells in peripheral blood. Acta Neurol Scand. 1994;90:160–6.
87. Botta-Orfila T, Sanchez-Pla A, Fernandez M, Carmona F, Ezquerra M, Tolosa E. Brain transcriptomic profiling in idiopathic and LRRK2-associated Parkinson's disease. Brain Res. 2012;1466:152–7.
88. Wissemann WT, Hill-Burns EM, Zabetian CP, Factor SA, Patsopoulos N, Hoglund B, et al. Association of Parkinson's disease with structural and regulatory variants in the HLA region. Am J Hum Genet. 2013;93(5):984–93.
89. Bialecka M, Kurzawski M, Klodowska-Duda G, Opala G, Juzwiak S, Kurzawski G, et al. CARD15 variants in patients with sporadic Parkinson's disease. Neurosci Res. 2007;57: 473–6.
90. Dobbs SM, Dobbs RJ, Weller C, Charlett A. Link between Helicobacter pylori infection and idiopathic parkinsonism. Med Hypotheses. 2000;55:93–8.
91. Woulfe J, Hoogendoorn H, Tarnopolsky M, Muñoz DG. Monoclonal antibodies against Epstein-Barr virus cross-react with alpha-synuclein in human brain. Neurology. 2000;55: 1398–401.
92. Shoji H, Watanabe M, Itoh S, Kuwahara H, Hattori F. Japanese encephalitis and parkinsonism. J Neurol. 1993;240:59–60.
93. Ogata A, Tashiro K, Nukuzuma S, Nagashima K, Hall WW. A rat model of Parkinson's disease induced by Japanese encephalitis virus. J Neurovirol. 1997;3:141–7.
94. Jang H, Boltz D, Sturm-Ramirez K, Shepherd KR, Jiao Y, Webster R, et al. Highly pathogenic H5N1 influenza virus can enter the central nervous system and induce neuroinflammation and neurodegeneration. Proc Natl Acad Sci U S A. 2009;106:14063–8.
95. Jang H, Boltz D, McClaren J, Pani AK, Smeyne M, Korff A, et al. Inflammatory effects of highly pathogenic H5N1 influenza virus infection in the CNS of mice. J Neurosci. 2012; 32:1545–59.
96. Cose S, Brammer C, Khanna KM, Masopust D, Lefrancois L. Evidence that a significant number of naive T cells enter non-lymphoid organs as part of a normal migratory pathway. Eur J Immunol. 2006;36:1423–33.

97. van der Most RG, Murali-Krishna K, Ahmed R. Prolonged presence of effector-memory CD8 T cells in the central nervous system after dengue virus encephalitis. Int Immunol. 2003;15:119–25.
98. Thomas HE, Trapani JA, Kay TW. The role of perforin and granzymes in diabetes. Cell Death Differ. 2010;17:577–85.
99. Joffre OP, Segura E, Savina A, Amigorena S. Cross-presentation by dendritic cells. Nat Rev Immunol. 2012;12:557–69.
100. Stevens CH, Rowe D, Morel-Kopp MC, Orr C, Russell T, Ranola M, et al. Reduced T helper and B lymphocytes in Parkinson's disease. J Neuroimmunol. 2012;252:95–9.
101. Bas J, Calopa M, Mestre M, Mollevi DG, Cutillas B, Ambrosio S, et al. Lymphocyte populations in Parkinson's disease and in rat models of parkinsonism. J Neuroimmunol. 2001; 113:146–52.
102. Amsen D, Backer RA, Helbig C. Decisions on the road to memory. Adv Exp Med Biol. 2013;7851:107–20.
103. Baba Y, Kuroiwa A, Uitti RJ, Wszolek ZK, Yamada T. Alterations of T-lymphocyte populations in Parkinson disease. Parkinsonism Relat Disord. 2005;11:493–8.
104. Saunders JA, Estes KA, Kosloski LM, Allen HE, Dempsey KM, Torres-Russotto DR, et al. CD4+ regulatory and effector/memory T cell subsets profile motor dysfunction in Parkinson's disease. J Neuroimmune Pharmacol. 2012;7:927–38.
105. Calopa M, Bas J, Callen A, Mestre M. Apoptosis of peripheral blood lymphocytes in Parkinson patients. Neurobiol Dis. 2010;38:1–7.
106. Niwa F, Kuriyama N, Nakagawa M, Imanishi J. Effects of peripheral lymphocyte subpopulations and the clinical correlation with Parkinson's disease. Geriatr Gerontol Int. 2012; 12:102–7.
107. Lehtimaki S, Lahesmaa R. Regulatory T cells control immune responses through their non-redundant tissue specific features. Front Immunol. 2013;4:294.
108. Fiszer U, Fredrikson S, Mix E, Olsson T, Link H. V region T cell receptor repertoire in Parkinson's disease. Acta Neurol Scand. 1996;93:25–9.
109. Alberio T, Pippione AC, Zibetti M, Olgiati S, Cecconi D, Comi C, et al. Discovery and verification of panels of T-lymphocyte proteins as biomarkers of Parkinson's disease. Sci Rep. 2012;2:953.
110. Migliore L, Petrozzi L, Lucetti C, Gambaccini G, Bernardini S, Scarpato R, et al. Oxidative damage and cytogenetic analysis in leukocytes of Parkinson's disease patients. Neurology. 2002;58:1809–15.
111. Cornetta T, Palma S, Aprile I, Padua L, Tonali P, Testa A, et al. Levodopa therapy reduces DNA damage in peripheral blood cells of patients with Parkinson's disease. Cell Biol Toxicol. 2009;25:321–30.
112. Blandini F, Mangiagalli A, Cosentino M, Marino F, Samuele A, Rasini E, et al. Peripheral markers of apoptosis in Parkinson's disease: the effect of dopaminergic drugs. Ann N Y Acad Sci. 2003;1010:675–8.
113. Kurkowska-Jastrzebska I, Wronska A, Kohutnicka M, Czlonkowski A, Czlonkowska A. The inflammatory reaction following 1-methyl-4-phenyl-1,2,3, 6-tetrahydropyridine intoxication in mouse. Exp Neurol. 1999;156:50–61.
114. Lira A, Kulczycki J, Slack R, Anisman H, Park DS. Involvement of the Fc gamma receptor in a chronic N-methyl-4-phenyl-1,2,3,6-tetrahydropyridine mouse model of dopaminergic loss. J Biol Chem. 2011;286:28783–93.
115. Fleisher TA, Oliveira JB. Monogenic defects in lymphocyte apoptosis. Curr Opin Allergy Clin Immunol. 2012;12:609–15.
116. Choi C, Benveniste EN. Fas ligand/Fas system in the brain: regulator of immune and apoptotic responses. Brain Res Rev. 2004;44:65–81.
117. Benner EJ, Banerjee R, Reynolds AD, Sherman S, Pisarev VM, Tsiperson V, et al. Nitrated alpha-synuclein immunity accelerates degeneration of nigral dopaminergic neurons. PLoS One. 2008;3:e1376.

118. Shlomchik MJ, Weisel F. Germinal center selection and the development of memory B and plasma cells. Immunol Rev. 2012;247:52–63.
119. Besong-Agbo D, Wolf E, Jessen F, Oechsner M, Hametner E, Poewe W, et al. Naturally occurring α-synuclein autoantibody levels are lower in patients with Parkinson disease. Neurology. 2013;80:169–75.
120. Han M, Nagele E, DeMarshall C, Acharya N, Nagele R. Diagnosis of Parkinson's disease based on disease-specific autoantibody profiles in human sera. PLoS One. 2012;7:e32383.
121. Souto-Carneiro MM, Mahadevan V, Takada K, Fritsch-Stork R, Nanki T, Brown M, et al. Alterations in peripheral blood memory B cells in patients with active rheumatoid arthritis are dependent on the action of tumour necrosis factor. Arthritis Res Ther. 2009;11:R84.
122. Hansen A, Odendahl M, Reiter K, Jacobi AM, Feist E, Scholze J, et al. Diminished peripheral blood memory B cells and accumulation of memory B cells in the salivary glands of patients with Sjogren's syndrome. Arthritis Rheum. 2002;46:2160–71.
123. Fekete A, Soos L, Szekanecz Z, Szabo Z, Szodoray P, Barath S, et al. Disturbances in B- and T-cell homeostasis in rheumatoid arthritis: suggested relationships with antigen-driven immune responses. J Autoimmun. 2007;29:154–63.
124. Carvey PM, McRae A, Lint TF, Ptak LR, Lo ES, Goetz CG, et al. The potential use of a dopamine neuron antibody and a striatal-derived neurotrophic factor as diagnostic markers in Parkinson's disease. Neurology. 1991;41(5 Suppl 2):53–8.
125. Papachroni KK, Ninkina N, Papapanagiotou A, Hadjigeorgiou GM, Xiromerisiou G, Papadimitriou A, et al. Autoantibodies to alpha-synuclein in inherited Parkinson's disease. J Neurochem. 2007;101:749–56.
126. Orr CF, Rowe DB, Mizuno Y, Mori H, Halliday GM. A possible role for humoral immunity in the pathogenesis of Parkinson's disease. Brain. 2005;128:2665–74.
127. Chen S, Le WD, Xie WJ, Alexianu ME, Engelhardt JI, Siklos L, et al. Experimental destruction of substantia nigra initiated by Parkinson disease immunoglobulins. Arch Neurol. 1998; 55(8):1075–80.
128. He Y, Le W-D, Appel SH. Role of Fcγ receptors in nigral cell injury induced by Parkinson disease immunoglobulin injection into mouse substantia nigra. Exp Neurol. 2002;176: 322–7.
129. Cao S, Theodore S, Standaert DG. Fcgamma receptors are required for NF-kappaB signaling, microglial activation and dopaminergic neurodegeneration in an AAV-synuclein mouse model of Parkinson's disease. Mol Neurodegener. 2010;5:42.
130. Bae EJ, Lee HJ, Rockenstein E, Ho DH, Park EB, Yang NY, et al. Antibody-aided clearance of extracellular alpha-synuclein prevents cell-to-cell aggregate transmission. J Neurosci. 2012;32:13454–69.
131. Trinh J, Farrer M. Advances in the genetics of Parkinson disease. Nat Rev Neurol. 2013; 9:445–54.
132. Singleton AB, Farrer MJ, Bonifati V. The genetics of Parkinson's disease: progress and therapeutic implications. Mov Disord. 2013;28:14–23.
133. Lesage S, Brice A. Parkinson's disease: from monogenic forms to genetic susceptibility factors. Hum Mol Genet. 2009;18(R1):R48–59.
134. Ross OA. A prognostic view on the application of individualized genomics in Parkinson's disease. Curr Genet Med Rep. 2013;1:52–7.
135. Houlden H, Singleton AB. The genetics and neuropathology of Parkinson's disease. Acta Neuropathol. 2012;124:325–38.
136. Shin EC, Cho SE, Lee DK, Hur MW, Paik SR, Park JH, et al. Expression patterns of alpha-synuclein in human hematopoietic cells and in Drosophila at different developmental stages. Mol Cells. 2000;10:65–70.
137. Su AI, Wiltshire T, Batalov S, Lapp H, Ching KA, Block D, et al. A gene atlas of the mouse and human protein-encoding transcriptomes. Proc Natl Acad Sci U S A. 2004;101:6062–7.
138. Wu C, Orozco C, Boyer J, Leglise M, Goodale J, Batalov S, et al. BioGPS: an extensible and customizable portal for querying and organizing gene annotation resources. Genome Biol. 2009;10:R130.

139. Austin SA, Floden AM, Murphy EJ, Combs CK. Alpha-synuclein expression modulates microglial activation phenotype. J Neurosci. 2006;26:10558–63.
140. Austin SA, Rojanathammanee L, Golovko MY, Murphy EJ, Combs CK. Lack of alpha-synuclein modulates microglial phenotype in vitro. Neurochem Res. 2011;36:994–1004.
141. Tanji K, Mori F, Imaizumi T, Yoshida H, Matsumiya T, Tamo W, et al. Upregulation of alpha-synuclein by lipopolysaccharide and interleukin-1 in human macrophages. Pathol Int. 2002;52:572–7.
142. Lu JV, Walsh CM. Programmed necrosis and autophagy in immune function. Immunol Rev. 2012;249:205–17.
143. Alessandri C, Barbati C, Vacirca D, Piscopo P, Confaloni A, Sanchez M, et al. T lymphocytes from patients with systemic lupus erythematosus are resistant to induction of autophagy. FASEB J. 2012;26:4722–32.
144. Zimprich A, Biskup S, Leitner P, Lichtner P, Farrer M, Lincoln S, et al. Mutations in LRRK2 cause autosomal-dominant parkinsonism with pleomorphic pathology. Neuron. 2004;44:601–7.
145. Latourelle JC, Sun M, Lew MF, Suchowersky O, Klein C, Golbe LI, et al. The Gly2019Ser mutation in LRRK2 is not fully penetrant in familial Parkinson's disease: the GenePD study. BMC Med. 2008;6:32.
146. Goldwurm S, Zini M, Mariani L, Tesei S, Miceli R, Sironi F, et al. Evaluation of LRRK2 G2019S penetrance: relevance for genetic counseling in Parkinson disease. Neurology. 2007;68(14):1141–3.
147. Simon-Sanchez J, Schulte C, Bras JM, Sharma M, Gibbs JR, Berg D, et al. Genome-wide association study reveals genetic risk underlying Parkinson's disease. Nat Genet. 2009;41:1308–12.
148. Melrose H, Lincoln S, Tyndall G, Dickson D, Farrer M. Anatomical localization of leucine-rich repeat kinase 2 in mouse brain. Neuroscience. 2006;139:791–4.
149. Taymans JM, Van den Haute C, Baekelandt V. Distribution of PINK1 and LRRK2 in rat and mouse brain. J Neurochem. 2006;98:951–61.
150. Westerlund M, Belin AC, Anvret A, Bickford P, Olson L, Galter D. Developmental regulation of leucine-rich repeat kinase 1 and 2 expression in the brain and other rodent and human organs: implications for Parkinson's disease. Neuroscience. 2008;152:429–36.
151. Galter D, Westerlund M, Carmine A, Lindqvist E, Sydow O, Olson L. LRRK2 expression linked to dopamine-innervated areas. Ann Neurol. 2006;59:714–9.
152. Liu Z, Lee J, Krummey S, Lu W, Cai H, Lenardo MJ. The kinase LRRK2 is a regulator of the transcription factor NFAT that modulates the severity of inflammatory bowel disease. Nat Immunol. 2011;12:1063–70.
153. West AB, Moore DJ, Biskup S, Bugayenko A, Smith WW, Ross CA, et al. Parkinson's disease-associated mutations in leucine-rich repeat kinase 2 augment kinase activity. Proc Natl Acad Sci U S A. 2005;102:16842–7.
154. West AB, Moore DJ, Choi C, Andrabi SA, Li X, Dikeman D, et al. Parkinson's disease-associated mutations in LRRK2 link enhanced GTP-binding and kinase activities to neuronal toxicity. Human Molecular Genet. 2007;16:223–32.
155. Greggio E, Jain S, Kingsbury A, Bandopadhyay R, Lewis P, Kaganovich A, et al. Kinase activity is required for the toxic effects of mutant LRRK2/dardarin. Neurobiol Dis. 2006;23:329–41.
156. Smith WW, Pei Z, Jiang H, Dawson VL, Dawson TM, Ross CA. Kinase activity of mutant LRRK2 mediates neuronal toxicity. Nat Neurosci. 2006;9:1231–3.
157. Lee BD, Shin JH, VanKampen J, Petrucelli L, West AB, Ko HS, et al. Inhibitors of leucine-rich repeat kinase-2 protect against models of Parkinson's disease. Nat Med. 2010;16:998–1000.
158. Li X, Patel JC, Wang J, Avshalumov MV, Nicholson C, Buxbaum JD, et al. Enhanced striatal dopamine transmission and motor performance with LRRK2 overexpression in mice is eliminated by familial Parkinson's disease mutation G2019S. J Neurosci. 2010;30:1788–97.

159. Lin X, Parisiadou L, Gu XL, Wang L, Shim H, Sun L, et al. Leucine-rich repeat kinase 2 regulates the progression of neuropathology induced by Parkinson's-disease-related mutant alpha-synuclein. Neuron. 2009;64:807–27.
160. Li Y, Liu W, Oo TF, Wang L, Tang Y, Jackson-Lewis V, et al. Mutant LRRK2(R1441G) BAC transgenic mice recapitulate cardinal features of Parkinson's disease. Nat Neurosci. 2009; 12:826–8.
161. Wang L, Xie C, Greggio E, Parisiadou L, Shim H, Sun L, et al. The chaperone activity of heat shock protein 90 is critical for maintaining the stability of leucine-rich repeat kinase 2. J Neurosci. 2008;28:3384–91.
162. Hakimi M, Selvanantham T, Swinton E, Padmore RF, Tong Y, Kabbach G, et al. Parkinson's disease-linked LRRK2 is expressed in circulating and tissue immune cells and upregulated following recognition of microbial structures. J Neural Transm. 2011;118:795–808.
163. Miklossy J, Arai T, Guo JP, Klegeris A, Yu S, McGeer EG, et al. LRRK2 expression in normal and pathologic human brain and in human cell lines. J Neuropathol Exp Neurol. 2006; 65:953–63.
164. Gardet A, Benita Y, Li C, Sands BE, Ballester I, Stevens C, et al. LRRK2 is involved in the IFN-gamma response and host response to pathogens. J Immunol. 2010;185:5577–85.
165. Moehle MS, Webber PJ, Tse T, Sukar N, Standaert DG, DeSilva TM, et al. LRRK2 inhibition attenuates microglial inflammatory responses. J Neurosci. 2012;32:1602–11.
166. Barrett JC, Hansoul S, Nicolae DL, Cho JH, Duerr RH, Rioux JD, et al. Genome-wide association defines more than 30 distinct susceptibility loci for Crohn's disease. Nat Genet. 2008;40:955–62.
167. Zhang FR, Huang W, Chen SM, Sun LD, Liu H, Li Y, et al. Genomewide association study of leprosy. N Engl J Med. 2009;361:2609–18.
168. Bonifati V. Autosomal recessive parkinsonism. Parkinsonism Relat Disord. 2012;18:S4–6.
169. Walden H, Martinez-Torres RJ. Regulation of Parkin E3 ubiquitin ligase activity. CMLS. 2012;69:3053–67.
170. Narendra D, Tanaka A, Suen DF, Youle RJ. Parkin is recruited selectively to impaired mitochondria and promotes their autophagy. J Cell Biol. 2008;183:795–803.
171. Shimura H, Hattori N, Kubo S, Mizuno Y, Asakawa S, Minoshima S, et al. Familial Parkinson disease gene product, parkin, is a ubiquitin-protein ligase. Nat Genet. 2000;25:302–5.
172. Vincow ES, Merrihew G, Thomas RE, Shulman NJ, Beyer RP, MacCoss MJ, et al. The PINK1-Parkin pathway promotes both mitophagy and selective respiratory chain turnover in vivo. Proc Natl Acad Sci U S A. 2013;110:6400–5.
173. Alves da Costa C, Checler F. Parkin: much more than a simple ubiquitin ligase. Neurodgener Dis. 2012;10:9–51.
174. Goldberg MS, Fleming SM, Palacino JJ, Cepeda C, Lam HA, Bhatnagar A, et al. Parkin-deficient mice exhibit nigrostriatal deficits but not loss of dopaminergic neurons. J Biol Chem. 2003;278:43628–35.
175. Zhu XR, Maskri L, Herold C, Bader V, Stichel CC, Gunturkun O, et al. Non-motor behavioural impairments in parkin-deficient mice. Eur J Neurosci. 2007;26:1902–11.
176. Frank-Cannon TC, Tran T, Ruhn KA, Martinez TN, Hong J, Marvin M, et al. Parkin deficiency increases vulnerability to inflammation-related nigral degeneration. J Neurosci. 2008;28:10825–34.
177. Tran TA, Nguyen AD, Chang J, Goldberg MS, Lee JK, Tansey MG. Lipopolysaccharide and tumor necrosis factor regulate Parkin expression via nuclear factor-kappa B. PLoS One. 2011;6:e23660.
178. Ali S, Vollaard AM, Widjaja S, Surjadi C, van de Vosse E, van Dissel JT. PARK2/PACRG polymorphisms and susceptibility to typhoid and paratyphoid fever. Clin Exp Immunol. 2006;144:425–31.
179. Mira MT, Alcais A, Nguyen VT, Moraes MO, Di Flumeri C, Vu HT, et al. Susceptibility to leprosy is associated with PARK2 and PACRG. Nature. 2004;427:636–40.
180. Manzanillo PS, Ayres JS, Watson RO, Collins AC, Souza G, Rae CS, et al. The ubiquitin ligase parkin mediates resistance to intracellular pathogens. Nature. 2013;501:512–6.

181. Johnston J, So TY. First-line disease-modifying therapies in paediatric multiple sclerosis: a comprehensive overview. Drugs. 2012;72:1195–211.
182. Boska MD, Lewis TB, Destache CJ, Benner EJ, Nelson JA, Uberti M, et al. Quantitative 1H magnetic resonance spectroscopic imaging determines therapeutic immunization efficacy in an animal model of Parkinson's disease. J Neurosci. 2005;25:1691–700.
183. Benner EJ, Mosley RL, Destache CJ, Lewis TB, Jackson-Lewis V, Gorantla S, et al. Therapeutic immunization protects dopaminergic neurons in a mouse model of Parkinson's disease. Proc Natl Acad Sci U S A. 2004;101:9435–40.
184. Steed PM, Tansey MG, Zalevsky J, Zhukovsky EA, Desjarlais JR, Szymkowski DE, et al. Inactivation of TNF signaling by rationally designed dominant-negative TNF variants. Science. 2003;301:1895–8.
185. McCoy MK, Martinez TN, Ruhn KA, Szymkowski DE, Smith CG, Botterman BR, et al. Blocking soluble tumor necrosis factor signaling with dominant-negative tumor necrosis factor inhibitor attenuates loss of dopaminergic neurons in models of Parkinson's disease. J Neurosci. 2006;26:9365–75.
186. McCoy MK, Ruhn KA, Martinez TN, McAlpine FE, Blesch A, Tansey MG. Intranigral lentiviral delivery of dominant-negative TNF attenuates neurodegeneration and behavioral deficits in hemiparkinsonian rats. Mol Ther. 2008;16:1572–9.
187. Harms AS, Barnum CJ, Ruhn KA, Varghese S, Trevino I, Blesch A, et al. Delayed dominant-negative TNF gene therapy halts progressive loss of nigral dopaminergic neurons in a rat model of Parkinson's disease. Mol Ther. 2011;19:46–52.
188. Masliah E, Rockenstein E, Adame A, Alford M, Crews L, Hashimoto M, et al. Effects of alpha-synuclein immunization in a mouse model of Parkinson's disease. Neuron. 2005;46: 857–68.
189. Masliah E, Rockenstein E, Mante M, Crews L, Spencer B, Adame A, et al. Passive immunization reduces behavioral and neuropathological deficits in an alpha-synuclein transgenic model of Lewy body disease. PLoS One. 2011;6:e19338.
190. Greenamyre JT, Cannon JR, Drolet R, Mastroberardino PG. Lessons from the rotenone model of Parkinson's disease. Trends Pharmacol Sci. 2010;31:141–2. author reply 2–3.
191. Salama M, Ellaithy A, Helmy B, El-Gamal M, Tantawy D, Mohamed M, et al. Colchicine protects dopaminergic neurons in a rat model of Parkinson's disease. CNS Neurol Disord Drug Targets. 2012;11:836–43.
192. Yao S, Zhu Y, Chen L. Advances in targeting cell surface signalling molecules for immune modulation. Nat Rev Drug Discov. 2013;12(2):130–46.
193. Larsen CP, Grinyó J, Medina-Pestana J, Vanrenterghem Y, Vincenti F, Breshahan B, et al. Belatacept-based regimens versus a cyclosporine A-based regimen in kidney transplant recipients: 2-year results from the BENEFIT and BENEFIT-EXT studies. Transplantation. 2010;90:1528–35.
194. Schiff M. Subcutaneous abatacept for the treatment of rheumatoid arthritis. Rheumatology. 2013;52:986–97.
195. Rudick R, Polman C, Clifford D, Miller D, Steinman L. Natalizumab: bench to bedside and beyond. JAMA Neurol. 2013;70:172–82.
196. Park TS, Rosenberg SA, Morgan RA. Treating cancer with genetically engineered T cells. Trends Biotechnol. 2011;29:550–7.
197. Furtado J, Isenberg DA. B cell elimination in systemic lupus erythematosus. Clin Immunol. 2013;146:90–103.
198. Schwab I, Nimmerjahn F. Intravenous immunoglobulin therapy: how does IgG modulate the immune system? Nature Rev Immunol. 2013;13:176–89.

"Good" and "Bad" Microglia in Parkinson's Disease: An Understanding of Homeostatic Mechanisms in Immunomodulation

Yu Tang and Weidong Le

Parkinson's Disease and Neuroinflammation

Parkinson's disease (PD) is the second most common neurodegenerative disease, manifesting with motor and non-motor symptoms, and the incidence increases markedly with age [1]. It is pathologically characterized by the intracellular inclusions containing α-synuclein called Lewy bodies (LBs) and the progressive loss of dopaminergic (DA) neurons in the substantia nigra (SN) of the midbrain [2]. It is now widely accepted that PD pathogenesis is driven by combined genetic and environmental factors. As the vast majority of PD cases are sporadic (>95 %), environmental factors that interact with common susceptibility genes are most likely to influence the onset of most cases of sporadic PD.

PD is also a chronic inflammation disease, with extensive neuroinflammation and "reactive microgliosis" defined by the microglial response secondary to direct neuronal lesions [3, 4]. The involvement of neuroinflammation in DA neuronal death in PD can be briefly accounted for by the following evidence: (1) prominent reactive microgliosis in the SN of patients and animal models of PD is revealed in postmortem and imaging analysis; (2) DNA polymorphisms in

Y. Tang, Ph.D.
Institute of Health Sciences, Shanghai Institutes for Biological Sciences, Chinese Academy of Sciences, Shanghai, China

W. Le, M.D., Ph.D. (✉)
Institute of Health Sciences, Shanghai Institutes for Biological Sciences, Chinese Academy of Sciences, Shanghai, China

The First Affiliated Hospital of Dalian Medical University, Translational Research Institutes of Medicine, Dalian, China
e-mail: wdle@sibs.ac.cn

M. Thomas (ed.), *Inflammation in Parkinson's Disease: Scientific and Clinical Aspects*,
DOI 10.1007/978-3-319-08046-8_4,

several inflammatory cytokines are studied as risk factors for PD, whereas deficiency of pro-inflammatory factors can produce protective effects; (3) experimental evidence shows that the suppression of inflammatory processes mitigates neuronal impairment in both in vitro and in vivo models; (4) long-term use of non-steroidal anti-inflammatory drugs (NSAIDs) in PD manifests a possible beneficial effect [5]. Although neuroinflammation may not typically represent an initiating factor, current scientific evidence demonstrates that sustained inflammatory responses involving microglia and astrocytes definitely contribute to progression of PD.

Microglia Involvement in PD Pathogenesis

The main executors of neuroinflammation, microglia, are the resident innate immune cells in the central nervous system (CNS), providing the first line of defense of the innate immune system whenever injury or disease occurs [6]. Microglia density varies in brain regions of both adult human and mice, with the highest concentrations being found in the hippocampus, olfactory telencephalon, basal ganglia, and SN [7, 8]. Thus, DA neurons in the SN might be particularly vulnerable to inflammatory insults compared with other regions, owing to the co-localization with a large increased number of microglia in the SN [7, 9].

In the early stage of PD, positron emission tomography (PET) imaging shows an increase of microglial activation, and the level of activation is inversely correlated with density of DA terminals, whereas it positively correlates with motor impairment [10]. Postmortem analysis of PD patients also reveals activated microglia presenting upregulated surface molecules and increased accumulation of inflammatory mediators in the SN [11, 12]. In addition, increased levels of cytokines in the cerebrospinal fluid (CSF) in PD have also been reported [4].

"Good" Microglia and "Bad" Microglia

Although microglial activation has been described extensively in PD, its impact on disease pathogenesis remains controversial. Until recent years, neuroinflammation was thought to be a double-edged sword. For a long time, we considered microglial activation as a monophasic process that contributes to neuronal death. Microglia rapidly sense a wide range of stimuli and produce a series of pro-inflammatory cytokines, numerous toxins, including reactive oxygen species (ROS), free radicals, proteases, and chemokines to destroy infectious organisms and infected neurons [13]. These inflammatory mediators together with the neuron debris, in turn, induce more widespread damage to neighboring neurons (reactive microgliosis).

Consequently, a vicious cycle between injured neurons and uncontrolled inflammation inevitably occurs [13] (Fig. 1).

In 2005, Heppner et al. [14] generated CD11b-HSVTK transgenic mice, in which microglial release of nitrite, pro-inflammatory cytokines, and chemokines was specifically abolished. Interestingly, this "microglial paralysis" was able to repress the development of experimental autoimmune encephalomyelitis (EAE), a mouse model of multiple sclerosis (MS), and repress EAE-associated inflammatory infiltrates [14]. This finding suggests that microglial activation might be detrimental to development of MS, and this also provides insights into the therapy of other immune-mediated CNS diseases, including PD, by targeting microglia.

It is important to understand the complexity of microglial activation in the healthy brain. Under physiological conditions, microglia exhibit a quiescent phenotype surveying the microenvironment and secrete anti-inflammatory and neurotrophic factors that are seemingly not toxic, but protective [15]. The primary objective of microglial activation is to engulf invading viruses, bacteria, or other foreign materials and promote clearance of toxic proteins and cell debris in the injury site through phagocytosis [5, 16, 17]. However, pro-inflammatory cytokines released upon microglial activation are also reported to inhibit microglial phagocytosis that can be relieved by co-incubation with anti-inflammatory cytokines or cyclooxygenase (COX) inhibitors, suggesting that microglia in different states of activation behave differently while removing pathogens or dead cells [18].

In addition to eliminating harmful stimuli, inflammation is also critical for repairing damaged tissue. Glial-derived neurotrophic factor (GDNF) has been reported to promote neuronal survival and rescue injured DA neurons [19, 20]. Microglia also secrete multiple anti-inflammatory cytokines and promote gene expression related to tissue recovery and regeneration. Moreover, microglia facilitate repair by directing the migration of stem cells to the site of inflammation and injury and instruct neurogenesis in the neurogenic niches in various areas [21, 22]. Therefore, without neuroinflammation, removal of offending pathogens and recovery from CNS injuries become impossible.

Regulatory Mechanisms of "Good" and "Bad" Microglia

Microglia exist in two differentiated states: "bad," or neurotoxic, microglia and "good," or neurorestorative, microglia. These two yin and yang states are interchangeable depending on the milieu of the affected region. "Bad" microglia are not bad as described, which is also necessary and crucial for host defense. Both "good" and "bad" microglia are required for keeping the homeostasis of the CNS.

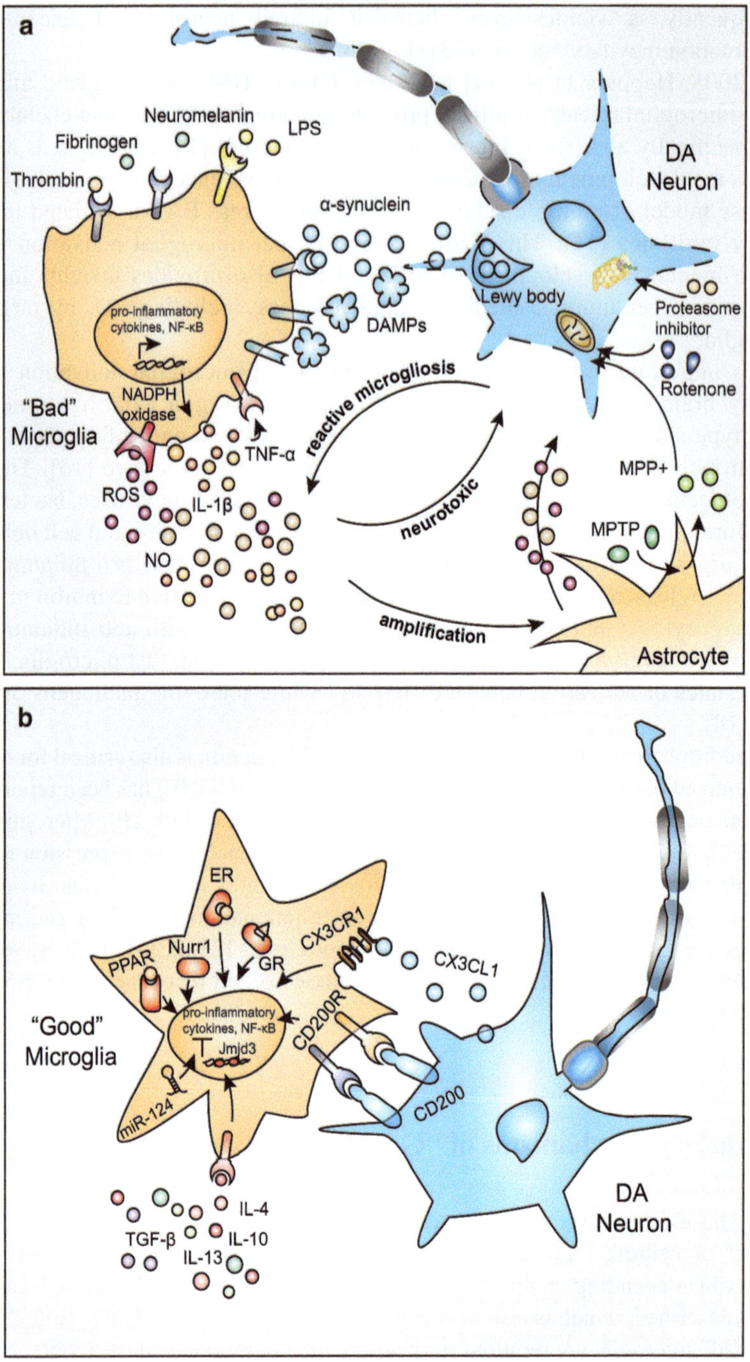

Fig. 1 Illustration of involvement of "bad" microglia and "good" microglia in PD. (**a**) Illustration of the vicious cycle between "bad" microglia and neurons. Microglia can rapidly sense a wide range of stimuli including released endogenous proteins such as α-synuclein, damaged cell debris,

Inducers and Effectors of "Bad" Microglia

Inducers of "Bad" Microglia

Activation of "bad" microglia produces a variety of pro-inflammatory factors, chemokines, and cytokines. There are different outcomes in microglia corresponding to different inducers. Briefly, these inducers are involved in aggregation of proteins such as α-synuclein [23, 24], matrix metalloproteinase-3 (MMP-3) [25], neuromelanin [26, 27], substance P [28], fibrinogen [29], thrombin [30], and various pro-inflammatory cytokines, as well as a variety of environmental cues (Table 1).

α-Synuclein Aggregates

α-Synuclein as a pathological gene alters neuropathological behaviors in sporadic PD and in most forms of familial PD, and it is initially thought to function mostly as an intracellular component. It is interesting to find out that the release of aggregated α-synuclein (the major component of LBs) from neurons into the extracellular space can induce microglial activation [23, 24]. α-Synuclein, when it is nitratized and oxidized, is more prone to induce microglial activation [31, 32]. Extracellular α-synuclein aggregates are sensed and internalized by microglia, followed by activation of nicotinamide adenine dinucleotide phosphate (NADPH) oxidase, production of ROS, and release of pro-inflammatory cytokines [23].

Interestingly, Rojanathammanee et al. [33] have found that overexpression of mutant α-synuclein solely in microglia was able to change microglia into a form of

Fig. 1 (continued) and cytosolic components (DAMPs, etc.) and a variety of environmental cues. All these pathways eventually converge into the common effectors including NADPH oxidase, ROS, superoxide, and multiple pro-inflammatory cytokines that are neurotoxic to neurons. The inflammatory mediators together with the neuron debris, in turn, induce more widespread damage to neighboring neurons (reactive microgliosis). Those inducers of microglia are deleterious through direct stimulation of microglia (e.g., α-synuclein, DAMPs, LPS, etc.) or indirectly revoke reactive microgliosis after neuronal lesions (e.g., MPTP, rotenone, etc.). Additionally, secreted inflammatory mediators can also act on astrocytes to induce secondary inflammatory responses and amply neurotoxic effects. Consequently, a vicious cycle between injured neurons and uncontrolled inflammation inevitably occurs. (**b**) Illustration of mechanisms or pathways in "good" microglia. The mechanisms employed by "good" microglia are mainly involving (1) transrepression pathways through multiple receptors such as GRs, ERs, Nurr1, and PPARs; (2) anti-inflammatory cytokines (IL-4, IL-10, IL-13, TGF-β); (3) neuron-microglia cross-talk (CX3CL1–CX3CR1 and CD200–CD200R pairing); (4) microRNAs (e.g., miR-124); and (5) epigenetic modifications (e.g., Jmjd3). All those mechanisms render "good" microglia immunosuppressive or quiescent by repressing pro-inflammatory cytokines, NF-κB, and related genes, whereas enhancing the expression of repair genes, trophic genes, and anti-inflammatory genes. The general effects of "good" microglia are neuroprotective, immunosuppressive, promoting tissue rebuilding, and possibly neurogenesis

Table 1 Inducers and effectors of "bad" microglia

Major inducers and effectors	Direct or indirect on microglial activation	Major references
Proteins		
α-Synuclein	Direct	[23, 24, 31–33]
Neuromelanin	Direct	[26, 27]
MMP-3	Direct	[25]
Substance P	Direct	[28]
Fibrinogen	Direct	[29]
Thrombin	Direct	[30]
Environmental toxins		
LPS	Direct	[34, 35, 60–64]
MPTP	Indirect	[43–55, 65]
Rotenone	Indirect	[38, 39]
Paraquat	Direct	[40–42]
Pesticides	Indirect	[36, 37]
Proteasome inhibitors	Indirect	[56, 57]
Heavy metals	Indirect	[58, 59]
Effectors		
NADPH oxidase	–	[23, 28, 38, 40, 43, 44, 68–70]
ROS and superoxide	–	[13, 23, 25, 27, 31, 43, 44]
Pro-inflammatory cytokines	Direct	[12, 50–53, 67–75]

reactive phenotype characterized by elevated levels of pro-inflammatory cytokines including tumor necrosis factor-α (TNF-α) and interleukin-6 (IL-6), as well as increased nitric oxide (NO) production and reactive nitrogen species (RNS) secretion. Their study shows that microglial activation in transgenic mice with *α-synuclein* mutation does not cause neurodegeneration. Of note, other components in LBs or cytosol proteins and membrane breakdown products released from dying neurons also have the potential to trigger microglial activation [5].

Environmental Factors

Apart from genetic factors, environmental factors are strongly implicated in PD development. The cumulative influence of environmental exposures on microglial activation has been reported. Among those, lipopolysaccharide (LPS) [34, 35], pesticides [36, 37], rotenone [38, 39], paraquat [40–42], 1-methyl-4-phenyl-1,2,3,6-tetrahydropyridine (MPTP) [43–55], proteasome inhibitors [56, 57], and heavy metals [58, 59] have been implicated in PD progression. Generally, the environment is implicated as a source for compounds that are both deleterious through direct stimulation of microglia (e.g., LPS, etc.) or indirectly revoke reactive microgliosis after neuronal lesions (e.g., MPTP, rotenone, etc.) (see Table 1).

LPS

Bacterial LPS, the polysaccharide component of the cell walls of gram-negative bacteria, is used to model microglia-induced loss of DA neurons in rodents. Various studies have demonstrated that LPS is neurotoxic to neurons only in the presence of microglia and inhibition of microglial activation has been shown to be neuroprotective [60–62]. Embryonic exposure to LPS leads to long-term microglial activation persistent into adulthood and progressive neuron loss [34, 63]. After chronic infusion into the SN, or a single systemic injection, LPS is capable of triggering a chronic inflammatory process and induces a delayed, progressive degeneration of DA neurons in rodents [35, 64]. Moreover, LPS-induced inflammation can also synergize with mutations in *α-synuclein* and *Parkin* that are associated with familial PD to potentiate the loss of DA neurons in animal models [32].

MPTP

Although not directly sensed by microglia, neurotoxin widely used in PD animal models, MPTP is known to induce neuronal degeneration that provokes reactive microgliosis, which exacerbates neurotoxicity. MPTP is metabolized to 1-methyl-4-phenylpyridinium (MPP^+) by glial cells, which is then taken up by DA neurons via the dopamine transporter (DAT), leading to mitochondrial damage and neuronal cell death [1]. Reactive microgliosis is then initiated and a series of pro-inflammatory cytokines are released.

Mounting evidence in animal model experiments shows that MPTP toxicity is markedly reduced in mutant mice deficient in inflammatory mediators including NADPH oxidase [43, 44], myeloperoxidase [45], COX-2 [46, 48], inducible nitric oxide (iNOS) [50], interferon-γ (IFN-γ) [51], and TNF-α [52, 53]. Studies have also applied anti-inflammatory drugs in the MPTP-models, in an attempt to discover or confirm any drugs that may alleviate DA neuron death and repress microglial activation [44, 54, 55, 65]. Overall, these studies indicate that MPTP-treated animals are good models for studying immunopathogenesis of PD.

Effectors of "Bad" Microglia

Microglia have evolved to express multiple, diverse membrane receptors, also termed pattern recognition receptors (PRRs), which are generally constitutively expressed to identify and bind pathogen-associated molecular patterns (PAMPs) associated with microbial pathogens, as well as damage-associated molecular patterns (DAMPs) associated with cell components released during cell damage [66]. There is increasing evidence to indicate that protein aggregates or neurotoxins could interact with multiple PRRs, including toll-like receptors (TLRs), scavenger receptors (SRs), macrophage antigen complex 1 (MAC1) receptor or through receptor complexes [13]. Although different combinations of receptors might be involved in the recognition of toxic and dangerous inducers, there are common deleterious downstream effectors that both induce neuronal death and amplify ongoing microglial activation. These effectors are NADPH oxidase, pro-inflammatory factors, ROS, superoxide, and so forth (see Table 1).

NADPH Oxidase

NADPH oxidase is a membrane-bound enzyme that catalyzes the production of superoxide free radicals from oxygen and a robust source of extracellular ROS and pro-inflammatory signaling in microglia [67]. NADPH oxidase is activated by various stimuli, including bacterial PAMPs, inflammatory mediators, and multiple neurotoxins, which are associated with PD and neuronal damage. It is found to be activated in the brains of patients with PD and the catalytic subunit (gp91) is upregulated [43]. The crucial role of NADPH oxidase in mediating inflammation-related neurotoxicity has been extensively studied. Genetic ablation of NADPH oxidase attenuates the neurodegeneration induced by diverse challenges both in vivo and in vitro, including LPS [68], rotenone [38], paraquat [40], MPTP [43, 44, 69], substance P [28], and α-synuclein aggregates [23, 70]. It appears that NADPH oxidase is at the very center of the downstream pathway and is the major source of effectors including pro-inflammatory factors, NO, ROS, and other factors in activated microglia in PD. Thus, NADPH oxidase could be a potential therapeutic target for PD [13].

Pro-inflammatory Factors

Pro-inflammatory factors are important aspects of elucidating pathogenesis of PD. After exposure to stimuli such as LPS or other inducers, microglia produce various pro-inflammatory mediators including TNF-α, IL-1β, and iNOS and thereby modulate the progression of neuronal cell death in PD [12, 67]. Microglia are the major sources of pro-inflammatory cytokines, which were then transferred to stimulate astrocytes and amplify inflammatory responses, leading to the extensive death of DA neurons [71]. Therefore, the combination of factors that are produced by activated microglia and astrocytes promote neurotoxicity.

Pro-inflammatory cytokines are extremely critical for neurodegeneration. Genetic analyses show that the DNA polymorphism of several pro-inflammatory cytokines including IL-1α, IL-1β, IL-6, and iNOS are a risk factor for PD [72–74]. Mangano et al. [41] have reported that knockout of IFN-γ prevents the paraquat-induced microglial activation and expression of key NADPH oxidase subunits, meanwhile reduces the time-dependent changes in pro-inflammatory enzymes iNOS, IL-1β, TNF-α, and signaling factors such as NF-κB. Similarly, IFN-γ-deficient mice also display protection against MPTP (in vivo) or rotenone (in vitro)-induced DA neuron loss [51], whereas overexpression of IFN-γ is able to induce progressive nigrostriatal degeneration [75]. Of note, these secreted inflammatory mediators should be considered as new inducers of "bad" microglia.

ROS and Superoxide

Activated microglia also release superoxide free radicals and extracellular ROS, which are mainly produced by the help of NADPH oxidase [67]. Excessive production of superoxide and its downstream products are highly reactive and can damage proteins, lipids, nucleotides, leading to cell dysfunction and death. Extracellular α-synuclein or neuromelanin is phagocytosed by microglia and leads to activation of NADPH oxidase, ROS production, and NF-κB regulated genes [23, 27, 31]. Lack of NADPH oxidase in mice makes them resistant to the toxic effects by α-synuclein or active recombinant MMP-3 exposure with reduced production of ROS and superoxide [23, 25]. In the MPTP-injected mice, MMP-3 deficiency attenuates microglial activation and superoxide generation, which contributes to neuron survival [25].

Regulation of "Good" Microglia

Regulatory mechanisms in microglia attenuate excessive inflammatory response to bad microglia and promote recovery and repair. Briefly, the mechanisms in "good" microglia that may be relevant to PD pathology are involved in Table 2. Eventually, these mechanisms of "good" microglia converge into counteraction with "bad" microglia by repressing pro-inflammatory cytokines, NF-κB, and other factors (Fig. 1).

Table 2 Mechanisms or pathways in "good" microglia

Mechanisms	Major references
Counter-regulation or transrepression pathways	
GRs	[76–79]
ERs	[81–84]
Nurr1	[71, 89]
PPARs	[90–96]
Anti-inflammatory factors	
IL-4	[96–100, 120]
IL-10	[98]
TGF-β	[98, 101, 120, 121]
G-CSF	[102–105]
Neuron-microglia cross-talk	
CX3CL1–CX3CR1	[107–110, 121]
CD200–CD200R	[113–115]
MicroRNA	
miR-124	[116]
Epigenetics	
Jmjd3	[123]

Counter-Regulation or Transrepression Pathways

A spectrum of endogenous protective receptors that mediated transrepression to counter-regulate pro-inflammation in the brain have been identified, these are glucocorticoid receptors, estrogen receptors, NR4A2, peroxisome proliferator-activated receptors, and others as shown (see Table 2).

Glucocorticoid Receptors

Glucocorticoids (GCs) predominantly are released during stressful states to maintain homeostasis and are the most efficient endocrine molecules that exert anti-inflammatory and immunosuppressive effects via glucocorticoid receptors (GRs). Upon binding, GRs translocate into the nucleus and regulate gene expression, resulting in suppression of NF-κB and downregulation of a wide variety of pro-inflammatory cytokines and immune mediators [76, 77]. In PD patients and MPTP-intoxicated mice, GR level is found to be decreased in the SN, suggesting the potential role of GRs in PD pathogenesis [78]. Various studies have showed that absence of GRs augments microglial reactivity and leads to persistent microglial activation; GR-deficient microglia produce higher nitrite level that precedes the loss of DA neurons and are resistant to the inhibitory effects of GCs [78, 79]. Furthermore, GR-deficient microglia also express higher level of pro-inflammatory genes (e.g., TNF-α) with a concomitant downregulation of anti-inflammatory genes (e.g., IL-1R2) [78]. GRs play an important role in suppression of microglial activity and deregulation of this leads to inflammation-mediated neuronal injury.

Estrogen Receptors

PD is more prevalent in men than in women and studies suggest a differential response to dopaminergic therapy between men and women raising the possibility of involvement of estrogen receptors (ERs) [80]. The protective effects of estrogen on the onset and severity of PD symptoms have been extensively evaluated. Numerous studies have showed that estrogens act through ERα or ERβ to suppress the production of several pro-inflammatory mediators including iNOS, TNF-α, as well as other secretory products induced by LPS in vitro and render neuroprotection to cultured neurons [81–83]. Notably, these protective effects could be blocked by treatment of ER antagonists, suggesting ER as a critical mediator of anti-inflammatory function of promoting neuron survival [82, 83]. Similarly, Tripanichkul et al. [84] have also reported that estrogen could decrease microglial activation and attenuate DA neuron loss in the MPTP intoxicated male mice in vivo. It is important to explore the role of estrogen in microglial activation and specific mechanism in pathophysiology of PD.

NR4A2

NR4A2 (Nurr1) belongs to the orphan nuclear receptors NR4A subfamily and is required for differentiation and maintenance of midbrain DA neurons [85, 86]. Reduced Nurr1 expression causes increased vulnerability of DA neurons to MPTP-induced injury in mice, and mutation in the gene has been reported in familial PD [87, 88]. Nurr1 is expressed both in neuronal and microglial cells. In recent years, Nurr1 has attracted increasing attention to its effect on neuroinflammation by mechanism of transrepression. After exposure to LPS express of Nurr1 gene expression increases, and it has been shown that nuclear translocation of Nurr1 occurs in the in vitro model [89]. In 2008, Saijo et al. [71] have demonstrated a Nurr1-mediated transrepression mechanism in LPS-induced PD model. In their study, Nurr1 is able to inhibit the expression of pro-inflammatory neurotoxic mediators and NF-κB targeted genes in microglia. Reduced Nurr1 expression initiates exaggerated inflammatory response in microglia in addition to astrocyte activation, leading to the extensive death of DA neurons [71]. Based on this evidence Nurr1 could be a potential therapeutic target.

Peroxisome Proliferator-Activated Receptors

Peroxisome proliferator-activated receptors (PPARs) are members of the steroid hormone nuclear receptor superfamily, which have been extensively studied in the regulation of genes involved in lipid metabolism, energy homeostasis, and macrophage differentiation. Numerous studies have shown that PPARs play a very important role in the regulation of brain inflammation through mechanisms involving transrepression pathways. Activation of PPARs inhibits the synthesis of NO, TNF-α, COX-2, and chemokines in microglia [90, 91]. One of the major natural PPAR-γ agonists, 15-deoxy-$\Delta^{12,14}$-prostaglandin J_2 (15d-PGJ_2), contributes to inhibition of LPS-induced microglial activation [90]. Similarly, synthetic agonists of PPAR-γ including ciglitazone, troglitazone, and pioglitazone could also reduce LPS-induced microglial activation and inhibit the excessive production of cytotoxic molecules, thereby preventing neuronal death [91, 92]. In addition, pioglitazone also attenuates DA neuron death in the MPTP model of PD, by blocking NF-κB and iNOS activation [93–95]. Interestingly, rosiglitazone, another agonist of PPAR-γ, possesses anti-inflammatory properties by increasing IL-4 expression [96], suggesting a cross-talk between counter-regulation and anti-inflammatory factors in the mechanisms of "good" microglia.

Anti-inflammatory Factors

IL-4, IL-13, IL-10, and transforming growth factor-β (TGF-β) are major anti-inflammatory cytokines that antagonize pro-inflammatory responses and promote the expression of genes involved in tissue reconstruction and repair. IL-4 is a well-described immune regulatory cytokine capable of suppressing inflammation. Its interaction with microglial IL-4 receptors suppresses superoxide production and NO release; reduces the production of pro-inflammatory cytokines such as IL-6, IL-8, and TNF-α; and alleviates LPS-induced neuron injury both in vitro and in vivo [97–100]. TGF-β is a pleiotropic cytokine with diverse functions including angiogenesis and increased extracellular matrix deposition and also plays a critical role in minimizing microglial responses and thus avoiding exacerbation of brain damage [101]. It is important to note that anti-inflammatory cytokines (IL-4, IL-10, and TGF-β) affect the production of inflammatory mediators in LPS-activated cocultures of microglial cells differentially [98]. Granulocyte-colony stimulating factor (G-CSF) is known to stimulate the proliferation of hematopoietic cells and has been reported to modulate the immune system by downregulating pro-inflammatory cytokines [102]. Two studies have shown that G-CSF administration provides neuroprotection against MPP^+-induced cell death in vitro and MPTP-induced DA neuron loss in vivo [103, 104]. Moreover, G-CSF could also enhance the recovery of nigrostriatal system from MPTP toxicity by modulating microglial responses [105].

Neuron-Microglia Cross-Talk

Fractalkine (CX3CL1) and Fractalkine Receptor (CX3CR1)

Microglia are the major CNS cells that express CX3CR1. CX3CL1, the exclusive ligand for CX3CR1, is synthesized as a transmembrane glycoprotein highly expressed in neurons [106]. CX3CL1 is cleaved from neuronal membranes in response to neurotoxic insults and subsequently attracts reactive immune cells as microglia cells by binding CX3CR1 [107]. Previous studies have supported that the interaction between CX3CL1 and CX3CR1 plays an important role in preserving microglia survival and attenuates neurodegeneration. For example, treatment of microglia with CX3CL1 maintains microglia survival and prevents from Fas-mediated apoptosis [108]. CX3CL1 also suppresses the production of NO, IL-6, and TNF-α from activated microglia upon LPS and IFN-γ insult that significantly suppresses neuronal death in vitro [109]. Importantly, Cardona et al. [110] have showed that CX3CR1 deficiency in vivo leads to enhanced microglial activation and exaggerates neuronal damage in response to systemic LPS treatment or augments DA neuron loss in the SN following MPTP administration, suggesting CX3CR1 signaling is critical to protect against microglial neurotoxicity.

CD200 and CD200R

CD200 receptor (CD200R), an inhibitory receptor present on microglia, actively maintains microglia in a quiescent state through its interaction with CD200, a member of the immunoglobulin superfamily expressed on the neuronal membrane surface [111, 112]. CD200–CD200R has been identified as one of the critical pathways in attenuating microglial activation. Microglia in CD200-deficient mice exhibit more characteristics of activation, which are less ramified with shorter processes. Moreover, this increased microglial activation is accompanied by enhanced expression of TNF-α and iNOS, demonstrating a loss of the neuronal inhibitory signal for microglial response [113]. Blocking CD200–CD200R engagement dramatically exacerbates DA neuron death in a primary neuron/microglia co-culture system [114]. Furthermore, deficits in the CD200–CD200R system also enhance microglial activation with elevated TNF-α and IL-6 production and thus exacerbate DA neuron loss in a 6-hydroxydopamine (6-OHDA)-induced rat model of PD [115]. Therefore, in the healthy brain, microglial activation is tightly restricted by signaling from neurons, whereas the progressive loss of DA neurons in the SN of PD patients might accelerate reactive microgliosis due to the lack of neuronal signals.

MicroRNA

Apart from CD200–CD200R, microRNAs have also been reported to promote microglia quiescence. Ponomarev et al. [116] published evidence that brain-specific miR-124 acts as a novel modulator of microglia and macrophage activation. There is downregulation of miR-124 in activated microglia and highly activated peripheral macrophages. Knockout modeling of miR-124 in microglia and macrophages results in activation of these cells both in vitro and in vivo. The administration of miR-124 before or after disease onset causes systemic deactivation and suppression of EAE [116]. This study offers insight into inhibition of microglial overactivation in PD.

Activation States of Microglia

The complexity of microglial activation states or phenotypes has been attracting increasing attention in recent years. As noted above, microglia exhibit a deactivated phenotype in the healthy brain helping in maintenance of tissue homeostasis through communication with other cells, analogous to homeostatic roles of "alternatively activated" macrophages in other tissues. Actually, increasing studies have reported that microglia, similar to peripheral macrophages, possess states of "classical activation," "alternative activation," and "acquired deactivation" [117, 118].

Classical activation is associated with the production and release of pro-inflammatory cytokines, proteases, superoxide anion, NO, and ROS/RNS that recapitulate the effects of "bad" microglia. Microglia in this state are also termed "M1 microglia" according to the studies on macrophages, whereas the term "M2 microglia" is used to include the states of both alternative activation and acquired deactivation that reflect the effects of "good" microglia [118]. Alternative activation is limited to microglia treated with IL-4 or IL-13 and is primarily associated with M2 genes that promote anti-inflammation, tissue repair, and extracellular matrix reconstruction, such as Arginase 1 (Arg1), Mannose receptor (CD206), Found in inflammatory zone 1 (FIZZ1), and Chitinase-3-Like-3 (Ym1) [117]. Acquired deactivation is another state to alleviate acute inflammation and is induced primarily by uptake of apoptotic cells or the insult of anti-inflammatory cytokines IL-10 and/or TGF-β [117, 118]. All three states could be transited into each other in different context that may contribute to pathogenic forms of inflammation in neurodegenerative diseases including PD.

However, molecular mechanisms that regulate M2 microglia are poorly understood and require further investigation. Nevertheless, the mechanisms of "good" microglia aforementioned can also converge into the elucidation of M2 microglia. For instance, it is reported that IL-4 production is essential for the maintenance of Ym1 expression and alternative activation in both microglia cells and peripheral infiltrating macrophages, thereby suppressing EAE clinical symptoms [119]. Treatment with the PPAR-γ agonist rosiglitazone increases IL-4 expression and attenuates the LPS-induced increase in IL-1β concentration in wild-type microglia while not $IL4^{-/-}$ microglia, suggesting that the anti-inflammatory actions of rosiglitazone are mediated by its ability to increase IL-4 expression [96]. More interestingly, since miR-124 is required for microglia quiescence, transfection of miR-124 results in downregulation of markers and cytokines associated with M1 microglia such as CD86 and iNOS, whereas cytokines and markers associated with M2 microglia including TGF-β, Arg1, and FIZZ1 are upregulated [116]. This is also consistent with the notion that quiescent microglia show properties of alternative activated microglia [116, 119].

It might be interesting to determine whether other molecules involving in the regulation of "good" microglia such as GRs, CX3CR1, ERs, and Nurr1 contribute to alternative activation of microglia.

Conclusion and Future Perspectives

In summary, "bad" microglia can be induced by endogenous proteins such as α-synuclein and a variety of environmental cues that eventually converge into the effectors including pro-inflammatory cytokines, ROS and superoxide, and especially NADPH oxidase (see Fig. 1). The function of "good" microglia is mainly involving transrepression pathways through multiple receptors such as GRs, ERs, Nurr1, and PPARs, anti-inflammatory cytokines, neuron-microglia cross-talk, and microRNAs that counteract with "bad" microglia by repressing pro-inflammatory cytokines, NF-κB, and other factors (see Fig. 1).

Notably, those mechanisms attributed by "bad" or "good" microglia are not in parallel pathways but in cross-talk with each other to amplify their effects. Activation of "bad" microglia produces a variety of pro-inflammatory factors, chemokines, and cytokines, which could then be involved as new inducers of "bad" microglia. This self-amplifying nature of neuroinflammation, together with secondary inflammatory responses mediated by astrocytes, partially underlies uncontrolled inflammation in PD [71]. Similarly, the various mechanisms that contributed to the resolution of inflammation by "good" microglia are not in parallel. Upon activation, they can promote expression of genes in other pathways and orchestrate each other against the pro-inflammation. This is already demonstrated by multiple studies on (1) IL-4 and TGF-β cross-talk [120]; (2) TGF-β and CX3CR1 cross-talk [121]; (3) IL-4 and PPARs cross-talk [96].

Depending on host environment microglial cells have dual responses and exist in differential states of activation. In most cases, these responses are self-limiting and well regulated to keep the balance between the pro-inflammation/injury and the resolution of inflammation/repair. However, it seems that the beneficial effects in PD are apparently either inadequate or ineffective due to the complex mechanisms involved. Because neural tissues have a restricted cell renewal and regenerative capacity, the CNS is extremely vulnerable to uncontrolled inflammatory processes. Deficits in generating those beneficial effects in response to CNS injuries might compromise important defense mechanisms of inflammation (e.g., the regulation of "good" microglia). In pathogenesis of PD there is a persistent stimulus resulting from the formation of endogenous factors especially α-synuclein aggregates or environmental factors (e.g., the inducers of "bad" microglia) that contribute to an excessive pro-inflammation. Thus, the persistence of pro-inflammation or a failure of normal protective mechanisms might lead to uncontrolled and sustained inflammation in the CNS. Uncontrolled inflammation acts either as an initiator or as a secondary reaction that drives the chronic and progressive neurodegenerative process in PD where detrimental effects of inflammation overwhelm beneficial effects.

Therefore, it becomes critical and urgent to investigate what determines the progressive nature of neuroinflammation in PD, i.e., a full understanding of the mechanisms of both "bad" microglia and "good" microglia. Focusing solely on "bad" microglia would not be sufficient or effective for PD therapy. Use of NSAIDs has shown mixed results with decreased risk of PD, but the same studies showed no benefit in Alzheimer's disease (AD) [13]. A major issue is whether inhibition of pro-inflammatory responses will be a safe and effective method for reversing or slowing the course of disease. Targeting any one of a large number of pro-inflammatory factors released from overactivated microglia is less efficacious.

A more detailed understanding of the transition of "bad/good" microglia or "M1/M2" microglia will be helpful in defining the molecular events and pathways to halt the progress of neuroinflammatory injury by switching the microglia states from M1 to M2 in an optimal therapeutic window, the concept of which has been demonstrated in the treatment of experimental autoimmune neuritis (EAN) disease [122]. More importantly, in a recent study of our lab, Tang et al. [123] have demonstrated that the histone H3K27me3 demethylase Jmjd3 is essential for M2 microglial activation. Suppression of Jmjd3 in microglia leads to defective M2 responses and augments M1 pro-inflammation that eventually accelerates DA neuron death [123], suggesting that switching microglia phenotypes is possible by epigenetic modification and any other mechanisms involved in this switch might be needed considering the complexity of microglia states. Moreover, it is important to monitor the microglial activation throughout the chronic progression of the disease that would present the dynamics of microglia states and give an indication of when to begin the treatment capable of altering disease progression.

Originally, activation of "bad" microglia is necessary and crucial for host defense. Targeting on "bad" microglia too early would not produce beneficial effects. Transrepression mechanisms are employed by "good" microglia to facilitate anti-inflammation and tissue reconstruction; however, abnormal prolongation of the same immunosuppressive and repair mechanisms is also associated with chronic disease with long-term "escape" of persistent parasites or pathogens from immune-mediated killing [124]. Further research is crucial to our understanding of mechanisms of microglial activation and regulatory homeostasis of microglial-mediated inflammatory processes.

References

1. Dauer W, Przedborski S. Parkinson's disease: mechanisms and models. Neuron. 2003;39(6): 889–909.
2. Braak H, Del Tredici K, Rub U, de Vos RA, Jansen Steur EN, Braak E. Staging of brain pathology related to sporadic Parkinson's disease. Neurobiol Aging. 2003;24(2):197–211.
3. Block ML, Hong JS. Chronic microglial activation and progressive dopaminergic neurotoxicity. Biochem Soc Trans. 2007;35(Pt 5):1127–32.
4. Nagatsu T, Sawada M. Inflammatory process in Parkinson's disease: role for cytokines. Curr Pharm Des. 2005;11(8):999–1016.
5. Gao HM, Hong JS. Why neurodegenerative diseases are progressive: uncontrolled inflammation drives disease progression. Trends Immunol. 2008;29(8):357–65.
6. Glass CK, Saijo K, Winner B, Marchetto MC, Gage FH. Mechanisms underlying inflammation in neurodegeneration. Cell. 2010;140(6):918–34.
7. Lawson LJ, Perry VH, Dri P, Gordon S. Heterogeneity in the distribution and morphology of microglia in the normal adult mouse brain. Neuroscience. 1990;39(1):151–70.
8. Mittelbronn M, Dietz K, Schluesener HJ, Meyermann R. Local distribution of microglia in the normal adult human central nervous system differs by up to one order of magnitude. Acta Neuropathol. 2001;101(3):249–55.
9. Kim WG, Mohney RP, Wilson B, Jeohn GH, Liu B, Hong JS. Regional difference in susceptibility to lipopolysaccharide-induced neurotoxicity in the rat brain: role of microglia. J Neurosci. 2000;20(16):6309–16.
10. Ouchi Y, Yoshikawa E, Sekine Y, Futatsubashi M, Kanno T, Ogusu T, et al. Microglial activation and dopamine terminal loss in early Parkinson's disease. Ann Neurol. 2005;57(2): 168–75.
11. McGeer PL, Itagaki S, Boyes BE, McGeer EG. Reactive microglia are positive for HLA-DR in the substantia nigra of Parkinson's and Alzheimer's disease brains. Neurology. 1988;38(8): 1285–91.
12. Hirsch EC, Hunot S. Neuroinflammation in Parkinson's disease: a target for neuroprotection? Lancet Neurol. 2009;8(4):382–97.
13. Block ML, Zecca L, Hong JS. Microglia-mediated neurotoxicity: uncovering the molecular mechanisms. Nat Rev Neurosci. 2007;8(1):57–69.
14. Heppner FL, Greter M, Marino D, Falsig J, Raivich G, Hovelmeyer N, et al. Experimental autoimmune encephalomyelitis repressed by microglial paralysis. Nat Med. 2005;11(2): 146–52.

15. Streit WJ. Microglia as neuroprotective, immunocompetent cells of the CNS. Glia. 2002; 40(2):133–9.
16. Schwartz M, Kipnis J. A common vaccine for fighting neurodegenerative disorders: recharging immunity for homeostasis. Trends Pharmacol Sci. 2004;25(8):407–12.
17. Glezer I, Simard AR, Rivest S. Neuroprotective role of the innate immune system by microglia. Neuroscience. 2007;147(4):867–83.
18. Koenigsknecht-Talboo J, Landreth GE. Microglial phagocytosis induced by fibrillar beta-amyloid and IgGs are differentially regulated by proinflammatory cytokines. J Neurosci. 2005;25(36):8240–9.
19. Kordower JH. *In vivo* gene delivery of glial cell line-derived neurotrophic factor for Parkinson's disease. Ann Neurol. 2003;53 Suppl 3:S120–32. discussion S32–4.
20. Ding YM, Jaumotte JD, Signore AP, Zigmond MJ. Effects of 6-hydroxydopamine on primary cultures of substantia nigra: specific damage to dopamine neurons and the impact of glial cell line-derived neurotrophic factor. J Neurochem. 2004;89(3):776–87.
21. Aarum J, Sandberg K, Haeberlein SL, Persson MA. Migration and differentiation of neural precursor cells can be directed by microglia. Proc Natl Acad Sci U S A. 2003;100(26): 15983–8.
22. Walton NM, Sutter BM, Laywell ED, Levkoff LH, Kearns SM, Marshall 2nd GP, et al. Microglia instruct subventricular zone neurogenesis. Glia. 2006;54(8):815–25.
23. Zhang W, Wang T, Pei Z, Miller DS, Wu X, Block ML, et al. Aggregated alpha-synuclein activates microglia: a process leading to disease progression in Parkinson's disease. FASEB J. 2005;19(6):533–42.
24. Roodveldt C, Christodoulou J, Dobson CM. Immunological features of alpha-synuclein in Parkinson's disease. J Cell Mol Med. 2008;12(5B):1820–9.
25. Kim YS, Choi DH, Block ML, Lorenzl S, Yang L, Kim YJ, et al. A pivotal role of matrix metalloproteinase-3 activity in dopaminergic neuronal degeneration via microglial activation. FASEB J. 2007;21(1):179–87.
26. Zecca L, Zucca FA, Wilms H, Sulzer D. Neuromelanin of the substantia nigra: a neuronal black hole with protective and toxic characteristics. Trends Neurosci. 2003;26(11):578–80.
27. Wilms H, Rosenstiel P, Sievers J, Deuschl G, Zecca L, Lucius R. Activation of microglia by human neuromelanin is NF-kappaB dependent and involves p38 mitogen-activated protein kinase: implications for Parkinson's disease. FASEB J. 2003;17(3):500–2.
28. Block ML, Li G, Qin L, Wu X, Pei Z, Wang T, et al. Potent regulation of microglia-derived oxidative stress and dopaminergic neuron survival: substance P vs dynorphin. FASEB J. 2006;20(2):251–8.
29. Piers TM, Heales SJ, Pocock JM. Positive allosteric modulation of metabotropic glutamate receptor 5 down-regulates fibrinogen-activated microglia providing neuronal protection. Neurosci Lett. 2011;505(2):140–5.
30. Lee DY, Oh YJ, Jin BK. Thrombin-activated microglia contribute to death of dopaminergic neurons in rat mesencephalic cultures: dual roles of mitogen-activated protein kinase signaling pathways. Glia. 2005;51(2):98–110.
31. Reynolds AD, Kadiu I, Garg SK, Glanzer JG, Nordgren T, Ciborowski P, et al. Nitrated alpha-synuclein and microglial neuroregulatory activities. J Neuroimmune Pharmacol. 2008;3(2):59–74.
32. Gao HM, Kotzbauer PT, Uryu K, Leight S, Trojanowski JQ, Lee VM. Neuroinflammation and oxidation/nitration of alpha-synuclein linked to dopaminergic neurodegeneration. J Neurosci. 2008;28(30):7687–98.
33. Rojanathammanee L, Murphy EJ, Combs CK. Expression of mutant alpha-synuclein modulates microglial phenotype *in vitro*. J Neuroinflammation. 2011;8:44.
34. Ling Z, Zhu Y, Tong C, Snyder JA, Lipton JW, Carvey PM. Progressive dopamine neuron loss following supra-nigral lipopolysaccharide (LPS) infusion into rats exposed to LPS prenatally. Exp Neurol. 2006;199(2):499–512.
35. Qin L, Wu X, Block ML, Liu Y, Breese GR, Hong JS, et al. Systemic LPS causes chronic neuroinflammation and progressive neurodegeneration. Glia. 2007;55(5):453–62.

36. Elbaz A, Levecque C, Clavel J, Vidal JS, Richard F, Amouyel P, et al. CYP2D6 polymorphism, pesticide exposure, and Parkinson's disease. Ann Neurol. 2004;55(3):430–4.
37. Jenner P. Parkinson's disease, pesticides and mitochondrial dysfunction. Trends Neurosci. 2001;24(5):245–7.
38. Gao HM, Liu B, Hong JS. Critical role for microglial NADPH oxidase in rotenone-induced degeneration of dopaminergic neurons. J Neurosci. 2003;23(15):6181–7.
39. Ling Z, Chang QA, Tong CW, Leurgans SE, Lipton JW, Carvey PM. Rotenone potentiates dopamine neuron loss in animals exposed to lipopolysaccharide prenatally. Exp Neurol. 2004;190(2):373–83.
40. Wu XF, Block ML, Zhang W, Qin L, Wilson B, Zhang WQ, et al. The role of microglia in paraquat-induced dopaminergic neurotoxicity. Antioxid Redox Signal. 2005;7(5–6):654–61.
41. Bonneh-Barkay D, Reaney SH, Langston WJ, Di Monte DA. Redox cycling of the herbicide paraquat in microglial cultures. Brain Res Mol Brain Res. 2005;134(1):52–6.
42. Mangano EN, Litteljohn D, So RM, Nelson E, Peters S, Bethune C, et al. Interferon-gamma plays a role in paraquat-induced neurodegeneration involving oxidative and proinflammatory pathways. Neurobiol Aging. 2012;33(7):1411–26.
43. Wu DC, Teismann P, Tieu K, Vila M, Jackson-Lewis V, Ischiropoulos H, et al. NADPH oxidase mediates oxidative stress in the 1-methyl-4-phenyl-1,2,3,6-tetrahydropyridine model of Parkinson's disease. Proc Natl Acad Sci U S A. 2003;100(10):6145–50.
44. Zhang W, Wang T, Qin L, Gao HM, Wilson B, Ali SF, et al. Neuroprotective effect of dextromethorphan in the MPTP Parkinson's disease model: role of NADPH oxidase. FASEB J. 2004;18(3):589–91.
45. Choi DK, Pennathur S, Perier C, Tieu K, Teismann P, Wu DC, et al. Ablation of the inflammatory enzyme myeloperoxidase mitigates features of Parkinson's disease in mice. J Neurosci. 2005;25(28):6594–600.
46. Feng ZH, Wang TG, Li DD, Fung P, Wilson BC, Liu B, et al. Cyclooxygenase-2-deficient mice are resistant to 1-methyl-4-phenyl-1, 2, 3, 6-tetrahydropyridine-induced damage of dopaminergic neurons in the substantia nigra. Neurosci Lett. 2002;329(3):354–8.
47. Teismann P, Vila M, Choi DK, Tieu K, Wu DC, Jackson-Lewis V, et al. COX-2 and neurodegeneration in Parkinson's disease. Ann N Y Acad Sci. 2003;991:272–7.
48. Vijitruth R, Liu M, Choi DY, Nguyen XV, Hunter RL, Bing G. Cyclooxygenase-2 mediates microglial activation and secondary dopaminergic cell death in the mouse MPTP model of Parkinson's disease. J Neuroinflammation. 2006;3:6.
49. Wang T, Pei Z, Zhang W, Liu B, Langenbach R, Lee C, et al. MPP^+-induced COX-2 activation and subsequent dopaminergic neurodegeneration. FASEB J. 2005;19(9):1134–6.
50. Liberatore GT, Jackson-Lewis V, Vukosavic S, Mandir AS, Vila M, McAuliffe WG, et al. Inducible nitric oxide synthase stimulates dopaminergic neurodegeneration in the MPTP model of Parkinson disease. Nat Med. 1999;5(12):1403–9.
51. Mount MP, Lira A, Grimes D, Smith PD, Faucher S, Slack R, et al. Involvement of interferon-gamma in microglial-mediated loss of dopaminergic neurons. J Neurosci. 2007;27(12): 3328–37.
52. Sriram K, Matheson JM, Benkovic SA, Miller DB, Luster MI, O'Callaghan JP. Mice deficient in TNF receptors are protected against dopaminergic neurotoxicity: implications for Parkinson's disease. FASEB J. 2002;16(11):1474–6.
53. Sriram K, Matheson JM, Benkovic SA, Miller DB, Luster MI, O'Callaghan JP. Deficiency of TNF receptors suppresses microglial activation and alters the susceptibility of brain regions to MPTP-induced neurotoxicity: role of TNF-alpha. FASEB J. 2006;20(6):670–82.
54. Wu DC, Jackson-Lewis V, Vila M, Tieu K, Teismann P, Vadseth C, et al. Blockade of microglial activation is neuroprotective in the 1-methyl-4-phenyl-1,2,3,6-tetrahydropyridine mouse model of Parkinson disease. J Neurosci. 2002;22(5):1763–71.
55. Ghosh A, Roy A, Liu X, Kordower JH, Mufson EJ, Hartley DM, et al. Selective inhibition of NF-kappaB activation prevents dopaminergic neuronal loss in a mouse model of Parkinson's disease. Proc Natl Acad Sci U S A. 2007;104(47):18754–9.

56. Miwa H, Kubo T, Suzuki A, Nishi K, Kondo T. Retrograde dopaminergic neuron degeneration following intrastriatal proteasome inhibition. Neurosci Lett. 2005;380(1–2):93–8.
57. McNaught KS, Perl DP, Brownell AL, Olanow CW. Systemic exposure to proteasome inhibitors causes a progressive model of Parkinson's disease. Ann Neurol. 2004;56(1):149–62.
58. Sadek AH, Rauch R, Schulz PE. Parkinsonism due to manganism in a welder. Int J Toxicol. 2003;22(5):393–401.
59. Hudnell HK. Effects from environmental Mn exposures: a review of the evidence from non-occupational exposure studies. Neurotoxicology. 1999;20(2–3):379–97.
60. Gibbons HM, Dragunow M. Microglia induce neural cell death via a proximity-dependent mechanism involving nitric oxide. Brain Res. 2006;1084(1):1–15.
61. Le WD, Rowe D, Xie WJ, Ortiz I, He Y, Appel SH. Microglial activation and dopaminergic cell injury: an *in vitro* model relevant to Parkinson's disease. J Neurosci. 2001;21(21):8447–55.
62. Li R, Huang YG, Fang D, Le WD. (−)-Epigallocatechin gallate inhibits lipopolysaccharide-induced microglial activation and protects against inflammation-mediated dopaminergic neuronal injury. J Neurosci Res. 2004;78(5):723–31.
63. Carvey PM, Chang Q, Lipton JW, Ling Z. Prenatal exposure to the bacteriotoxin lipopolysaccharide leads to long-term losses of dopamine neurons in offspring: a potential, new model of Parkinson's disease. Front Biosci. 2003;8:s826–37.
64. Gao HM, Jiang J, Wilson B, Zhang W, Hong JS, Liu B. Microglial activation-mediated delayed and progressive degeneration of rat nigral dopaminergic neurons: relevance to Parkinson's disease. J Neurochem. 2002;81(6):1285–97.
65. Thomas M, Le WD. Minocycline: neuroprotective mechanisms in Parkinson's disease. Curr Pharm Des. 2004;10(6):679–86.
66. Akira S, Uematsu S, Takeuchi O. Pathogen recognition and innate immunity. Cell. 2006;124(4):783–801.
67. Hunot S, Boissiere F, Faucheux B, Brugg B, Mouatt-Prigent A, Agid Y, et al. Nitric oxide synthase and neuronal vulnerability in Parkinson's disease. Neuroscience. 1996;72(2):355–63.
68. Qin L, Liu Y, Wang T, Wei SJ, Block ML, Wilson B, et al. NADPH oxidase mediates lipopolysaccharide-induced neurotoxicity and proinflammatory gene expression in activated microglia. J Biol Chem. 2004;279(2):1415–21.
69. Gao HM, Liu B, Zhang W, Hong JS. Critical role of microglial NADPH oxidase-derived free radicals in the *in vitro* MPTP model of Parkinson's disease. FASEB J. 2003;17(13):1954–6.
70. Zhang W, Dallas S, Zhang D, Guo JP, Pang H, Wilson B, et al. Microglial PHOX and Mac-1 are essential to the enhanced dopaminergic neurodegeneration elicited by A30P and A53T mutant alpha-synuclein. Glia. 2007;55(11):1178–88.
71. Saijo K, Winner B, Carson CT, Collier JG, Boyer L, Rosenfeld MG, et al. A Nurr1/CoREST pathway in microglia and astrocytes protects dopaminergic neurons from inflammation-induced death. Cell. 2009;137(1):47–59.
72. Schulte T, Schols L, Muller T, Woitalla D, Berger K, Kruger R. Polymorphisms in the interleukin-1 alpha and beta genes and the risk for Parkinson's disease. Neurosci Lett. 2002;326(1):70–2.
73. Levecque C, Elbaz A, Clavel J, Richard F, Vidal JS, Amouyel P, et al. Association between Parkinson's disease and polymorphisms in the nNOS and iNOS genes in a community-based case-control study. Hum Mol Genet. 2003;12(1):79–86.
74. Hakansson A, Westberg L, Nilsson S, Buervenich S, Carmine A, Holmberg B, et al. Interaction of polymorphisms in the genes encoding interleukin-6 and estrogen receptor beta on the susceptibility to Parkinson's disease. Am J Med Genet B Neuropsychiatr Genet. 2005;133B(1):88–92.
75. Chakrabarty P, Ceballos-Diaz C, Lin WL, Beccard A, Jansen-West K, McFarland NR, et al. Interferon-gamma induces progressive nigrostriatal degeneration and basal ganglia calcification. Nat Neurosci. 2011;14(6):694–6.
76. Scheinman RI, Cogswell PC, Lofquist AK, Baldwin Jr AS. Role of transcriptional activation of I kappa B alpha in mediation of immunosuppression by glucocorticoids. Science. 1995;270(5234):283–6.

77. Auphan N, DiDonato JA, Rosette C, Helmberg A, Karin M. Immunosuppression by glucocorticoids: inhibition of NF-kappa B activity through induction of I kappa B synthesis. Science. 1995;270(5234):286–90.
78. Ros-Bernal F, Hunot S, Herrero MT, Parnadeau S, Corvol JC, Lu L, et al. Microglial glucocorticoid receptors play a pivotal role in regulating dopaminergic neurodegeneration in parkinsonism. Proc Natl Acad Sci U S A. 2011;108(16):6632–7.
79. Morale MC, Serra PA, Delogu MR, Migheli R, Rocchitta G, Tirolo C, et al. Glucocorticoid receptor deficiency increases vulnerability of the nigrostriatal dopaminergic system: critical role of glial nitric oxide. FASEB J. 2004;18(1):164–6.
80. Shulman LM. Is there a connection between estrogen and Parkinson's disease? Parkinsonism Relat Disord. 2002;8(5):289–95.
81. Vegeto E, Pollio G, Ciana P, Maggi A. Estrogen blocks inducible nitric oxide synthase accumulation in LPS-activated microglia cells. Exp Gerontol. 2000;35(9–10):1309–16.
82. Vegeto E, Bonincontro C, Pollio G, Sala A, Viappiani S, Nardi F, et al. Estrogen prevents the lipopolysaccharide-induced inflammatory response in microglia. J Neurosci. 2001;21(6):1809–18.
83. Liu X, Fan XL, Zhao Y, Luo GR, Li XP, Li R, et al. Estrogen provides neuroprotection against activated microglia-induced dopaminergic both estrogen receptor-alpha in neuronal injury through receptor-beta and estrogen microglia. J Neurosci Res. 2005;81(5):653–65.
84. Tripanichkul W, Sripanichkulchai K, Finkelstein DI. Estrogen down-regulates glial activation in male mice following 1-methyl-4-phenyl-1,2,3,6-tetrahydropyridine intoxication. Brain Res. 2006;1084:28–37.
85. Jankovic J, Chen S, Le WD. The role of Nurr1 in the development of dopaminergic neurons and Parkinson's disease. Prog Neurobiol. 2005;77(1–2):128–38.
86. Kadkhodaei B, Ito T, Joodmardi E, Mattsson B, Rouillard C, Carta M, et al. Nurr1 is required for maintenance of maturing and adult midbrain dopamine neurons. J Neurosci. 2009;29(50):15923–32.
87. Le W, Conneely OM, He Y, Jankovic J, Appel SH. Reduced Nurr1 expression increases the vulnerability of mesencephalic dopamine neurons to MPTP-induced injury. J Neurochem. 1999;73(5):2218–21.
88. Le W, Xu P, Jankovic J, Jiang H, Appel SH, Smith RG, et al. Mutations in NR4A2 associated with familial Parkinson disease (vol 33, pg 85, 2003). Nat Genet. 2003;33(2):214.
89. Fan X, Luo G, Ming M, Pu P, Li L, Yang D, et al. Nurr1 expression and its modulation in microglia. Neuroimmunomodulation. 2009;16(3):162–70.
90. Bernardo A, Levi G, Minghetti L. Role of the peroxisome proliferator-activated receptor-gamma (PPAR-gamma) and its natural ligand 15-deoxy-Delta(12,14)-prostaglandin J(2) in the regulation of microglial functions. Eur J Neurosci. 2000;12(7):2215–23.
91. Kim EJ, Kwon KJ, Park JY, Lee SH, Moon CH, Baik EJ. Effects of peroxisome proliferator-activated receptor agonists on LPS-induced neuronal death in mixed cortical neurons: associated with iNOS and COX-2. Brain Res. 2002;941(1–2):1–10.
92. Hunter RL, Dragicevic N, Seifert K, Choi DY, Liu M, Kim HC, et al. Inflammation induces mitochondrial dysfunction and dopaminergic neurodegeneration in the nigrostriatal system. J Neurochem. 2007;100(5):1375–86.
93. Dehmer T, Heneka MT, Sastre M, Dichgans J, Schulz JB. Protection by pioglitazone in the MPTP model of Parkinson's disease correlates with I kappa B alpha induction and block of NF kappa B and iNOS activation. J Neurochem. 2004;88(2):494–501.
94. Breidert T, Callebert J, Heneka MT, Landreth G, Launay JM, Hirsch EC. Protective action of the peroxisome proliferator-activated receptor-gamma agonist pioglitazone in a mouse model of Parkinson's disease. J Neurochem. 2002;82(3):615–24.
95. Quinn L, Crook B, Hows M, Vidgeon-Hart M, Chapman H, Upton N, et al. The PPARgamma agonist pioglitazone is effective in the MPTP mouse model of Parkinson's disease through inhibition of monoamine oxidase B. Br J Pharmacol. 2008;154(1):226–33.
96. Loane DJ, Deighan BF, Clarke RM, Griffin RJ, Lynch AM, Lynch MA. Interleukin-4 mediates the neuroprotective effects of rosiglitazone in the aged brain. Neurobiol Aging. 2009;30(6):920–31.

97. Butovsky O, Talpalar AE, Ben-Yaakov K, Schwartz M. Activation of microglia by aggregated beta-amyloid or lipopolysaccharide impairs MHC-II expression and renders them cytotoxic whereas IFN-gamma and IL-4 render them protective. Mol Cell Neurosci. 2005;29(3): 381–93.
98. Ledeboer A, Breve JJP, Poole S, Tilders FJH, Van Dam AM. Interleukin-10, interleukin-4, and transforming growth factor-beta differentially regulate lipopolysaccharide-induced production of pro-inflammatory cytokines and nitric oxide in co-cultures of rat astroglial and microglial cells. Glia. 2000;30(2):134–42.
99. Zhao WH, Xie WJ, Xiao Q, Beers DR, Appel SH. Protective effects of an anti-inflammatory cytokine, interleukin-4, on motoneuron toxicity induced by activated microglia. J Neurochem. 2006;99(4):1176–87.
100. Park KW, Lee DY, Joe EH, Kim SU, Jin BK. Neuroprotective role of microglia expressing interleukin-4. J Neurosci Res. 2005;81(3):397–402.
101. Boche D, Cunningham C, Docagne F, Scott H, Perry VH. TGFbeta1 regulates the inflammatory response during chronic neurodegeneration. Neurobiol Dis. 2006;22(3):638–50.
102. Hartung T. Anti-inflammatory effects of granulocyte colony-stimulating factor. Curr Opin Hematol. 1998;5(3):221–5.
103. Cao XQ, Arai H, Ren YR, Oizumi H, Zhang N, Seike S, et al. Recombinant human granulocyte colony-stimulating factor protects against MPTP-induced dopaminergic cell death in mice by altering Bcl-2/Bax expression levels. J Neurochem. 2006;99(3):861–7.
104. Meuer K, Pitzer C, Teismann P, Kruger C, Goricke B, Laage R, et al. Granulocyte-colony stimulating factor is neuroprotective in a model of Parkinson's disease. J Neurochem. 2006;97(3):675–86.
105. Sanchez-Ramos J, Sava V, Rowe A, Li KY, Zesiewicz T, Mori T, et al. The hematopoietic growth factor G-CSF enhances recovery in the MPTP mouse model of PD. Neurology. 2010;74(9):A82–A82.
106. Cook DN, Chen SC, Sullivan LM, Manfra DJ, Wiekowski MT, Prosser DM, et al. Generation and analysis of mice lacking the chemokine fractalkine. Mol Cell Biol. 2001;21(9): 3159–65.
107. Chapman GA, Moores K, Harrison D, Campbell CA, Stewart BR, Strijbos PJLM. Fractalkine cleavage from neuronal membranes represents an acute event in the inflammatory response to excitotoxic brain damage. J Neurosci. 2000;20(15):RC87.
108. Boehme SA, Lio FM, Maciejewski-Lenoir D, Bacon KB, Conlon PJ. The chemokine fractalkine inhibits Fas-mediated cell death of brain microglia. J Immunol. 2000;165(1):397–403.
109. Mizuno T, Kawanokuchi J, Numata K, Suzumura A. Production and neuroprotective functions of fractalkine in the central nervous system. Brain Res. 2003;979(1–2):65–70.
110. Cardona AE, Pioro EP, Sasse ME, Kostenko V, Cardona SM, Dijkstra IM, et al. Control of microglial neurotoxicity by the fractalkine receptor. Nat Neurosci. 2006;9(7):917–24.
111. Gorczynski R, Chen Z, Kai Y, Lee L, Wong S, Marsden PA. CD200 is a ligand for all members of the CD200R family of immunoregulatory molecules. J Immunol. 2004;172(12): 7744–9.
112. Vieites JM, de la Torre R, Ortega MA, Montero T, Peco JM, Sanchez-Pozo A, et al. Characterization of human cd200 glycoprotein receptor gene located on chromosome 3q12-13. Gene. 2003;311:99–104.
113. Deckert M, Sedgwick JD, Fischer E, Schluter D. Regulation of microglial cell responses in murine toxoplasma encephalitis by CD200/CD200 receptor interaction. Acta Neuropathol. 2006;111(6):548–58.
114. Wang XJ, Zhang S, Yan ZQ, Zhao YX, Zhou HY, Wang Y, et al. Impaired CD200–CD200R-mediated microglia silencing enhances midbrain dopaminergic neurodegeneration: roles of aging, superoxide, NADPH oxidase, and p38 MAPK. Free Radic Biol Med. 2011;50(9): 1094–106.
115. Zhang S, Wang XJ, Tian LP, Pan J, Lu GQ, Zhang YJ, et al. CD200–CD200R dysfunction exacerbates microglial activation and dopaminergic neurodegeneration in a rat model of Parkinson's disease. J Neuroinflammation. 2011;8:154.

116. Ponomarev ED, Veremeyko T, Barteneva N, Krichevsky AM, Weiner HL. MicroRNA-124 promotes microglia quiescence and suppresses EAE by deactivating macrophages via the C/EBP-alpha-PU.1 pathway. Nat Med. 2011;17(1):64–70.
117. Colton CA. Heterogeneity of microglial activation in the innate immune response in the brain. J Neuroimmune Pharmacol. 2009;4(4):399–418.
118. Colton CA, Wilcock DM. Assessing activation states in microglia. CNS Neurol Disord Drug Targets. 2010;9(2):174–91.
119. Ponomarev ED, Maresz K, Tan Y, Dittel BN. CNS-derived interleukin-4 is essential for the regulation of autoimmune inflammation and induces a state of alternative activation in microglial cells. J Neurosci. 2007;27(40):10714–21.
120. Zhou XL, Spittau B, Krieglstein K. TGF beta signalling plays an important role in IL4-induced alternative activation of microglia. J Neuroinflammation. 2012;9:210.
121. Chen SZ, Luo DF, Streit WJ, Harrison JK. TGF-beta 1 upregulates CX3CR1 expression and inhibits fractalkine-stimulated signaling in rat microglia. J Neuroimmunol. 2002;133(1–2):46–55.
122. Zhang ZR, Zhang ZY, Schluesener HJ. Compound A, a plant origin ligand of glucocorticoid receptors, increases regulatory T cells and M2 macrophages to attenuate experimental autoimmune neuritis with reduced side effects. J Immunol. 2009;183(5):3081–91.
123. Tang Y, Li T, Li J, Yang J, Liu H, Zhang XJ, et al. Jmjd3 is essential for the epigenetic modulation of microglia phenotypes in the immune pathogenesis of Parkinson's disease. Cell Death Differ. 2014;21(3):369–80.
124. Bogdan C. Mechanisms and consequences of persistence of intracellular pathogens: leishmaniasis as an example. Cell Microbiol. 2008;10(6):1221–34.

The Role of Astrocytes in Parkinson's Disease

Claire Stevens and Glenda Halliday

Astrocytes: Structure and Function in the Healthy Brain

Two main types of astrocytes tile the brain in a contiguous and non-overlapping manner: protoplasmic astrocytes in gray matter, which wrap neuronal cell bodies and synapses (estimates suggest a single human astrocyte wraps more than 270,000 synapses [1]), and fibrous astrocytes in white matter, which wrap nodes of Ranvier and oligodendroglia [2]. Once considered to be only passive support cells for neurons, astrocytes are now known to have an active regulatory role in the brain. They form part of the basic functional element, the neurovascular unit, which is comprised of astrocytes, neurons (which are contacted by astrocyte processes), and blood vessels (which are contacted by astrocyte end feet) [3]. Due to their strategic position, astrocytes are able to directly influence neuronal electrical excitability, neurogenesis, synaptogenesis and plasticity, synaptic transmission, ion homeostasis, neurotransmitter uptake, production of neurotrophic factors, glial scar formation, blood flow regulation, and maintenance of the blood–brain barrier (reviewed in [2]). Their function is achieved via the calcium-dependent release of chemical transmitters, or gliotransmitters such as glutamate, adenosine triphosphate, and gamma-aminobutyric acid, and also by their removal through uptake of potentially toxic neurotransmitters that are released into the extracellular space during neuronal activity (reviewed in [2]). A number of neurodegenerative conditions including Alzheimer's disease and epilepsy show abnormalities in calcium signaling, highlighting the importance of astrocytes in normal brain functioning [4].

Astrocytic release of chemicals, including prostaglandins and nitric oxide, controls blood flow by restricting or expanding the diameter of blood vessels [5, 6]. In addition, astrocyte end feet in contact with blood vessels contain the water channel protein aquaporin-4 [7]. Aquaporin-4 is critical to the regulation of water movement

C. Stevens, B.Med.Sci. (Hons), Ph.D. • G. Halliday, B.Sc. (Hons), Ph.D. (✉)
Department of Medicine, and Neuroscience Research Australia,
University of New South Wales, Randwick, NSW, Australia

M. Thomas (ed.), *Inflammation in Parkinson's Disease: Scientific and Clinical Aspects*, DOI 10.1007/978-3-319-08046-8_5,

in the CNS [7, 8] and also maintains ion homeostasis through the transport of ions such as K^+ [9]. Astrocytes can regulate neural stem/progenitor cell differentiation and proliferation [10] by the secretion of factors through Wnt signaling [11] and the release of the cytokines interleukin 1-β and interleukin-6 [12]. It is also becoming increasingly recognized that astrocytes are actively involved in the formation and elimination of synapses and synaptic transmission [13]. Astrocyte-derived factors are important in synaptogenesis [14, 15] and include thrombospondins [16–18] and cholesterol bound to apolipoprotein-E-containing particles [19], while astrocytes and the complement cascade factor C1q appear to have a role in synaptic pruning [20]. Finally, astrocytes are also important in synaptic transmission through physical contact with neurons and the release of substances including glutamate and acetylcholine-binding protein [21–23].

Although the CNS was once considered to be an immune-privileged site, it is now recognized that both innate (nonspecific) and adaptive (antigen-specific response) immune responses occur in the CNS [24]. While research in the field of CNS immunity has concentrated on the role of the resident immune cells microglia, it is becoming increasingly recognized that astrocytes are also active players in the CNS immune response and are implicated in the initiation and development of immune-mediated mechanisms in a number of brain diseases [25]. Astrocytes release an extensive array of both pro- and anti-inflammatory cytokines and chemokines and may also be targets for these inflammatory mediators [25]. They express pattern-recognition receptors including toll-like receptors and complement factors, receptors, and inhibitors, which are critical components of innate immunity [25]. These receptors recognize pathogens and markers of cells damage, and dampening of their activation has been implicated in a number of CNS diseases including meningitis, encephalitis, Alzheimer's disease, multiple sclerosis, and prion disease [25].

Typically, astrocytes respond to brain tissue changes (whether it be due to injury, infection, or disease) by undergoing astrogliosis, a process involving the upregulation of the intermediate filament protein glial fibrillary acidic protein (GFAP), cell body enlargement, and proliferation [2] (Fig. 1). Astrogliosis has a graded response with progressive morphological enlargement that may eventually culminate in the formation of a glial scar (for review see [2]) (see Fig. 1). Interestingly, this process may have both protective and harmful effects. Protective effects include the release of neuroprotective substances, containment of inflammation or infection in the affected area, and repair of damaged tissue [2]. However, there is increasing evidence that astrocytes contribute to the progression of CNS disorders through the loss of their normal protective roles or a gain of abnormal function, resulting in a range of detrimental effects including the release of toxic substances and proinflammatory cytokines and subsequent exacerbation of inflammatory processes (for review see [2]).

The importance of astrocytes in the brain and their capacity to have both a neuroprotective and neurodegenerative role are further illustrated in mouse models with altered astrocyte protein function (reviewed in [26]). After lesioning of the entorhinal cortex the reactive astrocytes in mice lacking the intermediate filaments GFAP and vimentin show a reduction in process hypertrophy but significantly improved

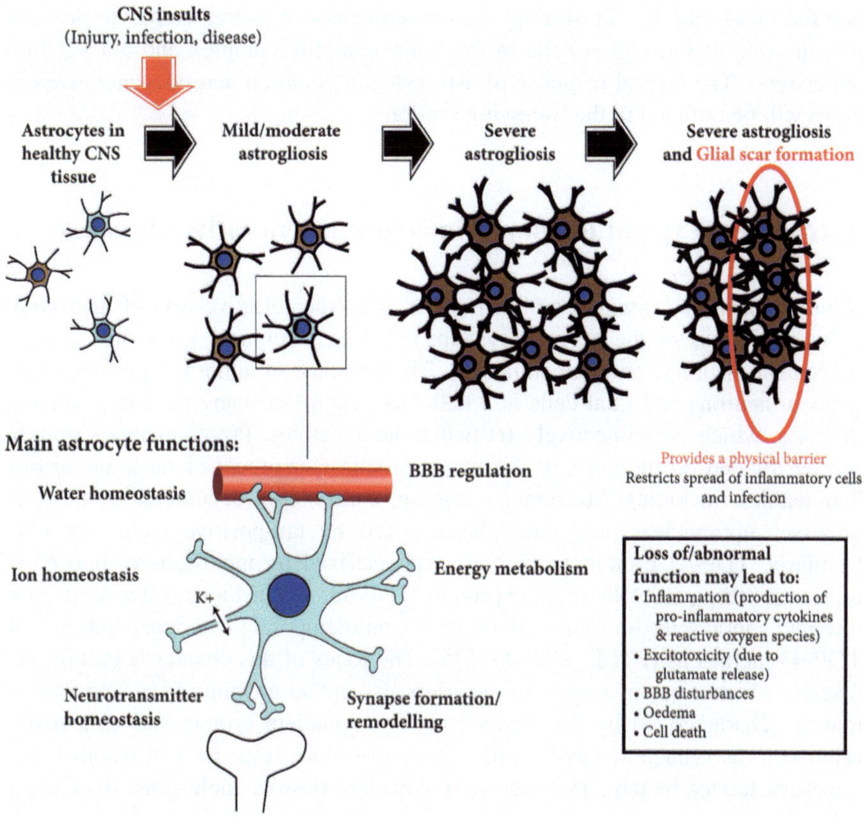

Fig. 1 Schematic representation of the main functions of astrocytes, their response to CNS insults, and the consequences of disrupted or abnormal astrocyte function. If astrocytes sense a disturbance in brain tissue, they undergo a graded process known as astrogliosis, which involves the upregulation of the intermediate filament protein glial fibrillary acid protein (*brown*), cell body enlargement, and proliferation, and may eventually culminate in the formation of a glial scar (*at right*). *BBB* blood–brain barrier, *CNS* central nervous system

synaptic regeneration [27]. Similarly, after unilateral hemisection of the spinal cord, mice deficient in these filaments show improved axonal sprouting and functional recovery [28], suggesting that reactive astrocytes actually impair neuroregeneration. Furthermore, the survival and integration of grafted neurons and neural progenitor cells is dramatically improved in GFAP and vimentin knockout mouse models [29, 30]. In contrast, mice overexpressing the human GFAP gene show abnormal astrocyte morphology, increased stress proteins, and the formation of filaments identical to Rosenthal fibers (hallmark pathology of the neurodegenerative disease Alexander disease) [31]. Similarly, mice lacking the astrocytic glutamate transporter GLT-1 show hippocampal neuron loss, severe and eventually lethal seizures, and an increased susceptibility to acute cortical injury, most likely due to raised levels of glutamate [32]. It is clear from the extensive array of functions outlined, and the mouse models illustrating the consequences of altered astrocyte proteins, that the role of these glial cells in the brain is highly complex and not yet fully understood. The typical response of astrocytes in common neurodegenerative diseases will be outlined in the following section.

Astrocytes: Typical Response in Neurodegenerative Diseases

Neurodegenerative diseases are characterized by the selective loss of neurons in vulnerable areas of the nervous system, resulting in clinical symptoms such as movement disorders and dementia [33]. The presence of abnormal protein aggregates in neurons and glial cells is a hallmark feature of many neurodegenerative diseases, which are collectively termed proteinopathies. Proteinopathies may be further divided on the basis of the major protein constituent of these inclusions. Tauopathies, including Alzheimer's disease, corticobasal degeneration, and progressive supranuclear palsy, are characterized by tau-positive inclusions [34]. Similarly, TDP-43 proteinopathies are characterized by inclusions composed of transactive response DNA-binding protein (TDP-43) and include the disorders amyotrophic lateral sclerosis and a subgroup of frontotemporal lobar degeneration with TDP-43 inclusions (FTLD-TDP-43) [35]. The focus of this chapter is Parkinson's disease, which is one of a group of disorders also including multiple system atrophy that are characterized by the deposition of α-synuclein protein and collectively referred to as synucleinopathies [36]. These disorders, regardless of whether they are characterized by tau-, TDP-43-, or α-synuclein-positive inclusions, show astrocytic gliosis in regions associated with degeneration, suggesting a typical astrocyte response to disease, with the exception of Parkinson's disease (see "Astrocytes: Role in Parkinson's Disease").

Alzheimer's disease is the most common cause of dementia and is characterized by two hallmark pathologies, tau-positive neurofibrillary tangles and β-amyloid (Aβ)-positive plaques [37]. Astrogliosis is a pathological feature of Alzheimer's disease, with activated astrocytes commonly observed in close proximity to hallmark Aβ plaque pathology (Fig. 2a) in postmortem brain tissue from patients with Alzheimer's disease [38–41]. There is also evidence that astrocytes may contribute to Aβ-induced neurotoxicity through altered glucose metabolism [42], by releasing proinflammatory substances and mediating neuronal tau phosphorylation [43]. In addition, a number of studies suggest that astrocytes, but not microglia, may be involved in the uptake of Aβ protein [44, 45]. Corticobasal degeneration and progressive supranuclear palsy, which clinically display variable disturbances in gait, balance, vision, and cognition, are also pathologically characterized by up-regulated astrocytes (see Fig. 2b, c) that correlate with the severity of neurodegeneration and disease stage [46]. Interestingly, in all three diseases some astrocytes accumulate abnormal tau protein [46–50]; however, the type of inclusion varies between diseases. GFAP-positive thorn-shaped astrocytes with cytoplasmic tau staining are observed in brain regions with up-regulated fibrous astrocytes in all

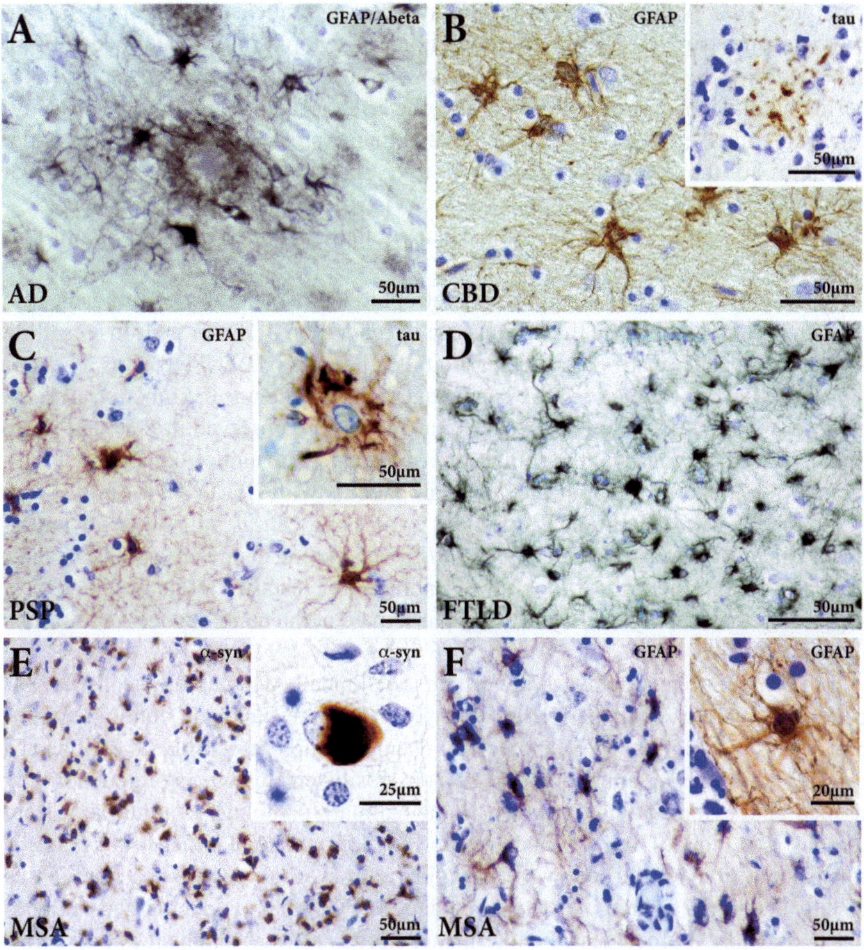

Fig. 2 Photomicrographs showing the typical astrocyte response in common neurodegenerative disorders. *α-syn* α-synuclein, *GFAP* glial fibrillary acidic protein. (**a**) Reactive GFAP-positive astrocytes around an Aβ plaque in Alzheimer's disease (AD) (double-labeling immunoperoxidase with GFAP in *black* and Aβ in *brown* and with cresyl violet counterstain). (**b**) Reactive GFAP-positive astrocytes in corticobasal degeneration (CBD) (immunoperoxidase with cresyl violet counterstain). Inset of tau-immunopositive astrocytic plaque in CBD (immunoperoxidase with cresyl violet counterstain). (**c**) Reactive GFAP-positive astrocytes in progressive supranuclear palsy (PSP) (immunoperoxidase with cresyl violet counterstain). Inset of tau-immunopositive tufted astrocyte in PSP (immunoperoxidase with cresyl violet counterstain). (**d**) Reactive GFAP-positive astrocytes in frontotemporal lobar degeneration (FTLD) (enhanced immunoperoxidase with cresyl violet counterstain). (**e**) Unlike in Parkinson's disease (see Fig. 3), α-synuclein does not accumulate in astrocytes in multiple system atrophy (MSA), but forms inclusions in oligodendroglia known as glial cytoplasmic inclusions (α-synuclein immunohistochemistry with cresyl violet counterstain). (**f**) Reactive GFAP-positive astrocytes in MSA (immunoperoxidase with cresyl violet counterstain)

three diseases [49]. However, in progressive supranuclear palsy gray matter protoplasmic astrocytes show accumulations of cytoplasmic tau termed tufts of abnormal fibers, while astrocytic plaques with tau-positive processes characterize corticobasal degeneration [49]. To assess the effect of tau pathology in astrocytes, transgenic mouse models have been created that express human tau protein under the control of the GFAP promoter. These mice show considerable accumulation of abnormal tau in astrocytes, blood–brain barrier disruption, and neuron degeneration [51], as well as loss of neuromuscular strength and altered expression of glutamate transporters [52].

Of the TDP-43 proteinopathies, amyotrophic lateral sclerosis or motor neuron disease is characterized by the progressive degeneration of motor neurons resulting in muscle weakness, atrophy, and spasticity [53], while FTLD-TDP-43 is a heterogeneous disorder characterized by language and/or behavior dysfunction [54]. In postmortem human brain tissue, reactive astrocytes are observed in gray and white matter cortical regions and the spinal cord of patients with amyotrophic lateral sclerosis [55–57] and throughout the cortex in patients with FTLD-TDP-43 [58] (see Fig. 2d). Interestingly, human astrocytes expressing causal mutations for amyotrophic lateral sclerosis in the enzyme Cu/Zn-superoxide dismutase (SOD1) confer toxicity to motor neurons through the generation of reactive oxygen species [59], suggesting that astrocytes may actively participate in the neurodegeneration of this disorder.

Finally, multiple system atrophy, which is a clinically and pathologically heterogeneous disease, is characterized by changes in executive and autonomic functions and usually a predominance of either parkinsonian symptoms (similar to Parkinson's disease) or cerebellar signs [60]. α-Synuclein-positive inclusions in oligodendroglia termed glial cytoplasmic inclusions are the hallmark pathology of multiple system atrophy (see Fig. 2e), but α-synuclein does not accumulate in either fibrous or protoplasmic astrocytes [46]. However, a typical astrocyte response is observed in this disease (see Fig. 2f), involving the upregulation of GFAP protein, enlarged cell bodies, and distorted processes of white matter fibrous astrocytes, changes that correlate with measures of neurodegeneration in this disease [46].

Although only discussed here briefly, astrocytes are clearly implicated throughout the progression of these common neurodegenerative diseases. Although these disorders are characterized by the accumulation of different proteins in variable cell types, they each exhibit a typical reactive astrocyte response to disease (see Fig. 2). In contrast, there is evidence that this response is very different in Parkinson's disease, and this will be discussed in the following section.

Astrocytes: Role in Parkinson's Disease

The role of astrocytes in Parkinson's disease is not well understood, mainly due to the limited number of studies that have been performed in the human disease and the discrepancies observed between these studies and those performed in animal models of the disease. As will be discussed in detail below, current evidence suggests that astrocytes are involved in the earliest stages of Parkinson's disease, where they accumulate α-synuclein in their cytoplasm, but do not undergo substantial reactive astrogliosis, making Parkinson's disease unique amongst most brain disorders, including other parkinsonian conditions (see "Astrocytes: Typical Response in Neurodegenerative Diseases").

The Role of Astrocytes in Animal Models of Parkinson's Disease

The majority of toxin-induced, inflammatory and genetic animal models of Parkinson's disease display varying degrees of astrocyte activation [61, 62]. However, there are two key issues that need to be considered with regard to the astrocyte response in animal models: (1) the accuracy of the model at recapitulating the pathological features of Parkinson's disease and (2) whether the results reflect those reported from studies using postmortem tissue from patients with Parkinson's disease. Nonetheless, assessing astrocytes in animal models of Parkinson's disease can provide important information, particularly relating to the timing of astrocyte involvement in Parkinson's disease that can be difficult to determine in human patients.

In humans there are two essential features required for a pathological diagnosis of Parkinson's disease, the severe loss of pigmented neurons in the substantia nigra and the presence of α-synuclein-positive inclusions in neuronal perikarya and axons known as Lewy bodies and Lewy neurites, respectively [63]. Common animal models of Parkinson's disease (such as those generated by the neurotoxins 1-Methyl-4-phenyl-1,2,3,6-tetrahydropyridine (MPTP), 6-Hydroxydopamine (6-OHDA), and rotenone and genetic models that overexpress human α-synuclein or express common mutations in the α-synuclein gene such as A53T) pathologically show a loss of nigral neurons; however only the rotenone-induced and α-synuclein genetic models also show cytoplasmic inclusion bodies resembling Lewy bodies [64, 65], potentially making these more accurate models of the pathological process occurring in Parkinson's disease.

While a number of different neurotoxins may be used to generate mouse models of Parkinson's disease (MPTP, 6-OHDA, rotenone), they all show dopaminergic cell death that is associated with oxidative stress and inflammation including, in most models, severe astrocyte and microglial activation and consequent production of toxic inflammatory mediators that contribute to cell death [62]. The treatment of astrocytes from these models with inhibitors for the various proinflammatory molecules secreted results in the downregulation of their expression and associated cell damage [62], suggesting that astrocyte upregulation is an important contributor to the pathogenesis of Parkinson's disease. However, it also important to consider whether such an acute insult resulting in the rapid activation of both microglia and astrocytes truly reflects the chronic nature of the human disease which develops over years, if not decades. In line with this, MPTP use in humans, while inducing a clinical phenotype similar to Parkinson's disease (levodopa-responsive parkinsonism) together with the loss of dopaminergic neurons in the substantia nigra, is associated with a significant glial response involving both astrocytes and microglia that is observed in patients with drug use ranging from 3 to 16 years [66]. However, many of these cases do not have substantial Lewy body formation [66], similar to the toxin-induced animal models and different from classic Parkinson's disease. In this aspect, it is interesting to note the effect different rotenone administration methods have on the astrocyte response in mice. A single unilateral infusion of rotenone in the medial forebrain bundle resulted in the loss of tyrosine hydroxylase neurons in the substantia nigra and fibers in the striatum and was accompanied by a significant glial reaction involving both astrocytes and microglia [67]. In contrast, mice undergoing chronic rotenone infusion every day for up to 4 weeks also showed selective degeneration of dopaminergic neurons, α-synuclein aggregates, severe microglial activation but only minimal if any upregulation of astrocytes [68], reflecting pathological observations in postmortem tissue from patients with Parkinson's disease (see the following section).

Since the discovery of mutations in the gene encoding α-synuclein, a number of mouse models have been developed that overexpress human α-synuclein or express common mutations in the α-synuclein gene [61]. Importantly, these mice (unlike the majority of toxin-induced models) show the abnormal accumulation of insoluble α-synuclein aggregates in neuronal cell bodies and processes, recapitulating the human Lewy pathology [61]. Astrogliosis is consistently observed in these models, but appears to occur early in the disease process, when there is minimal neuronal α-synuclein deposition and no significant neuronal loss [61, 69]. As will be discussed in more detail in the following section, studies in postmortem tissue from patients with Parkinson's disease reveal the accumulation of α-synuclein inclusions in gray matter protoplasmic astrocytes in Parkinson's disease [46, 70]. The suggestion is that astrocytes can take up altered α-synuclein released from axon terminals [70], and direct experiments confirm the transfer of α-synuclein from neurons to astrocytes [71]. It has been suggested that astrocytes may be neuroprotective in the earliest stages of Parkinson's disease, but over time with increasing exposure to toxic α-synuclein aggregates may lose their protective effect or might be aberrantly activated [61]. Supporting this, retracted astrocyte processes have been observed in postmortem brain tissue from patients with Parkinson's disease [72], and proliferating nonreactive astrocytes with sparse and significantly smaller processes have been identified in neurotoxin-induced models [73, 74]. A study in mice expressing A53T mutant α-synuclein directly addressed the question of the pathological consequences of selective astrocytic accumulation of α-synuclein and found that astrocytic α-synuclein initiates noncell autonomous killing of neurons, producing a rapidly progressive paralysis [75]. In these mice, there was increasing presymptomatic and symptomatic accumulation of α-synuclein aggregates and astrocyte dysregulation of the blood–brain barrier and glutamate transporters [75]. Similar accumulation of α-synuclein aggregates in astrocytes has been observed in transgenic mice with nonselective α-synuclein expression where astrocytes produced proinflammatory cytokines and chemokines [71]. These astrocytic changes led directly to microglial activation in the midbrain, brainstem, and spinal cord, where a significant loss of dopaminergic and motor neurons was observed [75]. Suppression of this subsequent microglial activity extended mice survival, suggesting that the excess microglial responses elicited by α-synuclein-containing astrocytes directly contribute to the degeneration of neurons [75].

Assessment of Astrocytes in Parkinson's Disease

As discussed in the preceding section, the typical response of astrocytes to tissue changes involves GFAP upregulation. Only a small number of studies have assessed the astrocyte response in brain tissue from patients with Parkinson's disease. While a variable increase in GFAP in select regions has been reported [76], most studies observe only minimal, if any, astrocyte activation [46, 77], in direct contrast to the severe astrogliosis observed in the majority of rodent models of Parkinson's disease (see preceding section). Song et al. assessed the number of GFAP-immunopositive cells in different parkinsonian conditions (Parkinson's disease, multiple system atrophy, corticobasal disease, and progressive supranuclear palsy) with classic reactive astrocytes reported in the gray matter regions examined (substantia nigra and putamen) in all diseases except Parkinson's disease [46]. Gray matter protoplasmic astrocytes did not display any morphological changes in Parkinson's disease (Fig. 3); however the astrocytes were abnormal with approximately 45 % displaying immunoreactivity for α-synuclein (see Fig. 3), with no obvious changes in white matter fibrous astrocytes [46]. The distribution of α-synuclein-immunoreactive protoplasmic astrocytes not only parallels the distribution of Lewy bodies but also occurs more broadly in regions without Lewy bodies (striatum, dorsal thalamus) where terminals are likely to be dysfunctional [70].

Protoplasmic astrocytes normally envelope all neurons and synapses, and astrocytes continue to do so around healthy neurons in Parkinson's disease [72]. However, in patients with Parkinson's disease, these protective protoplasmic astrocytic processes withdraw from around damaged neurons and are replaced by phagocytic microglia [72]. Astrocytes in other neurodegenerative conditions express growth factor receptors in response to microglial-secreted brain-derived growth factors with the downstream consequences of the perpetuation of neurodegeneration [78]. In contrast, in Alzheimer's disease protoplasmic astrocytes themselves produce brain-derived growth factors following their contact with β-amyloid, and the astrocytic production of this growth factor has been shown to rescue neurons from β-amyloid toxicity [79]. Although speculative, the abnormal accumulation of α-synuclein in protoplasmic astrocytes may impact on their ability to produce brain-derived growth factors in the same manner (note this abnormality has been recently described for astrocytes abnormally accumulating huntingtin [80]). This could assist with explaining the marked difference in the reactivity of the protoplasmic astrocytes in Parkinson's disease versus similar neurodegenerative conditions and the loss of their primary protective function in this disease.

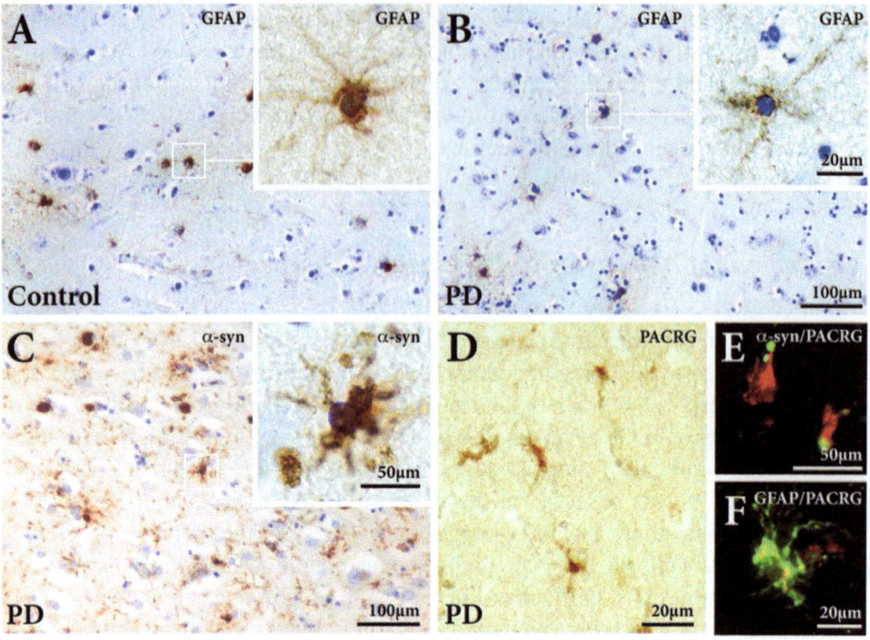

Fig. 3 Photomicrographs showing the unique astrocyte response in Parkinson's disease (PD). *α-syn* α-synuclein, *GFAP* glial fibrillary acidic protein, *PACRG* parkin-coregulated gene protein. (**a**) GFAP-immunoreactive protoplasmic astrocytes in healthy brain tissue (immunoperoxidase with cresyl violet counterstain). (**b**) GFAP-immunoreactive protoplasmic astrocytes in PD show minimal, if any, upregulation of GFAP compared to controls (**a**) (immunoperoxidase with cresyl violet counterstain). *Scale bars* in (**b**) are equivalent for (**a**). (**c, d**) Protoplasmic astrocytes in PD accumulate α-synuclein in the cytoplasm (**c**) (immunoperoxidase with cresyl violet counterstain) and show constitutive, but not increased expression of PACRG (**d**) (immunoperoxidase). (**e, f**) Double-labeling immunofluorescence shows the co-localization of α-synuclein (*green*) with PACRG (*red*) in the same astrocytes in patients with PD, with PACRG-immunopositive protoplasmic astrocytes (*red*) also expressing GFAP (*green, overlap seen as yellow*)

In addition to these observed structural alterations in astrocytes, identifying any changes in other constituent proteins could assist with understanding the role of protoplasmic astrocytes in the etiology of Parkinson's disease. Increased levels of S100B, an astrocytic calcium-binding protein shown to cause neuronal death directly or through microglial activation [81–83], have been found in the substantia nigra and cerebrospinal fluid of patients with Parkinson's disease and in MPTP mice [84]. S100B knockout mice show reduced numbers of activated microglia and expression of molecules including the proinflammatory cytokine tumor necrosis factor-α [84]. Furthermore, in the human brain, protoplasmic astrocytes express most of the recessive gene products involved in Parkinson's disease (PINK-1, parkin, and DJ-1) [85–88], and their production is usually increased in association with astrogliosis in disease states [46, 85, 86, 88, 89]. In particular, protoplasmic but not fibrous astrocytes constitutively express *parkin-coregulated gene* (PACRG) (see Fig. 3), which has the same promoter as the *parkin gene* and is upregulated with parkin in neurodegenerative conditions other than Parkinson's disease [46]. Genetic alterations in the *parkin-coregulated gene* have also been identified in early-onset recessive cases of Parkinson's disease [90]. It is of interest that these proteins are not up-regulated in astrocytes in Parkinson's disease [46, 85, 86] providing further evidence to suggest a dramatically different response to the α-synuclein protein accumulation and degeneration that occurs in this disease.

All astrocytes from parkin knockout mice exhibit damaged mitochondria (disintegration and reduction of mitochondrial cristae, mitochondrial enlargement, and formation of protrusions or even disruption of the outer membrane) from 3 months of age, although some even have damage at 16 days [91]. Similarly, astrocytes from PINK-1 knockout mice have mitochondrial defects (decreased mitochondrial mass and membrane potential, increased levels of intracellular reactive oxygen species, decreased glucose-uptake capacity, and decreased ATP production) [92]. Of interest, PINK-1-deficient astrocytes are incapable of wound healing [92], similar to astrocytes in the brain of patients with Parkinson's disease, and DJ-1-deficient astrocytes have a neurotoxic effect by enhancing brain inflammation [93–95]. DJ-1 knockout astrocytes show increased expression of proinflammatory substances [95] including cyclooxygenase-2 and interleukin-6, have reduced capacity to support neuronal cells resulting in neuronal death or damage [93], and are less able to mount a protective response against oxidative stress induced by the neurotoxin 6-OHDA [94], effects that could be due to defective mitochondria. Of interest, similar astrocytic mitochondrial defects are also observed in transgenic mice where α-synuclein is overexpressed only in neurons as well as in transgenic mice where α-synuclein is expressed in astrocytes and other glia [92]. The uptake of α-synuclein into human astrocytes impairs their mitochondria leading to cell degeneration and death [96]. Furthermore, mitochondrial uncoupling proteins (UCP) (which dissociate ATP synthesis from oxygen consumption in mitochondria and suppress free-radical production) are reduced in astrocytes resulting in endoplasmic reticulum stress and neuroinflammation [97], and changes in UCP proteins are associated with the causal mutations for Parkinson's disease in both DJ-1 [98] and LRRK2 [99]. While speculative, it appears that the loss of function of these Parkinson's disease-associated proteins in astrocytes precipitates early mitochondrial defects that are likely to have significant consequences for both normal astrocytic and neuronal functions.

The recessive gene products constitutively expressed by astrocytes (PINK-1, parkin, and DJ-1) are also found in Lewy bodies [85, 86, 100–102], providing additional evidence for a role of astrocytes in Parkinson's disease. Furthermore, astrocyte-concentrating proteins such as Pael-R (substrate for Parkin) [102], DnaJ/Hsp40 homologue, subfamily B, member 6 (DnaJB6) [103], and nonselenium glutathione peroxidase [104] are found in the cores of Lewy bodies, suggesting astrocyte involvement at the earliest disease stages. Interestingly, a number of these proteins are also found to be up-regulated in astrocytes in patients with Parkinson's disease. DnaJB6, a molecular chaperone with an important role in the maintenance of normal cellular functions, has been shown to be up-regulated in astrocytes in both the substantia nigra and frontal cortex [103], possibly in an attempt to prevent or suppress α-synuclein accumulation in a manner similar to that described for huntingtin in Huntington's disease [105]. Similarly, the metal-binding proteins metallothioneins, which are associated with neuroprotection, show a variable increase in substantia nigra astrocytes [106], possibly in response to mitochondrial oxidative stress [107]. Finally, increased expression of the antioxidant enzyme non-selenium glutathione peroxidase is observed predominantly in the unaffected white matter astrocytes but also in gray matter astrocytes in the frontal cortex and cingulate cortex of patients with Parkinson's disease [104]. In contrast, no significant immunoreactivity for this enzyme is observed in substantia nigra astrocytes [104], and reduced levels of glutathione (an enzyme that protects against protein oxidation) are reported in the substantia nigra of patients with Parkinson's disease [108], again supporting the evidence that protoplasmic astrocytes are unable to maintain their normal protective functions in regions highly affected by degeneration in Parkinson's disease.

Of major interest is the recent study examining how L-DOPA, the most commonly used dopamine replacement therapy for Parkinson's disease [109], enters the brain, particularly as astrocyte end feet surround brain blood vessels [110]. This study showed that L-DOPA accumulates mainly in astrocyte cell bodies, astrocytic end feet surrounding blood vessels, and pericytes and that the pattern of monoamine oxidase type B staining (enzyme that catabolizes L-DOPA to dopamine) in pericytes and astrocytic end feet was similar to that of L-DOPA [110]. The study concluded that astrocytes control L-DOPA uptake and metabolism and, therefore, play a key role in regulating brain dopamine levels during dopamine-associated diseases [110]. If this is applicable to human astrocytes, then any astrocytic dysregulation, as discussed above, would have consequences for the long-term success of dopamine replacement therapies, and dysfunction of astrocytes in Parkinson's disease could underlie difficulties with dopamine medication use over time.

Conclusion

The astrocyte response in Parkinson's disease is clearly unique from most neurodegenerative conditions, including other parkinsonian disorders. Instead of a typical reactive astrogliosis, protoplasmic astrocytes in Parkinson's disease accumulate α-synuclein, withdraw their processes from around damaged neurons, and show altered expression of constituent proteins, suggesting that they have reduced neuronal support and protection capabilities, particularly in regions associated with significant degeneration. In contrast, the majority of work in rodent models of Parkinson's disease has reported severe astrogliosis occurring in the brain. This combined with the link between dopamine replacement medication and astrocytes highlights the need for a greater understanding of the role of these glial cells in the human disease.

References

1. Oberheim NA, Takano T, Han X, He W, Lin JH, Wang F, et al. Uniquely hominid features of adult human astrocytes. J Neurosci. 2009;29:3276–87.
2. Sofroniew MV, Vinters HV. Astrocytes: biology and pathology. Acta Neuropathol. 2010; 119:7–35.
3. Lecrux C, Hamel E. The neurovascular unit in brain function and disease. Acta Physiol (Oxf). 2011;203:47–59.
4. Rossi D, Martorana F, Brambilla L. Implications of gliotransmission for the pharmacotherapy of CNS disorders. CNS Drugs. 2011;25:641–58.
5. Gordon GR, Mulligan SJ, MacVicar BA. Astrocyte control of the cerebrovasculature. Glia. 2007;55:1214–21.
6. Iadecola C, Nedergaard M. Glial regulation of the cerebral microvasculature. Nat Neurosci. 2007;10:1369–76.
7. Iacovetta C, Rudloff E, Kirby R. The role of aquaporin 4 in the brain. Vet Clin Pathol. 2012; 41:32–44.
8. Jung JS, Bhat RV, Preston GM, Guggino WB, Baraban JM, Agre P. Molecular characterization of an aquaporin cDNA from brain: candidate osmoreceptor and regulator of water balance. Proc Natl Acad Sci U S A. 1994;91:13052–6.
9. Jin BJ, Zhang H, Binder DK, Verkman AS. Aquaporin-4-dependent K(+) and water transport modeled in brain extracellular space following neuroexcitation. J Gen Physiol. 2013;141: 119–32.
10. Song H, Stevens CF, Gage FH. Astroglia induce neurogenesis from adult neural stem cells. Nature. 2002;417:39–44.
11. Lie DC, Colamarino SA, Song HJ, Desire L, Mira H, Consiglio A, et al. Wnt signalling regulates adult hippocampal neurogenesis. Nature. 2005;437:1370–5.
12. Barkho BZ, Song H, Aimone JB, Smrt RD, Kuwabara T, Nakashima K, et al. Identification of astrocyte-expressed factors that modulate neural stem/progenitor cell differentiation. Stem Cells Dev. 2006;15:407–21.
13. Stevens B. Neuron-astrocyte signaling in the development and plasticity of neural circuits. Neurosignals. 2008;16:278–88.
14. Ullian EM, Sapperstein SK, Christopherson KS, Barres BA. Control of synapse number by glia. Science. 2001;291:657–61.
15. Nagler K, Mauch DH, Pfrieger FW. Glia-derived signals induce synapse formation in neurones of the rat central nervous system. J Physiol. 2001;533:665–79.
16. Liauw J, Hoang S, Choi M, Eroglu C, Choi M, Sun GH, et al. Thrombospondins 1 and 2 are necessary for synaptic plasticity and functional recovery after stroke. J Cereb Blood Flow Metab. 2008;28:1722–32.
17. Risher WC, Eroglu C. Thrombospondins as key regulators of synaptogenesis in the central nervous system. Matrix Biol. 2012;31:170–7.
18. Christopherson KS, Ullian EM, Stokes CC, Mullowney CE, Hell JW, Agah A, et al. Thrombospondins are astrocyte-secreted proteins that promote CNS synaptogenesis. Cell. 2005;120:421–33.
19. Mauch DH, Nagler K, Schumacher S, Goritz C, Muller EC, Otto A, et al. CNS synaptogenesis promoted by glia-derived cholesterol. Science. 2001;294:1354–7.
20. Stevens B, Allen NJ, Vazquez LE, Howell GR, Christopherson KS, Nouri N, et al. The classical complement cascade mediates CNS synapse elimination. Cell. 2007;131:1164–78.
21. Iino M, Goto K, Kakegawa W, Okado H, Sudo M, Ishiuchi S, et al. Glia-synapse interaction through Ca^{2+}-permeable AMPA receptors in Bergmann glia. Science. 2001;292:926–9.
22. Oliet SH, Piet R, Poulain DA. Control of glutamate clearance and synaptic efficacy by glial coverage of neurons. Science. 2001;292:923–6.
23. Smit AB, Syed NI, Schaap D, van Minnen J, Klumperman J, Kits KS, et al. A glia-derived acetylcholine-binding protein that modulates synaptic transmission. Nature. 2001;411:261–8.

24. Becker K. Innate and adaptive immune responses in CNS disease. Clin Neurosci Res. 2006;6:227–36.
25. Farina C, Aloisi F, Meinl E. Astrocytes are active players in cerebral innate immunity. Trends Immunol. 2007;28:138–45.
26. Maragakis NJ, Rothstein JD. Mechanisms of disease: astrocytes in neurodegenerative disease. Nat Clin Pract Neurol. 2006;2:679–89.
27. Wilhelmsson U, Li L, Pekna M, Berthold CH, Blom S, Eliasson C, et al. Absence of glial fibrillary acidic protein and vimentin prevents hypertrophy of astrocytic processes and improves post-traumatic regeneration. J Neurosci. 2004;24:5016–21.
28. Menet V, Prieto M, Privat A, Gimenez y Ribotta M. Axonal plasticity and functional recovery after spinal cord injury in mice deficient in both glial fibrillary acidic protein and vimentin genes. Proc Natl Acad Sci U S A. 2003;100:8999–9004.
29. Kinouchi R, Takeda M, Yang L, Wilhelmsson U, Lundkvist A, Pekny M, et al. Robust neural integration from retinal transplants in mice deficient in GFAP and vimentin. Nat Neurosci. 2003;6:863–8.
30. Widestrand A, Faijerson J, Wilhelmsson U, Smith PL, Li L, Sihlbom C, et al. Increased neurogenesis and astrogenesis from neural progenitor cells grafted in the hippocampus of GFAP–/– Vim–/– mice. Stem Cells. 2007;25:2619–27.
31. Eng LF, Lee YL, Kwan H, Brenner M, Messing A. Astrocytes cultured from transgenic mice carrying the added human glial fibrillary acidic protein gene contain Rosenthal fibers. J Neurosci Res. 1998;53:353–60.
32. Tanaka K, Watase K, Manabe T, Yamada K, Watanabe M, Takahashi K, et al. Epilepsy and exacerbation of brain injury in mice lacking the glutamate transporter GLT-1. Science. 1997;276:1699–702.
33. Double KL, Reyes S, Werry EL, Halliday GM. Selective cell death in neurodegeneration: why are some neurons spared in vulnerable regions? Prog Neurobiol. 2010;92:316–29.
34. Tolnay M, Probst A. The neuropathological spectrum of neurodegenerative tauopathies. IUBMB Life. 2003;55:299–305.
35. Kwong LK, Uryu K, Trojanowski JQ, Lee VM. TDP-43 proteinopathies: neurodegenerative protein misfolding diseases without amyloidosis. Neurosignals. 2008;16:41–51.
36. Jellinger KA. Neuropathological spectrum of synucleinopathies. Mov Disord. 2003;18 Suppl 6:S2–12.
37. Selkoe DJ. Alzheimer's disease: genes, proteins, and therapy. Physiol Rev. 2001;81:741–66.
38. Beach TG, McGeer EG. Lamina-specific arrangement of astrocytic gliosis and senile plaques in Alzheimer's disease visual cortex. Brain Res. 1988;463:357–61.
39. Griffin WS, Stanley LC, Ling C, White L, MacLeod V, Perrot LJ, et al. Brain interleukin 1 and S-100 immunoreactivity are elevated in down syndrome and Alzheimer disease. Proc Natl Acad Sci U S A. 1989;86:7611–5.
40. Kashon ML, Ross GW, O'Callaghan JP, Miller DB, Petrovitch H, Burchfiel CM, et al. Associations of cortical astrogliosis with cognitive performance and dementia status. J Alzheimers Dis. 2004;6:595–604. discussion 73–81.
41. Wisniewski HM, Wegiel J. Spatial relationships between astrocytes and classical plaque components. Neurobiol Aging. 1991;12:593–600.
42. Allaman I, Gavillet M, Belanger M, Laroche T, Viertl D, Lashuel HA, et al. Amyloid-beta aggregates cause alterations of astrocytic metabolic phenotype: impact on neuronal viability. J Neurosci. 2010;30:3326–38.
43. Garwood CJ, Pooler AM, Atherton J, Hanger DP, Noble W. Astrocytes are important mediators of Abeta-induced neurotoxicity and tau phosphorylation in primary culture. Cell Death Dis. 2011;2:e167.
44. Matsunaga W, Shirokawa T, Isobe K. Specific uptake of Abeta1-40 in rat brain occurs in astrocyte, but not in microglia. Neurosci Lett. 2003;342:129–31.
45. Funato H, Yoshimura M, Yamazaki T, Saido TC, Ito Y, Yokofujita J, et al. Astrocytes containing amyloid beta-protein (Abeta)-positive granules are associated with Abeta40-positive diffuse plaques in the aged human brain. Am J Pathol. 1998;152:983–92.

46. Song YJ, Halliday GM, Holton JL, Lashley T, O'Sullivan SS, McCann H, et al. Degeneration in different parkinsonian syndromes relates to astrocyte type and astrocyte protein expression. J Neuropathol Exp Neurol. 2009;68:1073–83.
47. Dickson DW, Ksiezak-Reding H, Liu WK, Davies P, Crowe A, Yen SH. Immunocytochemistry of neurofibrillary tangles with antibodies to subregions of tau protein: identification of hidden and cleaved tau epitopes and a new phosphorylation site. Acta Neuropathol. 1992;84: 596–605.
48. Papasozomenos SC, Binder LI. Phosphorylation determines two distinct species of tau in the central nervous system. Cell Motil Cytoskeleton. 1987;8:210–26.
49. Komori T. Tau-positive glial inclusions in progressive supranuclear palsy, corticobasal degeneration and Pick's disease. Brain Pathol. 1999;9:663–79.
50. Ikeda K, Akiyama H, Arai T, Nishimura T. Glial tau pathology in neurodegenerative diseases: their nature and comparison with neuronal tangles. Neurobiol Aging. 1998;19:S85–91.
51. Forman MS, Lal D, Zhang B, Dabir DV, Swanson E, Lee VM, et al. Transgenic mouse model of tau pathology in astrocytes leading to nervous system degeneration. J Neurosci. 2005;25:3539–50.
52. Dabir DV, Robinson MB, Swanson E, Zhang B, Trojanowski JQ, Lee VM, et al. Impaired glutamate transport in a mouse model of tau pathology in astrocytes. J Neurosci. 2006;26: 644–54.
53. Gordon PH. Amyotrophic lateral sclerosis: an update for 2013 clinical features, pathophysiology, management and therapeutic trials. Aging Dis. 2013;4:295–310.
54. Warren JD, Rohrer JD, Rossor MN. Clinical review. Frontotemporal dementia. BMJ. 2013;347:f4827.
55. Kushner PD, Stephenson DT, Wright S. Reactive astrogliosis is widespread in the subcortical white matter of amyotrophic lateral sclerosis brain. J Neuropathol Exp Neurol. 1991;50: 263–77.
56. Nagy D, Kato T, Kushner PD. Reactive astrocytes are widespread in the cortical gray matter of amyotrophic lateral sclerosis. J Neurosci Res. 1994;38:336–47.
57. Schiffer D, Cordera S, Cavalla P, Migheli A. Reactive astrogliosis of the spinal cord in amyotrophic lateral sclerosis. J Neurol Sci. 1996;139(Suppl):27–33.
58. Lin WL, Castanedes-Casey M, Dickson DW. Transactivation response DNA-binding protein 43 microvasculopathy in frontotemporal degeneration and familial Lewy body disease. J Neuropathol Exp Neurol. 2009;68:1167–76.
59. Marchetto MC, Muotri AR, Mu Y, Smith AM, Cezar GG, Gage FH. Non-cell-autonomous effect of human SOD1 G37R astrocytes on motor neurons derived from human embryonic stem cells. Cell Stem Cell. 2008;3:649–57.
60. Gilman S, Wenning GK, Low PA, Brooks DJ, Mathias CJ, Trojanowski JQ, et al. Second consensus statement on the diagnosis of multiple system atrophy. Neurology. 2008;71: 670–6.
61. Sekiyama K, Sugama S, Fujita M, Sekigawa A, Takamatsu Y, Waragai M, et al. Neuroinflammation in Parkinson's disease and related disorders: a lesson from genetically manipulated mouse models of alpha-synucleinopathies. Parkinsons Dis. 2012;2012:271732.
62. Niranjan R. The role of inflammatory and oxidative stress mechanisms in the pathogenesis of Parkinson's disease: focus on astrocytes. Mol Neurobiol. 2014;49(1):28–38.
63. Gelb DJ, Oliver E, Gilman S. Diagnostic criteria for Parkinson disease. Arch Neurol. 1999;56:33–9.
64. Betarbet R, Sherer TB, Greenamyre JT. Animal models of Parkinson's disease. Bioessays. 2002;24:308–18.
65. Schober A. Classic toxin-induced animal models of Parkinson's disease: 6-OHDA and MPTP. Cell Tissue Res. 2004;318:215–24.
66. Langston JW, Forno LS, Tetrud J, Reeves AG, Kaplan JA, Karluk D. Evidence of active nerve cell degeneration in the substantia nigra of humans years after 1-methyl-4-phenyl-1,2,3,6-tetrahydropyridine exposure. Ann Neurol. 1999;46:598–605.

67. Norazit A, Meedeniya AC, Nguyen MN, Mackay-Sim A. Progressive loss of dopaminergic neurons induced by unilateral rotenone infusion into the medial forebrain bundle. Brain Res. 2010;1360:119–29.
68. Sherer TB, Betarbet R, Kim JH, Greenamyre JT. Selective microglial activation in the rat rotenone model of Parkinson's disease. Neurosci Lett. 2003;341:87–90.
69. Halliday GM, Stevens CH. Glia: initiators and progressors of pathology in Parkinson's disease. Mov Disord. 2011;26:6–17.
70. Braak H, Sastre M, Del Tredici K. Development of alpha-synuclein immunoreactive astrocytes in the forebrain parallels stages of intraneuronal pathology in sporadic Parkinson's disease. Acta Neuropathol. 2007;114:231–41.
71. Lee HJ, Suk JE, Patrick C, Bae EJ, Cho JH, Rho S, et al. Direct transfer of alpha-synuclein from neuron to astroglia causes inflammatory responses in synucleinopathies. J Biol Chem. 2010;285:9262–72.
72. Knott C, Wilkin GP, Stern G. Astrocytes and microglia in the substantia nigra and caudate-putamen in Parkinson's disease. Parkinsonism Relat Disord. 1999;5:115–22.
73. Nomura T, Yabe T, Rosenthal ES, Krzan M, Schwartz JP. PSA-NCAM distinguishes reactive astrocytes in 6-OHDA-lesioned substantia nigra from those in the striatal terminal fields. J Neurosci Res. 2000;61:588–96.
74. Wachter B, Schurger S, Rolinger J, von Ameln-Mayerhofer A, Berg D, Wagner HJ, et al. Effect of 6-hydroxydopamine (6-OHDA) on proliferation of glial cells in the rat cortex and striatum: evidence for de-differentiation of resident astrocytes. Cell Tissue Res. 2010; 342:147–60.
75. Gu XL, Long CX, Sun L, Xie C, Lin X, Cai H. Astrocytic expression of Parkinson's disease-related A53T alpha-synuclein causes neurodegeneration in mice. Mol Brain. 2010;3:12.
76. Mythri RB, Venkateshappa C, Harish G, Mahadevan A, Muthane UB, Yasha TC, et al. Evaluation of markers of oxidative stress, antioxidant function and astrocytic proliferation in the striatum and frontal cortex of Parkinson's disease brains. Neurochem Res. 2011;36: 1452–63.
77. Mirza B, Hadberg H, Thomsen P, Moos T. The absence of reactive astrogliosis is indicative of a unique inflammatory process in Parkinson's disease. Neuroscience. 2000;95:425–32.
78. Colombo E, Cordiglieri C, Melli G, Newcombe J, Krumbholz M, Parada LF, et al. Stimulation of the neurotrophin receptor TrkB on astrocytes drives nitric oxide production and neurodegeneration. J Exp Med. 2012;209:521–35.
79. Kimura N, Takahashi M, Tashiro T, Terao K. Amyloid beta up-regulates brain-derived neurotrophic factor production from astrocytes: rescue from amyloid beta-related neuritic degeneration. J Neurosci Res. 2006;84:782–9.
80. Wang L, Lin F, Wang J, Wu J, Han R, Zhu L, et al. Truncated N-terminal huntingtin fragment with expanded-polyglutamine (htt552-100Q) suppresses brain-derived neurotrophic factor transcription in astrocytes. Acta Biochim Biophys Sin (Shanghai). 2012;44:249–58.
81. Hu J, Ferreira A, Van Eldik LJ. S100beta induces neuronal cell death through nitric oxide release from astrocytes. J Neurochem. 1997;69:2294–301.
82. Li Y, Barger SW, Liu L, Mrak RE, Griffin WS. S100beta induction of the proinflammatory cytokine interleukin-6 in neurons. J Neurochem. 2000;74:143–50.
83. Sorci G, Bianchi R, Riuzzi F, Tubaro C, Arcuri C, Giambanco I, et al. S100B protein, a damage-associated molecular pattern protein in the brain and heart, and beyond. Cardiovasc Psychiatry Neurol. 2010;2010.
84. Sathe K, Maetzler W, Lang JD, Mounsey RB, Fleckenstein C, Martin HL, et al. S100B is increased in Parkinson's disease and ablation protects against MPTP-induced toxicity through the RAGE and TNF-alpha pathway. Brain. 2012;135:3336–47.
85. Gandhi S, Muqit MM, Stanyer L, Healy DG, Abou-Sleiman PM, Hargreaves I, et al. PINK1 protein in normal human brain and Parkinson's disease. Brain. 2006;129:1720–31.
86. Bandopadhyay R, Kingsbury AE, Cookson MR, Reid AR, Evans IM, Hope AD, et al. The expression of DJ-1 (PARK7) in normal human CNS and idiopathic Parkinson's disease. Brain. 2004;127:420–30.

87. Zarate-Lagunes M, Gu WJ, Blanchard V, Francois C, Muriel MP, Mouatt-Prigent A, et al. Parkin immunoreactivity in the brain of human and non-human primates: an immunohistochemical analysis in normal conditions and in Parkinsonian syndromes. J Comp Neurol. 2001;432:184–96.
88. Ledesma MD, Galvan C, Hellias B, Dotti C, Jensen PH. Astrocytic but not neuronal increased expression and redistribution of parkin during unfolded protein stress. J Neurochem. 2002; 83:1431–40.
89. Mullett SJ, Hamilton RL, Hinkle DA. DJ-1 immunoreactivity in human brain astrocytes is dependent on infarct presence and infarct age. Neuropathology. 2009;29:125–31.
90. Taylor JM, Wu RM, Farrer MJ, Delatycki MB, Lockhart PJ. Analysis of PArkin co-regulated gene in a Taiwanese-ethnic Chinese cohort with early-onset Parkinson's disease. Parkinsonism Relat Disord. 2009;15:417–21.
91. Schmidt S, Linnartz B, Mendritzki S, Sczepan T, Lubbert M, Stichel CC, et al. Genetic mouse models for Parkinson's disease display severe pathology in glial cell mitochondria. Hum Mol Genet. 2011;20:1197–211.
92. Choi I, Kim J, Jeong HK, Kim B, Jou I, Park SM, et al. PINK1 deficiency attenuates astrocyte proliferation through mitochondrial dysfunction, reduced AKT and increased p38 MAPK activation, and downregulation of EGFR. Glia. 2013;61:800–12.
93. Waak J, Weber SS, Waldenmaier A, Gorner K, Alunni-Fabbroni M, Schell H, et al. Regulation of astrocyte inflammatory responses by the Parkinson's disease-associated gene DJ-1. FASEB J. 2009;23:2478–89.
94. Lev N, Barhum Y, Ben-Zur T, Melamed E, Steiner I, Offen D. Knocking out DJ-1 attenuates astrocytes neuroprotection against 6-hydroxydopamine toxicity. J Mol Neurosci. 2013; 50:542–50.
95. Kim JH, Choi DJ, Jeong HK, Kim J, Kim DW, Choi SY, et al. DJ-1 facilitates the interaction between STAT1 and its phosphatase, SHP-1, in brain microglia and astrocytes: a novel anti-inflammatory function of DJ-1. Neurobiol Dis. 2013;60:1–10.
96. Braidy N, Gai WP, Xu YH, Sachdev P, Guillemin GJ, Jiang XM, et al. Uptake and mitochondrial dysfunction of alpha-synuclein in human astrocytes, cortical neurons and fibroblasts. Transl Neurodegener. 2013;2:20.
97. Lu M, Sun XL, Qiao C, Liu Y, Ding JH, Hu G. Uncoupling protein 2 deficiency aggravates astrocytic endoplasmic reticulum stress and nod-like receptor protein 3 inflammasome activation. Neurobiol Aging. 2014;35(2):421–30.
98. Inden M, Kitamura Y, Takahashi K, Takata K, Ito N, Niwa R, et al. Protection against dopaminergic neurodegeneration in Parkinson's disease-model animals by a modulator of the oxidized form of DJ-1, a wild-type of familial Parkinson's disease-linked PARK7. J Pharmacol Sci. 2011;117:189–203.
99. Papkovskaia TD, Chau KY, Inesta-Vaquera F, Papkovsky DB, Healy DG, Nishio K, et al. G2019S leucine-rich repeat kinase 2 causes uncoupling protein-mediated mitochondrial depolarization. Hum Mol Genet. 2012;21:4201–13.
100. Jin J, Meredith GE, Chen L, Zhou Y, Xu J, Shie FS, et al. Quantitative proteomic analysis of mitochondrial proteins: relevance to Lewy body formation and Parkinson's disease. Brain Res Mol Brain Res. 2005;134:119–38.
101. Schlossmacher MG, Frosch MP, Gai WP, Medina M, Sharma N, Forno L, et al. Parkin localizes to the Lewy bodies of Parkinson disease and dementia with Lewy bodies. Am J Pathol. 2002;160:1655–67.
102. Murakami T, Shoji M, Imai Y, Inoue H, Kawarabayashi T, Matsubara E, et al. Pael-R is accumulated in Lewy bodies of Parkinson's disease. Ann Neurol. 2004;55:439–42.
103. Durrenberger PF, Filiou MD, Moran LB, Michael GJ, Novoselov S, Cheetham ME, et al. DnaJB6 is present in the core of Lewy bodies and is highly up-regulated in parkinsonian astrocytes. J Neurosci Res. 2009;87:238–45.
104. Power JH, Shannon JM, Blumbergs PC, Gai WP. Nonselenium glutathione peroxidase in human brain: elevated levels in Parkinson's disease and dementia with Lewy bodies. Am J Pathol. 2002;161:885–94.

105. Chuang JZ, Zhou H, Zhu M, Li SH, Li XJ, Sung CH. Characterization of a brain-enriched chaperone, MRJ, that inhibits Huntingtin aggregation and toxicity independently. J Biol Chem. 2002;277:19831–8.
106. Michael GJ, Esmailzadeh S, Moran LB, Christian L, Pearce RK, Graeber MB. Up-regulation of metallothionein gene expression in parkinsonian astrocytes. Neurogenetics. 2011;12: 295–305.
107. Futakawa N, Kondoh M, Ueda S, Higashimoto M, Takiguchi M, Suzuki S, et al. Involvement of oxidative stress in the synthesis of metallothionein induced by mitochondrial inhibitors. Biol Pharm Bull. 2006;29:2016–20.
108. Sian J, Dexter DT, Lees AJ, Daniel S, Agid Y, Javoy-Agid F, et al. Alterations in glutathione levels in Parkinson's disease and other neurodegenerative disorders affecting basal ganglia. Ann Neurol. 1994;36:348–55.
109. Fernandez HH. Updates in the medical management of Parkinson disease. Cleve Clin J Med. 2012;79:28–35.
110. Inyushin MY, Huertas A, Kucheryavykh YV, Kucheryavykh LY, Tsydzik V, Sanabria P, et al. L-DOPA uptake in astrocytic endfeet enwrapping blood vessels in rat brain. Parkinsons Dis. 2012;2012:321406.

Proinflammatory Chemical Signaling: Cytokines

Kumi Nagamoto-Combs and Colin K. Combs

Microglial Activation in Parkinson's Disease

For several decades, reactive microglia have been known to be associated with the histological changes that occur in Parkinson's disease brains. Stemming from an initial report of HLA-DR immunoreactive microglia in the substantia nigra of Parkinson's disease patient brains [1], multiple subsequent studies performed from autopsy brains have verified with a range of immunomarkers that microgliosis is a characteristic of diseased brains in not only the pars compacta region of the nigra but also the striatum, hippocampus, and various cortical areas [1–6]. Although microglial numbers are reportedly higher in the nigra than other brain regions [1, 7, 8] and some age-associated nigral microgliosis has been reported [9], it is generally assumed that some form of disease-relevant stimulus is still involved in driving microglia to acquire a particular reactive phenotype that contributes to neuron loss during disease.

Unfortunately, histologic data from autopsy brains does not allow for temporal assessment of microglial activation during disease course. Therefore, in spite of the convincing histologic evidence of microgliosis, a lingering question is whether or not microglial-mediated inflammatory changes contribute or simply respond to neuron death. It is clear that the degree of reactive microgliosis is increased proportionally to the degree of dopaminergic cell loss in the nigra. However, their activation state appears to be independent of the amount of Lewy bodies present [4]. In vivo imaging of microglia during disease using the positron emission tomography

K. Nagamoto-Combs, Ph.D. • C.K. Combs, Ph.D. (✉)
Department of Basic Sciences, University of North Dakota School of Medicine and Health Sciences, Grand Forks, ND, USA
e-mail: colin.combs@med.und.edu

M. Thomas (ed.), *Inflammation in Parkinson's Disease: Scientific and Clinical Aspects*,
DOI 10.1007/978-3-319-08046-8_6,

marker, [^{11}C](R)-PK11195, has demonstrated in a small study of 18 Parkinson's disease patients and 11 healthy, age-matched controls that levels of microglial activation in diseased brains were elevated in the basal ganglia, cerebral cortex, and brainstem compared to controls [10]. Longitudinal comparison in eight of these Parkinson's disease patients indicated that levels of reactive microgliosis remained stable over a 2-year period with no correlation with clinical severity [10]. The authors concluded from their findings that microglial activation may occur early in disease and simply remain, perhaps with altered phenotypes, for years [10]. On the other hand, additional in vivo imaging using [^{11}C](R)-PK11195 in ten early-stage Parkinson's disease patients and ten healthy, age-matched controls with a 4-year follow-up for four patients in each group demonstrated increased midbrain microgliosis in diseased brains that spread throughout the brain in correlation with loss of dopaminergic transporter density in the putamen and increased motor symptom severity [11]. As stated prior, it appears that the precise role of microglial activation in the ongoing process of dopaminergic cell loss in Parkinson's disease is still unclear.

Nevertheless, data from a variety of models of disease continue to support the notion that microgliosis may be something more than a reaction to cell death. The 1-methyl-4-phenyl-1,2,3,6-tetrahydropyridine (MPTP) toxin-induced model of Parkinson's disease provides support for a prolonged microglial-mediated inflammatory process during disease. Microgliosis is apparently maintained for years based upon data derived from MPTP-treated rhesus monkeys whose brains displayed reactive, persistent microgliosis resulting from drug exposure 5–14 years prior to death [12]. This correlates precisely with human data derived from patients with MPTP-induced Parkinsonism 3–16 years before death who also demonstrated robust microgliosis in their nigras [13].

This human and monkey data demonstrating the ability of the nigra to maintain prolonged microglial activation has been supplemented by data from rodent studies which provide mechanistic support for an active role of inflammatory changes in cell death. For example, several studies demonstrate that microgliosis correlates with ongoing dopaminergic cell loss using the rat 6-hydroxydopamine (6-OHDA) toxin injection paradigm [14, 15]. An additional in vivo rodent model of Parkinson's disease involving the use of intranigral injection of bacterial endotoxin, lipopolysaccharide (LPS), has also supported this idea. This paradigm similarly demonstrates microgliosis occurring with and potentially preceding dopaminergic cell death [16]. Moreover, the LPS-stimulated, microglial-associated cell death appears unique to dopaminergic neurons in the nigra with cholinergic and serotoninergic neurons unaffected [17]. MPTP injection into rodents also results in dramatic striatonigral microgliosis potentially preceding and certainly correlating with loss of dopaminergic cells [18–24]. Collectively, histologic findings from human brain and temporal analysis from rodent studies continue to support the idea that microglial activation and the associated inflammatory changes are a part of the disease process.

Peripheral Immune Cell Changes in Parkinson's Disease

Although abundant data supporting microglial activation during neuron loss have been generated from both human and animal models of disease, there are also a significant number of findings that report altered peripheral immune cell behavior during disease. This suggests that some communication exists between the peripheral immune system as well as the possibility that disease involves a more general alteration of immune function. For example, a report by Ton et al. examining patients from the Cardiovascular Health Study determined that the risk of prevalent Parkinson's disease was significantly higher with elevated IL-6 levels and white blood cell counts in women and men, respectively [25]. However, over a 13-year follow-up, the risk of incident disease did not correlate with higher levels of interleukin-6 (IL-6), fibrinogen, tumor necrosis factor-alpha (TNF-α), C-reactive protein, albumin, or white blood cell counts [25]. Based upon these data from 60 prevalent and 154 incident disease cases, it appears that peripheral inflammatory biomarkers are elevated during disease with unclear value for pre-diagnostic or progression assessments. However, a nested case-control study including 84 incident Parkinson's disease patients and 165 health age-matched controls prospectively examined blood for inflammatory markers on average 4.3 years before diagnosis to reveal that higher pre-diagnostic levels of IL-6 but not C-reactive protein, fibrinogen, or TNF-α receptor 1 or 2 (TNFR1 or TNFR2) were significantly associated with greater risk of disease after controlling for caffeine intake, age, smoking, and creatine and uric acid levels [26]. Another study of incident versus prevalent disease from Wong and colleagues compared 61 cases of Parkinson's disease and matched controls to demonstrate that high fibrinogen levels correlated significantly with both prevalent and incident disease in men after adjusting for age, smoking, and low-density lipoprotein cholesterol [27]. Elevated levels of interleukin-2 (IL-2) but not IL-6, cortisol, adrenocorticotropic hormone (ACTH), or interleukin-1β (IL-1β) have been reported in the serum of 21 non-drug-treated Parkinson's disease patients versus healthy, age-matched controls [28]. A similar study of cytokine serum concentrations from 78 idiopathic Parkinson's disease patients versus healthy controls aged 30–90 years demonstrated elevated TNF-α and IL-6 in disease patients with elevated TNF-α correlating with abnormal postural and psychomotor performance [29]. Hofmann et al. also quantified IL-6 levels from serum of 23 Parkinson's disease patients versus age-matched, healthy controls to demonstrate that IL-6 levels were not significantly elevated compared to controls but levels did increase with disease severity [30]. Comparison of 20 Parkinson's disease patients and 22 age-matched healthy controls by Bessler et al. found that isolated peripheral blood mononuclear cells had impaired ability to secrete IL-2 compared to controls [31]. Similar findings were reported by Kluter et al., who also found that mitogenically stimulated peripheral blood mononuclear cells from Parkinson's disease patients had impaired IL-2 secretion compared to cells isolated from controls [32]. Another cytokine comparison by Rentzos and colleagues found elevated serum RANTES (Regulated on Activation, Normal T Cell Expressed and Secreted) when comparing

41 Parkinson's disease patients to 19 matched controls that significantly correlated with the Unified Parkinson's Disease Rating Scale (UPDRS III) score of patients [33]. A subsequent study of 41 Parkinson's disease patients compared to 19 healthy age-matched controls demonstrated elevated IL-10 concentrations in serum of diseased individuals [34]. Quantitation of multiple cytokines, TNF-α, IL-1β, IL-1α, IL-6, and IFN-γ, secreted upon LPS stimulation of peripheral blood mononuclear cells demonstrated the Parkinson's disease patient cells secreted significantly lower amounts compared to both healthy age-matched controls and patients with cerebrovascular disease that paralleled disease progression [35]. Lindqvist and colleagues also measured select inflammatory markers from the blood of 86 Parkinson's disease and 40 healthy control patients to correlate with changes in fatigue, anxiety/depression, and sleep patterns [36]. They observed that elevated levels of soluble IL-2 receptor (sIL-2R) and TNF-α in the blood of Parkinson's disease patients significantly correlated with more severe symptoms of depression and anxiety [36]. In fact, after controlling for effects of age, gender, motor symptoms, and medications, sIL-2R increases were predictive of depression/anxiety scores [36]. Collectively, these data suggest that serum concentrations of a range of cytokines differ between Parkinson's disease patients and controls. However, outcome variability and differences in study design contribute to uncertainty in identifying a particular biomarker cytokine that is predictive of either disease risk or progression.

Beyond simply looking for a biomarker through quantifying cytokine differences in serum, a multitude of studies suggest that peripheral immune cells from Parkinson's disease patients have different phenotypes when compared to controls. For instance, mononuclear cells isolated from peripheral blood of Parkinson's disease patients demonstrate reduced immunoglobulin secretion basally and with mitogen stimulation [37]. Saunders and colleagues concluded that immune changes in 113 Parkinson's disease patients versus 96 age-matched caregiver controls correlated with UPDRS III severity but not disease duration by demonstrating increased effector/memory T cells with increased $CD45RO^+$ and FAS^+ $CD4^+$ T cells and decreased $CD31^+$ $\alpha 4\beta 7^+$ $CD4^+$ T cells in disease patients [38]. Fiszer et al. compared lymphocyte subpopulations from blood of Parkinson's disease patients versus age-matched patients with other neurologic disease or tension headache to find that Parkinson's disease patients had decreased $CD4^+$ $CD45RA^+$ cells as well as increased gamma delta+ T cells [39, 40]. Comparison of peripheral blood lymphocyte subsets from 32 drug-treated and 32 non-drug-treated Parkinson's disease patients with 38 healthy age-matched controls also found overall decreased T cells ($CD3^+$) and B cells ($CD19^+$) in both treated and untreated disease [41]. In particular, the number of naïve $CD4^+$ ($CD4^+$ $CD45RA^+$) helper (T_h) cells but not $CD8^+$ cells was decreased by disease [41]. However, the number of activated $CD4^+$ $CD25^+$ T cells was increased with disease although the number and percentage of lymphocyte subsets did not correlate with disease duration or severity as assessed by the UPDRS [41]. Chiba and colleagues also reported elevated numbers of activated peripheral T lymphocytes isolated from blood of Parkinson's disease patients compared to controls [42]. A study of 40 idiopathic Parkinson's disease patients compared to

22 age-matched healthy controls and 33 patients with mild cerebrovascular disease demonstrated that Parkinson's disease patients had increased $CD4^+$ $CD8dull^+$ T cells in peripheral blood compared to either of the other conditions similar to what is sometimes seen postinfection [43]. Baba and colleagues compared peripheral blood from 33 sporadic Parkinson's disease patients and 34 healthy age-matched controls to again find alteration of lymphocyte subsets. Parkinson's disease patients had significantly lower $CD4^+$ T cells and increased $CD8^+$ T cells demonstrating an increased $CD8^+$ suppressor/cytotoxic T cell to $CD4^+$ T cell ratio [44]. In addition T cells had an increased interferon gamma (IFN-γ) to IL-4 production ratio demonstrating a skew towards at T_h1 phenotype [44]. Although many of the studies have profiled changes in lymphocytes, other peripheral blood immune cells clearly are altered with disease as well. For instance, Luo et al. demonstrated impaired ability of monocyte-derived macrophages from Parkinson's disease patients to upregulate expression of CD200R upon stimulation compared to young as well as age-matched controls [45]. Moreover, impairment of induced CD200R expression correlated inversely with the age of onset of disease and ability of the cells to secrete TNF-α [45]. Although the evidence is not conclusive and somewhat variable, the trend certainly supports the idea that peripheral immune cells, particularly lymphocytes, have altered behavior during disease.

Further evidence of the possibility of peripheral immune cell behavior contributing to disease progression or neuron loss has been provided again, by rodent studies. Villaran et al. used a rat model of ulcerative colitis induced by dextran sulfate to produce elevations in levels of several serum as well as nigral cytokines including TNF-α, IL-1β, and IL-6 that correlated with increased permeability of the blood–brain barrier [46]. Moreover, ulcerative colitis potentiated the increase in nigral cytokine levels and the decrease in tyrosine hydroxylase-immunoreactive neurons induced by LPS injection [46]. This exacerbation of LPS-dependent change was attenuated by depleting peripheral macrophage from the ulcerative colitis animals by pretreating with clodronate encapsulated in liposomes [46]. This data suggested not only that peripheral immune cells and cytokine levels influence brain cytokine levels but they also directly contribute to nigral inflammatory degeneration. Pott Godoy et al. reported similar findings focusing on IL-1β-mediated loss of dopaminergic cells in the nigra. By injecting an adenoviral vector responsible for driving human IL-1β expression into the striatum of rats, they demonstrated not only decreased tyrosine hydroxylase-immunoreactive cell numbers in the nigra by 21 days but also potentiation of this loss if IL-1β was simultaneously overexpressed in the periphery [47]. This observation was consistent with prior work by this group demonstrating that peripheral IL-1β overexpression via adenoviral vector also potentiated 6-OHDA-induced decrease in nigral tyrosine hydroxylase cell numbers but had no effect on its own [48]. This suggests that peripheral inflammation, at least via IL-1β alone, was not sufficient to produce nigral neuron loss but instead exacerbates a brain challenge. Moreover, it appears that chronic rather than transient or acute exposure to IL-1β was required since at least 21 days of overexpression was required for significant changes to occur [47]. In addition, prior studies with single acute injections of TNF-α, IFN-γ, or IL-1β into the substantia nigra of rats produced no toxicity at least for 7 days [49]. Additional rodent studies have also lent significant support to the notion that elevated peripheral circulating cytokine levels or peripheral inflammatory stimuli may contribute to brain inflammation. For example, in a recent mouse study Skelly and colleagues compared brain effects following intraperitoneal injection of LPS, IL-1β, TNF-α, and IL-6. Systemic stimulation with LPS, IL-1β, and TNF-α but not IL-6 was sufficient to increase IL-1β and TNF-α mRNA in the hippocampus by 2 h of stimulation with only LPS able to increase IFN-β mRNA [50]. Although data from the substantia nigra was not reported, these changes in brain cytokine mRNA correlated with increased neuronal c-Fos immunoreactivity in the central nucleus of the amygdala [50]. This data again demonstrates that the peripheral cytokine changes clearly affect brain physiology consistent with the possibility that they may also exert neurotoxic effects. Finally, Engler and colleagues performed an elegant study in which they demonstrated that intrastriatal injection of 6-OHDA into rats lead to a transient increase in peripheral white blood cell counts that included T cells, B cells, and neutrophils during the periods of active dopaminergic degeneration [51]. In addition, LPS stimulation of whole blood cultures demonstrated impaired production of TNF-α, IL-6, and IL-1β from the 6-OHDA-injected animals although plasma levels of cytokines were not different from control rats [51]. On the other hand, hypoactivity of the dopaminergic system due to 6-OHDA injection superimposed upon a peripheral proinflammatory stimulus, intraperitoneal LPS injection, led to decreased numbers of peripheral white blood cells and a heightened proinflammatory response following intraperitoneal LPS injection [51]. 6-OHDA-injected mice had significantly higher plasma cytokine concentrations of IL-1β, TNF-α, and IL-6 following LPS injection [51]. These data suggest that inflammatory neurodegenerative changes in the substantia nigra directly influence the phenotype of circulating peripheral immune cells, and loss of dopaminergic cells exacerbates the peripheral response to immune challenge.

As reviewed above, it is important to keep in mind that numerous conflicting findings exist regarding the cytokine and immune cell changes during disease both in the periphery and in the brain. Moreover, animal models designed to allow more mechanistic dissection of the disease process have not yet provided conclusive evidence of inflammatory change driving or responding to dopaminergic degeneration during disease. Finally, it is also clear that the immune responses of mice and humans, particularly following peripheral LPS challenge, are characterized by unique genomic expression profile changes leading some investigators to conclude that mice poorly mimic human immune responses in general [52]. In an effort to determine whether a particular mechanistic contribution of inflammatory changes can be extracted from the extensive existing literature, we will focus on the immune cell-secreted inflammatory signaling molecules already mentioned, cytokines, to determine whether they are more than potential biomarkers of disease and perhaps represent molecular targets for therapeutic intervention.

Cytokines in Parkinson's Disease

In spite of the fact that the specific cause(s) and temporal phenotypes of microglia and peripheral immune cells during disease remain unclear, it is well known that either of these cell types rely upon secretion of a plethora of low molecular weight signaling molecules, termed cytokines, to act via both paracrine and autocrine cellular mechanisms. These critical signaling proteins not only regulate and coordinate the behavior of peripheral immune cells and brain microglia but also a multitude of cells throughout the brain and body. We will review, sequentially, evidence of particular cytokine changes reported in Parkinson's disease patients in either the brain or periphery for comparison to animal models of disease in an effort to determine whether particular changes can be mechanistically linked with disease progression or neuron loss. The focus of the remaining part of the chapter will be restricted to TNF-α and IL-1β not necessarily because they are the most important cytokines for disease processes but instead based upon the fact that they appear to be the more intensely studied with respect to Parkinson's disease.

Tumor Necrosis Factor-Alpha (TNF-α)

TNF-α was originally described as a lymphocyte-secreted toxin [53–56] and then later included as a macrophage-secreted protein with an ability to contribute to necrosis of tumors [57, 58]. Although it was identified outside of the brain, it is clear that it can be expressed by multiple cell types in the brain, particularly microglia [59–61], with receptor binding throughout the brain as assessed by radioiodinated TNF binding [62]. It is an approximately 17 kDa pleiotropic cytokine capable of stimulating a variety of cell types with a diverse set of consequences [63, 64]. Its effects on target cells occur via binding to a trimerized form of two distinct receptors, CD120a (p55, TNFRI) and CD120b (p75, TNFRII) [65]. Both neurons and glia have been reported to express these receptors [62, 66]. The cytoplasmic domain of TNFRI contains a death domain (DD) sequence of 60–80 amino acids responsible for recruiting the adaptor protein TRADD and leading to transduction of diverse signaling pathways including activation of IKK kinases and NFκB or the adapter protein Fas-associating protein with a death domain (FADD) and subsequent caspase activation [67–71]. Although TNFRII lacks the DD sequence, it contains a region of 78 amino acids responsible for recruiting the adaptor protein, TRAF2, also allowing subsequent activation of NFκB [72]. The extracellular portion of both TNF receptors contains four cysteine-rich domains termed, CRDs. TNF-α binds to CRD2 and 3, while CRD1 contains a self-association domain required for homotypic receptor trimerization in order for the receptors to be able to bind the TNF-α trimer [73, 74]. This has been termed the pre-ligand assembly domain (PLAD) since it is necessary for receptor trimerization independent of ligand binding. The PLAD sequence differs significantly between TNFRI and TNFRII, allowing the design of competing peptides that will attenuate trimerization of one and not the other. Indeed, these have already been synthesized and used in vitro and in vivo to selectively attenuate TNFRI versus TNFRII-mediated cell death and inflammation in rodents [75].

TNF-α in Parkinson's Disease

Perhaps due to its widely held role as a master regulatory cytokine, characterization of changes in TNF-α related biology, as compared to other cytokines, is best described in Parkinson's disease. Increased glial TNF-α immunoreactivity has been reported in the substantia nigra of Parkinson's disease brains compared to controls with both displaying robust neuronal immunoreactivity for TNFR1 [76]. Indeed, subsequent study has demonstrated robust TNF-α immunoreactivity localizing to particularly, microglia, in the Parkinson's disease brain [4]. Mogi and colleagues also demonstrated elevated TNFR1 levels in the substantia nigra of Parkinson's disease patients compared to controls suggesting a receptor subtype-specific change is involved in disease [77]. A microarray study from the substantia nigra of Parkinson's disease patients compared to controls again verified elevated TNF-α levels with disease [78]. Collectively, there appears significant evidence of elevated TNF-α levels in the brains of Parkinson's disease patients.

As already mentioned, abundant peripheral changes in TNF-α biology have also been documented during disease. For instance, serum TNF-α levels measured from 78 idiopathic Parkinson's disease patients compared to 140 health controls demonstrated elevated levels of the cytokine in Parkinson's disease patients with abnormal postural and psychomotor function compared to controls [29]. Mogi et al. reported similar data from both striatum and cerebrospinal fluid showing significantly increased TNF-α levels in Parkinsonian patients compared to controls [79]. An additional study by Scalzo and colleagues examined serum levels of soluble TNFRI and soluble TNFRII from 46 Parkinson's disease patients compared to 23 healthy age-matched controls to find that diseased patients had significantly higher levels of soluble TNFRI indicating again that changes in the cytokine as well as its receptors occur in the periphery during disease [80]. A comparison of peripheral blood mononuclear cells from 40 Parkinson's disease and 40 healthy, age-matched controls found that basal as well as LPS-stimulated TNF-α release (as well as numerous other cytokines) was elevated from Parkinson's disease patient cells [81]. This is consistent with data from Bongioanni et al. who demonstrated that peripheral blood T cells from Parkinson's disease patients had elevated TNF-α binding and therefore higher receptor expression compared to control cells [82]. A study of 60 idiopathic Parkinson's disease patients compared to 24 healthy controls again demonstrated significantly higher serum TNF-α levels with disease [83]. As mentioned above, Lindqvist and colleagues correlated increased non-motor symptoms such as depression and fatigue in Parkinson's disease patients with this elevation in serum TNF-α [36]. Similar data from Menza et al. also demonstrated that elevated serum TNF-α levels in Parkinson's disease patients with depression significantly correlated with deficits in cognition and depression [84].

TNF-α Polymorphisms in Parkinson's Disease

These changes in measured levels of TNF-α correlate well with single-nucleotide polymorphism analysis from Parkinson's disease patients. A comparison of 289 idiopathic Parkinson's disease patients and 269 matched controls examined a single-nucleotide polymorphism in the TNF-α promoter (G-308A) to find a 1.14-fold increased risk for heterozygous carriers and a 2.49-fold increased risk for homozygous carriers [85]. This is consistent with evidence that the polymorphism at −308 in the TNF-α promoter is associated with high TNF-α production [86]. A subsequent study by Bialecka et al. found that the T-308A polymorphism was significantly more frequent in early-onset Parkinson's disease patients than controls in a study comparing 102 early-onset patients to 214 late-onset patients [87]. Kruger and colleagues also found 1.56-fold relative increased risk in heterozygous carriers [88], while Ross et al. [89] as well as Passarelli et al. [90] failed to find such an association for the TNF-α-308 polymorphism. Nishimura and colleagues reported data from additional promoter polymorphism analysis studying 172 varying-age onset Parkinson's disease patients compared to 157 healthy controls to demonstrate that carriers of the T-1031C polymorphism, associated with elevated TNF-α levels, significantly correlated with early-onset PD [91]. Similar conclusions were reached by Wu et al. who analyzed 369 Parkinson's disease patients and 326 controls to find that individuals homozygous for the −1031 polymorphism had elevated risk of disease [92].

TNF-α in Animal Models of Parkinson's Disease and Neurodegeneration

In an effort to identify a mechanism by which TNF-α contributes to dopaminergic cell death, a number of animal model studies have been performed. Many of these mechanistic dissections have relied upon transgenic mouse studies that are deficient in either TNFRI or TNFRII. A study by Sriram et al. demonstrated increased TNF-α levels in the striatum of 1-methyl-4-phenyl-1,2,3,4-tetrahydropyridine (MPTP) mice prior to gliosis and a decrease in striatal dopamine and tyrosine hydroxylase levels [93]. However, animals deficient in both high- and low-affinity TNF-α receptors (TNFRI and TNFRII, respectively) were protected against this decrease [93]. A similar study by Rousselet and colleagues demonstrated that TNFRI/RII double-knockout mice, but not mice lacking only one receptor, had lower striatal dopamine levels basally and lower dopamine levels after MPTP injection compared to wild-type littermates correlating with increased turnover in the knockout animals [94]. In addition, the degree of nigral neuron loss was comparable in the TNFRI/RII double-knockout mice compared to single receptor deletion and wild-type mice [94]. This study concluded that TNF-α does not have a direct role in cell death in this particular mouse MPTP toxicity paradigm. Similar findings were reported by

Leng et al., who demonstrated that MPTP treatment also produced no difference in the toxin-induced decrease in striatal dopamine levels or nigral dopamine transporter immunoreactive neuron numbers between TNFRI knockout, TNFRII knockout, or wild-type mice [95]. Likely based upon experimental design differences, data from these toxin-based models of disease have not yet provided a cohesive argument for a particular TNF-α receptor in mediating neuron death or protection in Parkinson's disease.

Other studies have focused on TNF-α itself rather than its receptors in an effort to validate a role for the cytokine in Parkinson's disease-related neuron death. Using mice deficient in TNF-α, Ferger et al. demonstrated significant protection against MPTP-induced decreases in striatal dopamine levels and tyrosine hydroxylase immunoreactivity with no effect on toxin-induced changes in nigral tyrosine hydroxylase or dopamine transporter immunoreactivities [96]. McCoy and colleagues demonstrated that neutralizing secreted TNF-α with a dominant negative TNF-α inhibitor protected nigral neuron death in rats in response to both LPS infusion and 6-hydroxydopamine (6-OHDA) injection [97]. Consistent with the notion that chronic cytokine elevation is needed to produce dopaminergic loss, De Lella Ezcurra and colleagues demonstrated that adenoviral expression of high levels of TNF-α in the rat substantia nigra was sufficient to produce macrophage infiltration by day 7 and significant decrease in tyrosine hydroxylase-immunoreactive cell numbers by 14 days of overexpression [98]. However, a subsequent study by Chertoff et al. demonstrated that it is the level of TNF-α overexpression in the substantia nigra that dictates the effects of the cytokine [99]. In this study, low levels of adenoviral-mediated nigral TNF-α expression protected murine dopaminergic neurons from 6-OHDA-mediated toxicity, while overexpression again mediated neuron loss [99]. Therefore, in these studies focusing on the cytokine rather than any particular receptor, there may still be some dichotomy of behavior with respect to a role in protection or death. Nevertheless, the majority of data seems to indicate across several different paradigms that TNF-α can stimulate dopaminergic neuron death.

To better appreciate this dichotomous role that TNF-α appears capable of having in the brain, it is useful to remember, as already mentioned, that TNFRI and TNFRII have unique signaling responses, at least in nonneuronal cells, in which the two receptors are able to help mediate distinct cellular phenotypes. More importantly, a conflicting body of literature has demonstrated that neuronal stimulation via either TNF-α receptor mediates protection or death across a range of experimental paradigms well beyond the field of Parkinson's disease research. In fact, even using the same toxin can produce differing results with regard to a role for TNF-α in protection or not depending upon the particular experimental design [100, 101]. To add to the complexity of TNF-α biology in the brain, in several experimental systems, TNF-α stimulation mediates its toxicity in the context of a proinflammatory milieu suggesting that its effects are often superimposed upon responses initiated by a plethora of additional glial secreted stimuli [102–104]. For example, expression and secretion of TNF-α, particularly by microglia, has been observed in several neurotoxic paradigms including multiple sclerosis, Alzheimer's disease, stroke/ischemia, traumatically injured, and epileptic brains and implicated in mechanisms of neuron loss [105–111].

Some explanation for the varying effects of the cytokine on neuron behavior stems from the fact TNF-α not only operates through two different receptors on neurons but these receptors can also utilize a variety of signal transduction pathways to mediate phenotype changes. The more classic caspase and NFκB transduction responses have been mentioned already, but a growing body of literature demonstrates additional TNF-α-mediated responses that can control death or survival. For example, the potential neuroprotective or neurotoxic effects of TNF-α stimulation have been examined in the context of its ability to regulate synaptic scaling and ischemic tolerance. For several years now, glial secreted TNF-α has been implicated in the neuronal phenomenon of synaptic scaling, which describes the ability of TNF-α to stimulate increased cell surface localization of glutamatergic AMPA receptors to strengthen synapses [112, 113]. It appears that the particular localization of the receptors to synaptic or extrasynaptic compartments and the particular subunit composition of the receptors allow TNF-α to serve as more than a synaptic modulator capable of potentiating excitotoxicity or attenuating it as seen during ischemic preconditioning. For instance, to support a protective role of the cytokine, it has been shown that low-level TNF-α stimulation of neuron or organotypic slice cultures not only attenuates the intracellular calcium response of neurons to subsequent excitatory stimulation but also increases protein levels of excitatory amino acid transporter 3 (EAAT3) to increase glutamate uptake [114, 115]. More specifically, transient (15 min) murine hippocampal slice treatment with low-concentration (6 nM) TNF-α stimulates a rapid increase in neuronal cell surface localization of both GluR1 and GluR2 of the AMPA receptor [116]. Similar findings were observed by Rainey-Smith and colleagues using murine motor neuron cultures to demonstrate that 15-min stimulation with 10 ng/mL TNF-α resulted in increased GluR1 and GluR2 cell surface localization offering protection from subsequent calcium excitotoxicity [117]. This effect appears to be mediated by the high-affinity receptor, since TNFRI but not TNFRII knockout neurons are resistant to the effects of TNF-α to increase cell surface AMPA receptor subunit localization [118].

On the other hand, TNF-α stimulation can augment intracellular calcium signaling to contribute to cell death in other paradigms. Indeed, TNF-α can potentiate excitotoxic death via altering AMPA or NMDA excitatory neurotransmitter receptor activities [119–121]. A similar experiment using rat hippocampal neuron cultures demonstrated that TNF-α stimulation for 15 min was sufficient to increase GluR2-lacking AMPA receptor localization in the extrasynaptic compartment as well as GluR2-containing AMPA receptors but with a delayed time course that resulted in potentiation of excitotoxic death [122]. This role in potentiation of cell death was supported by in vivo data using a soluble TNF-α receptor in spinal cord injury.

To summarize the vast field of TNF-α-related neuron death and cite only a few of the many studies it appears that data from receptor-specific knockout mouse in vivo studies support a role for the high-affinity receptor, TNFRI, rather than the low-affinity receptor, TNFRII, in mediating TNF-α-stimulated neuron death [118, 123]. This mechanism has been linked to caspase-mediated apoptotic events based upon the understanding that TNF-α binding to TNFRI has the ability to stimulate caspase and/or NFκB activity. However, these signaling pathways have been almost exclusively characterized in nonneuronal cells, and it is largely assumed that these responses are also employed by neurons. There is mounting evidence that TNF-α receptors utilize atypical signaling pathways in neurons. In fact, Jarosinski et al. demonstrated in 2001 that TNF-α stimulation of primary neurons is unable to activate NFκB [124]. A more recent study indicates that TNF-α stimulation does increase NFκB activity but to a degree that is less than even constitutive activation in other cells. Moreover, transcription of many NFκB-responsive genes is not increased by stimulation in neurons again suggesting that typical TNF-α-stimulated signaling responses described in nonneuronal cells may not be relevant in neurons [125]. This paradoxical behavior of TNF-α in neurons was even the topic of a review by Massa et al. [126]. Adding even more complexity to the field is the fact that gene array analysis from the brains of TNFRI and TNFRII receptor knockout mice displays significant basal brain expression differences across a range of different protein classes compared to each other as well as wild-type mice, indicating clear phenotype changes simply from loss of receptor expression that are likely developmental changes [127, 128]. This suggests, as always, that caution must be applied when interpreting data derived from the use of transgenic models such as the TNFRI or TNFRII knockout mice when attempting mechanistic predictions for the contribution of TNF-α in Parkinson's disease.

Evidence of Particular TNF-α Signaling in Parkinson's Disease

Although a mechanism of particular TNF-α receptor-mediated death remains unclear, Hartmann and colleagues have demonstrated decreased FADD immunoreactivity in dopaminergic neurons within the substantia nigra pars compacta of Parkinson's disease brains, suggesting that a FADD-caspase-mediated mechanism of death might occur [129]. This is supported by work from Mogi and colleagues, which demonstrated elevated caspase 1 and caspase 3 activity, based on fluoropeptide substrate cleavage, in the substantia nigra of Parkinson's disease patients compared to controls [77]. Similarly, elevated caspase 3 and BAX immunoreactivity has been reported from neuromelanin-containing neurons from the Parkinson's disease brains compared to controls [130]. An additional piece of evidence supporting a possible role for TNFRI-mediated cell death is based upon the observation by Hunot and colleagues who compared 5 idiopathic Parkinson's disease patients and 7 matched controls to find a very significant increase in neuromelanin-containing neuronal nuclear NFκB immunoreactivity in diseased brains at least correlating with a proposed consequence of TNFRI-mediated signaling [131]. Rodent data seems to support this idea of apoptotic death as a component of the disease process. For instance, it is clear that caspase-3 activity is required for cell death and microgliosis in the mouse MPTP injection model as determined by comparison between wild-type and caspase 3 knockout mice [132]. These data provide some support for the notion that an apoptotic process may be one of the mechanisms of death during disease. However, based upon the scarcity of apoptotic death-related evidence reported from human disease brains, it is clear that other death mechanisms are likely involved [133] (Fig. 1).

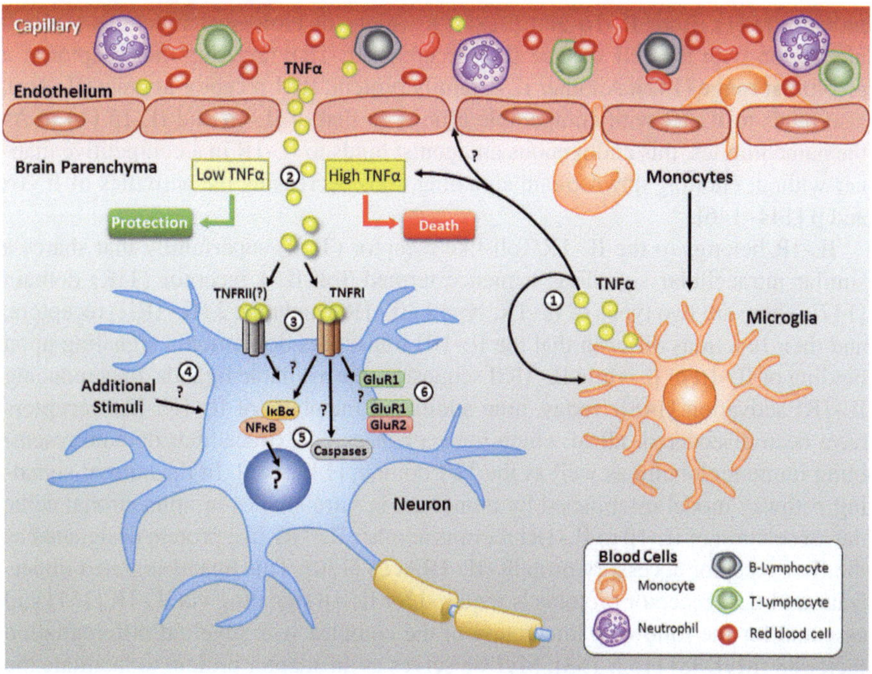

Fig. 1 Hypothesized signaling mechanism of TNF-α in Parkinson's disease. Following cleavage from its precursor form, secreted TNF-α can be released from numerous immune cells in the periphery as well as from microglia as has been reported from Parkinson's disease brains (1). It may act in an autocrine fashion to manipulate microglial phenotype or stimulate neurons where high concentrations of TNF-α are reportedly toxic to dopaminergic neurons, while low concentrations offer protective stimulation via interacting with a trimerized TNFR on the cell surface (2). Although it is not clear whether dopaminergic neurons express the low-affinity receptor, TNFRII, neurons in diseased brains have increased high-affinity receptor, TNFRI, immunoreactivity (3). Perhaps acting alone or with additional stimuli (4), TNF-α stimulation through interaction with one or both receptors may lead to the initiation of particular signaling events that are responsible for DA-neuron death or protection. Based upon signaling mechanisms defined in other cell types, TNF-α stimulation may initiate activation of NFκB-mediated transcriptional changes as well as caspase-mediated death in the dopaminergic neurons (5). In addition, based upon mechanisms defined in non-dopaminergic neurons, it is possible that TNF-α stimulates altered localization and subunit composition of AMPA receptors (GluR1/R2) to contribute to potentiate or attenuate excitotoxic death of the cells (6)

Interleukin 1-Beta (IL-1β)

Interleukin-1β (IL-1β) is one of the 11 interleukin-1 cytokine family members identified to date [134, 135] and shares 26 % sequence homology with its structurally and functionally similar but genetically distinct acidic relative, IL-1α [136–140]. Biologically active, mature form of 17-kDa IL-1β molecule is synthesized via proteolysis of its 31-kDa precursor by caspase-1, an inflammasome-associated cysteine protease [141]. Both IL-1α and β exert a variety of biological functions through interaction with the cell surface IL-1 receptor (IL-1R), targeting the receptor at a picomolar range [142]. Another IL-1 family protein, IL-1 receptor agonist (IL-1ra), also binds to IL-1R with comparable affinity to that of IL-1α and IL-1β [143]. As the name implies, this endogenous antagonist binds to IL-1R in a competitive manner without eliciting downstream signaling, thus decreasing the activities of IL-1α and β [144–146].

IL-1R belongs to the IL-1R/Toll-like receptor (TLR) superfamily that shares a similar intracellular signaling sequence termed Toll-IL-1 receptor (TIR) domain [147]. There are two types of IL-1R, type 1 (IL-1RI) and type 2 (IL-1RII) receptors, and their functions differ in that the IL-1RI transduces downstream signaling upon binding of IL-1α or β, while IL-1RII sequesters the available ligands, thus reducing IL-1RI activation [148]. Today, nine additional members of IL-1RI-like receptors have been discovered, all of which have a conserved extracellular domain resembling immunoglobulin as well as the TIR domain [147, 149]. In the current signaling pathway model established by numerous in vitro studies in nonneuronal cells, the association of IL-1β to IL-1RI recruits another IL-1RI-like protein designated as the IL-1 receptor accessory protein (IL-1RAcP) [150]. This ligand-initiated dimerization of IL-1 receptor proteins is required for IL-1β signaling via IL-1R [151] and essential for the following interaction of the complex with myeloid differentiation factor 88 (MyD88) [152, 153]. MyD88 serves as an adaptor protein to facilitate the recruitment of first IL-1 receptor-associated kinase 4 (IRAK4) and then IRAK1, after which the latter enzyme becomes phosphorylated by the former and by itself [147, 154, 155]. The phosphorylation of the IRAK1 prompts the kinase to interact with tumor necrosis factor receptor-associated factor 6 (TRAF6), leading to the ubiquitination of TRAF6 that proceeds the activation of transforming growth factor-β-activated protein kinase (TAK1) [156, 157]. This IL-1R pathway diverges to activate at least two distinct sets of transcription factors, NFκB and AP-1/c-Jun, via the activation of the inhibitor of NFκB (IκB) kinase (IKK) and mitogen-activated protein kinase kinases (MKKs), respectively [156, 157].

Since IL-1β was initially identified as a pyrogen in the 1940s, additional biological functions and characteristics were discovered following its purification and cloning as a recombinant protein [158]. IL-1β is produced and secreted primarily by the cells of myeloid origin including macrophages and dendritic cells, and its function as a proinflammatory mediator has been extensively documented in a variety of fields [158]. It is now well acknowledged that IL-1β is one of the major immune response mediators and it is identical to the factors previously referred to as endogenous pyrogen, leukocytic endogenous mediator [159, 160], lymphocyte-activating factor [160–162], hemopoietin-1 [163], mononuclear cell factor [164], proteolysis-inducing factor [165], catabolin [166], and osteoclast-activating factor [167]. Elevated levels of IL-1β are widely reported in the peripheral blood and tissues in inflammatory conditions such as bacterial infections, injury, leukemia, and autoimmune diseases [168, 169].

In the central nervous system, IL-1β is expressed and released by microglia. Moreover, IL-1R localization inferred by radioiodinated IL-1α binding has validated abundant neuronal receptor expression [170]. As in the periphery, increased expression of this cytokine is associated with central inflammatory conditions including Parkinson's disease [171–173], Alzheimer's disease [174], stroke/ischemia [175–180], traumatic brain and spinal cord injury [181–183], excitotoxicity [184, 185], and HIV-1 infection [186]. Therefore, IL-1β is thought to be one of the major cytokines utilized by activated microglia to mediate inflammatory responses [169].

IL-1β in Parkinson's Disease

In the mid-1990s, the involvement of IL-1β in Parkinson's disease was investigated in a few correlative studies with human patients. A pioneering study by Mogi et al. [171] quantified for the first time the levels of IL-1β and other cytokines in the brain tissues of Parkinson's disease patients using sandwich enzyme-linked immunosorbent assay (ELISA). They reported that the level of the cytokine was significantly increased by 3.5-fold in the striatum, but not in the cerebral cortex, of the Parkinson's disease patients when compared to their age- and gender-matched control brains [171]. IL-1β concentrations were also measured in the cerebrospinal fluid in subsequent studies by the same group and others. Blum-Degen and colleagues compared levels of IL-1β to additional cytokines, IL-2 and IL-6, in the cerebrospinal fluid versus plasma of 22 Parkinson's disease patients, 12 controls and 11 sporadic Alzheimer's disease patients to find no differences in IL-2 but elevated IL-6 and IL-1β in the cerebrospinal fluid but not plasma of both Parkinson's and Alzheimer's disease patients [172]. This observation was partly supported by another study in which IL-1β was measured in the ventricular cerebrospinal fluid of Parkinson's disease patients [173]. Results from this study showed a significant increase in IL-1β levels in patients diagnosed with juvenile Parkinsonism (age 39–55 years; mean age 48 years). However, the small increase in IL-1β levels observed in "classical" Parkinson's disease patient population (age 54–77 years; mean age 68 years) did not reach a statistically significant value [173]. These reported elevations in extracellular cytokine correlate well with increased glial IL-1β immunoreactivity reported in Parkinson's disease substantia nigra [187].

IL-1β Polymorphisms in Parkinson's Disease

Studying polymorphisms of the IL-1β gene (*IL-1B*) has provided some additional support for a role of IL-1β in the pathogenesis of Parkinson's disease. Single-nucleotide polymorphisms within the promoter region of *IL-1B* at position −511 have been repeatedly reported in population analyses, suggesting its association with increased risk [188–192] or earlier age at onset [193, 194] of Parkinson's disease. However, the results from these studies are inconsistent and even conflicting, perhaps due to multiple variables such as ethnicity, age groups, and genders of the subjects. Supporting this notion, a meta-analysis of eleven published studies during 2000–2008 from 2,803 PD patients and 2,593 controls showed no significant association of *IL-1B* polymorphism at −511 with the risk of Parkinson's disease [195]. Additional extensive population studies are warranted in order to evaluate the involvement of IL-1β at the genomic level.

IL-1β in Animal Models of Parkinson's Disease and Neurodegeneration

In accordance with the observations in human patients, upregulation of IL-1-β has also been reported in the brains of animal models of Parkinson's disease. Daily intraperitoneal injections of MPTP for 13 days resulted in over a 20-fold increase in IL-1β levels in the striatum of MPTP-treated mice compared to control animals [196]. Similarly, maximum of a 16-fold increase was detected 30 days after a single intrastriatal injection of 6-OHDA [197].

A significant literature derived from the rodent studies suggests that this increase in IL-1β is actually neuroprotective. For example, the increase in IL-1β in Parkinson's disease brain might be a compensatory mechanism activated by the nigral cell death whereby the cytokine functions in combination with TNF-α to elicit neurotrophic effects via stimulation of astrocyte proliferation [171, 198]. Moreover, findings from an animal model study demonstrate that pretreatment with 20 ng IL-1β via stereotaxic infusion prevented dopaminergic cell bodies within the substantia nigra from degenerating after the subsequent 6-OHDA challenge [199]. A few in vitro studies reported similar neuroprotective actions of IL-1β, demonstrating that pretreatment with IL-1β increases the neural growth and survival of rat superior cervical ganglia explants [200], and IL-1β stimulation of a human microglial cell line culture results in production and secretion of nerve growth factor (NGF) synergistically with TNF-α [201].

On the contrary, several lines of evidence suggest neurotoxic actions of IL-1β in various animal models. Koprich et al. [202] reported that increasing the level of IL-1β (approximately twofold, to 13.5 pg/mg substantia nigra protein) by preadministration of a nontoxic dose of LPS in the substantia nigra rendered the dopaminergic neurons more susceptible to a subsequent 6-OHDA treatment, indicating a role of IL-1β opposite from the neuroprotective function proposed earlier by Saura et al. [199]. In the MPTP animal model, inhibiting the synthesis of biologically active, mature IL-1β with a dominant negative form of caspase-1 abolished MPTP-mediated dopaminergic loss [203]. Furthermore, continuous adenovirus-driven IL-1β expression alone resulted in progressive dopaminergic neuron death accompanied by T cell infiltration into the substantia nigra and Parkinson's disease-like motor impairments in the rat [47, 204]. Conversely, pretreatment with recombinant IL-1ra was found to be neuroprotective, corroborating the involvement of IL-1β activity in neurodegeneration. Inhibition of LPS-induced IL-1β activity by administration of IL-1ra prior to a 6-OHDA challenge protected the dopaminergic cells [202].

Similar results with IL-1ra have also been documented with hippocampal neurons with ischemia [205] and excitotoxic insults [206], suggesting that counteracting IL-1β activity with IL-1ra is beneficial in minimizing neurodegeneration.

Interestingly, a review by Allen et al. [207] has pointed out that the IL-1β-mediated neuronal damages detected in these animal models might be a combined outcome occurring with administration of an inflammatory stimulus (e.g., 6-OHDA, MPTP, LPS). Such observations argue against the idea that IL-1β alone is sufficient for dopaminergic cell death in Parkinson's disease, but rather multiple factors are involved in the pathogenesis of the disease [208]. In this view, IL-1β significantly exacerbates neuronal damage when the nervous system has been previously exposed to or "primed" by inflammatory stimuli such as infections, neurotoxins, and trauma [209–211], or by "sterile inflammation" instigated by secretion of endogenous molecules due to aging or cell death [211]. Inversely, repeated or prolonged inflammation from previous infections or injury may contribute to the "priming" of microglia, therefore triggering the disease with aging and/or additional exposures to pathogens and toxins.

Evidence of Particular IL-1β Signaling in Parkinson's Disease

In spite of the elevations in brain IL-1β protein levels and increased glial immunoreactivity reported from Parkinson's disease brains and its mouse models, it is not clear what particular signaling response the cytokine may be eliciting on neurons and/or glia at this point. Indeed, reports of evidence for IL-1R expression are also lacking in the striatum and substantia nigra. As already mentioned, the potentially dual neuroprotective and neurotoxic actions of IL-1β further increase the complexity of its potential effects in Parkinson's disease. Based upon the lack of particular signaling dissection of the IL-1R in dopaminergic neurons, it is even difficult to hypothesize how the cytokine might be stimulating the cells. Nevertheless, as stated in the TNF-α discussion, some evidence of possible IL-1R-mediated signaling in neurons during disease may be suggested by data from Hunot and colleagues who found significantly increased nuclear NFκB immunoreactivity in neuromelanin-containing neurons of Parkinson's disease brains compared to controls [131] (Fig. 2).

Clearly, the mechanistic implications of any particular cytokine contributing to dopaminergic cell death or loss during Parkinson's disease remain unclear. We have attempted to review the literature related to at least two of the cytokines reported to be elevated with disease. It is likely that neither TNF-α nor IL-1β would be acting alone during the prolonged changes occurring in a diseased brain. Moreover, there are many remaining cytokines/chemokines that could change or have already been reported to change during disease that undoubtedly also affect dopaminergic neurons. Perhaps future efforts quantifying the efficacy of receptor-selective antagonists for each cytokine of interest that is tested in the most disease-relevant animal model will offer insight into whether or not manipulation of cytokine biology offers a valuable therapeutic strategy for Parkinson's disease.

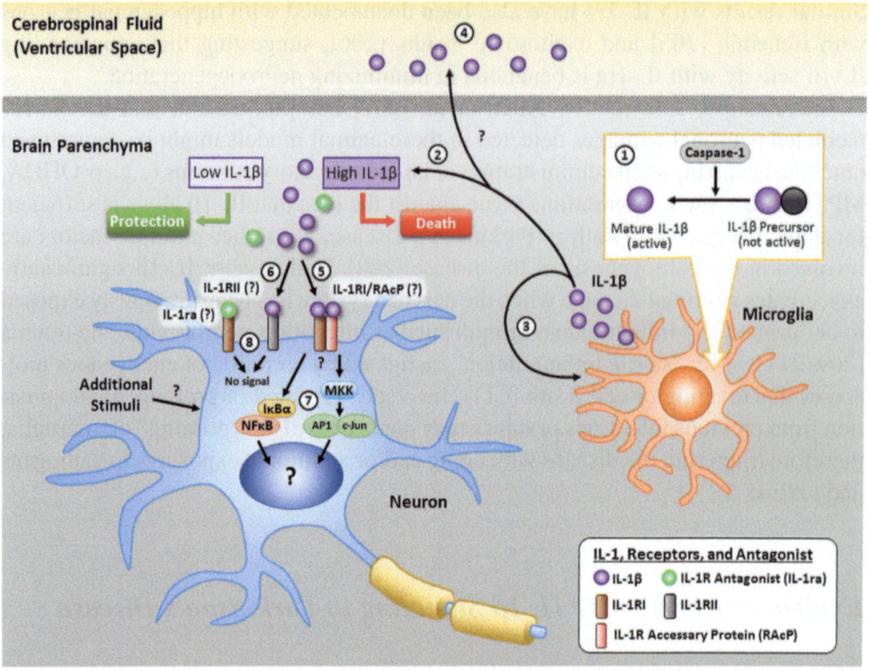

Fig. 2 Hypothesized signaling mechanism of IL-1β in Parkinson's disease. Upon inflammatory stimulation, microglia produce mature, biologically active IL-1β from a larger precursor molecule via activation of caspase-1 (1). Increased glial immunoreactivity in Parkinson's disease brains suggests that microglia may release IL-1β into the extracellular space where it could act as a paracrine (2) or autocrine (3) stimuli. IL-1β could also be released into the cerebrospinal fluid (4), where increased levels may be detected in Parkinson's disease patients. High levels of IL-1β are reportedly toxic to dopaminergic neurons, while low levels are toxic. Paracrine IL-1β may interact with IL-1RI (5) or IL-1RII (6), although only limited evidence exists for the presence of cell surface IL-1 receptors on dopaminergic neurons. Based upon mechanisms defined in non-dopaminergic cells, it is postulated that the association of IL-1β with IL-1RI prompts dimerization of the receptor-ligand complex with IL-1RAcP to initiate downstream intracellular signaling, ultimately leading to the activation NFκB and AP-1/c-Jun transcription factors via the IκB and MKK pathways, respectively (7). In contrast, the binding of IL-1β to IL-1RII or IL-1ra to IL1-RI does not lead to signal transduction (8)

References

1. McGeer PL, Itagaki S, Boyes BE, McGeer EG. Reactive microglia are positive for HLA-DR in the substantia nigra of Parkinson's and Alzheimer's disease brains. Neurology. 1988;38: 1285–91.
2. Banati RB, Daniel SE, Blunt SB. Glial pathology but absence of apoptotic nigral neurons in long-standing Parkinson's disease. Mov Disord. 1998;13:221–7.
3. Forno LS, DeLanney LE, Irwin I, Di Monte D, Langston JW. Astrocytes and Parkinson's disease. Prog Brain Res. 1992;94:429–36.

4. Imamura K, Hishikawa N, Sawada M, Nagatsu T, Yoshida M, Hashizume Y. Distribution of major histocompatibility complex class II-positive microglia and cytokine profile of Parkinson's disease brains. Acta Neuropathol. 2003;106:518–26.
5. Mirza B, Hadberg H, Thomsen P, Moos T. The absence of reactive astrocytosis is indicative of a unique inflammatory process in Parkinson's disease. Neuroscience. 2000;95:425–32.
6. Sawada M, Imamura K, Nagatsu T. Role of cytokines in inflammatory process in Parkinson's disease. J Neural Transm Suppl. 2006;70:373–81.
7. Lawson LJ, Perry VH, Dri P, Gordon S. Heterogeneity in the distribution and morphology of microglia in the normal adult mouse brain. Neuroscience. 1990;39:151–70.
8. Kim WG, Mohney RP, Wilson B, Jeohn GH, Liu B, Hong JS. Regional difference in susceptibility to lipopolysaccharide-induced neurotoxicity in the rat brain: role of microglia. J Neurosci. 2000;20:6309–16.
9. Beach TG, Sue LI, Walker DG, Lue LF, Connor DJ, Caviness JN, et al. Marked microglial reaction in normal aging human substantia nigra: correlation with extraneuronal neuromelanin pigment deposits. Acta Neuropathol. 2007;114:419–24.
10. Gerhard A, Pavese N, Hotton G, Turkheimer F, Es M, Hammers A, et al. In vivo imaging of microglial activation with [^{11}C](R)-PK11195 PET in idiopathic Parkinson's disease. Neurobiol Dis. 2006;21:404–12.
11. Ouchi Y, Yagi S, Yokokura M, Sakamoto M. Neuroinflammation in the living brain of Parkinson's disease. Parkinsonism Relat Disord. 2009;15 Suppl 3:S200–4.
12. McGeer PL, Schwab C, Parent A, Doudet D. Presence of reactive microglia in monkey substantia nigra years after 1-methyl-4-phenyl-1,2,3,6-tetrahydropyridine administration. Ann Neurol. 2003;54:599–604.
13. Langston JW, Forno LS, Tetrud J, Reeves AG, Kaplan JA, Karluk D. Evidence of active nerve cell degeneration in the substantia nigra of humans years after 1-methyl-4-phenyl-1,2,3,6-tetrahydropyridine exposure. Ann Neurol. 1999;46:598–605.
14. Akiyama H, McGeer PL. Microglial response to 6-hydroxydopamine-induced substantia nigra lesions. Brain Res. 1989;489:247–53.
15. Marinova-Mutafchieva L, Sadeghian M, Broom L, Davis JB, Medhurst AD, Dexter DT. Relationship between microglial activation and dopaminergic neuronal loss in the substantia nigra: a time course study in a 6-hydroxydopamine model of Parkinson's disease. J Neurochem. 2009;110:966–75.
16. Castano A, Herrera AJ, Cano J, Machado A. Lipopolysaccharide intranigral injection induces inflammatory reaction and damage in nigrostriatal dopaminergic system. J Neurochem. 1998;70:1584–92.
17. Herrera AJ, Castaño A, Venero JL, Cano J, Machado A. The single intranigral injection of LPS as a new model for studying the selective effects of inflammatory reactions on dopaminergic system. Neurobiol Dis. 2000;7:429–47.
18. Wu DC, Jackson-Lewis V, Vila M, Tieu K, Teismann P, Vadseth C, et al. Blockade of microglial activation is neuroprotective in the 1-methyl-4-phenyl-1,2,3,6-tetrahydropyridine mouse model of Parkinson disease. J Neurosci. 2002;22:1763–71.
19. Czlonkowska A, Kohutnicka M, Kurkowska-Jastrzebska I, Członkowski A. Microglial reaction in MPTP (1-methyl-4-phenyl-1,2,3,6-tetrahydropyridine) induced Parkinson's disease mice model. Neurodegeneration. 1996;5:137–43.
20. Kohutnicka M, Lewandowska E, Kurkowska-Jastrzebska I, Członkowski A, Członkowska A. Microglial and astrocytic involvement in a murine model of Parkinson's disease induced by 1-methyl-4-phenyl-1,2,3,6-tetrahydropyridine (MPTP). Immunopharmacology. 1998;39: 167–80.
21. Kurkowska-Jastrzebska I, Wrońska A, Kohutnicka M, Członkowski A, Członkowska A. MHC class II positive microglia and lymphocytic infiltration are present in the substantia nigra and striatum in mouse model of Parkinson's disease. Acta Neurobiol Exp (Wars). 1999;59:1–8.
22. Kurkowska-Jastrzebska I, Wrońska A, Kohutnicka M, Członkowski A, Członkowska A. The inflammatory reaction following 1-methyl-4-phenyl-1,2,3, 6-tetrahydropyridine intoxication in mouse. Exp Neurol. 1999;156:50–61.

23. Francis JW, Von Visger J, Markelonis GJ, Oh TH. Neuroglial responses to the dopaminergic neurotoxicant 1-methyl-4-phenyl-1,2,3,6-tetrahydropyridine in mouse striatum. Neurotoxicol Teratol. 1995;17:7–12.
24. Liang SM, Liang CM, Chiueh CC. Visualization of interleukin-2-like molecules in MPP(+)-lesioned rat brain. Biochem Biophys Res Commun. 1989;165:1312–8.
25. Ton TG, Jain S, Biggs ML, Thacker EL, Strotmeyer ES, Boudreau R, et al. Markers of inflammation in prevalent and incident Parkinson's disease in the cardiovascular health study. Parkinsonism Relat Disord. 2012;18:274–8.
26. Chen H, O'Reilly EJ, Schwarzschild MA, Ascherio A. Peripheral inflammatory biomarkers and risk of Parkinson's disease. Am J Epidemiol. 2008;167:90–5.
27. Wong KT, Grove JS, Grandinetti A, Curb JD, Yee M, Blanchette P, et al. Association of fibrinogen with Parkinson disease in elderly Japanese–American men: a prospective study. Neuroepidemiology. 2010;34:50–4.
28. Stypula G, Kunert-Radek J, Stepień H, Zylińska K, Pawlikowski M. Evaluation of interleukins, ACTH, cortisol and prolactin concentrations in the blood of patients with Parkinson's disease. Neuroimmunomodulation. 1996;3:131–4.
29. Dobbs RJ, Charlett A, Purkiss AG, Dobbs SM, Weller C, Peterson DW. Association of circulating TNF-alpha and IL-6 with ageing and parkinsonism. Acta Neurol Scand. 1999;100: 34–41.
30. Hofmann KW, Schuh AF, Saute J, Townsend R, Fricke D, Leke R, et al. Interleukin-6 serum levels in patients with Parkinson's disease. Neurochem Res. 2009;34:1401–4.
31. Bessler H, Djaldetti R, Salman H, Bergman M, Djaldetti M. IL-1 beta, IL-2, IL-6 and TNF-alpha production by peripheral blood mononuclear cells from patients with Parkinson's disease. Biomed Pharmacother. 1999;53:141–5.
32. Kluter H, Vieregge P, Stolze H, Kirchner H. Defective production of interleukin-2 in patients with idiopathic Parkinson's disease. J Neurol Sci. 1995;133:134–9.
33. Rentzos M, Nikolaou C, Andreadou E, Paraskevas GP, Rombos A, Zoga M, et al. Circulating interleukin-15 and RANTES chemokine in Parkinson's disease. Acta Neurol Scand. 2007; 116:374–9.
34. Rentzos M, Nikolaou C, Andreadou E, Paraskevas GP, Rombos A, Zoga M, et al. Circulating interleukin-10 and interleukin-12 in Parkinson's disease. Acta Neurol Scand. 2009;119: 332–7.
35. Hasegawa Y, Inagaki T, Sawada M, Suzumura A. Impaired cytokine production by peripheral blood mononuclear cells and monocytes/macrophages in Parkinson's disease. Acta Neurol Scand. 2000;101:159–64.
36. Lindqvist D, Kaufman E, Brundin L, Hall S, Surova Y, Hansson O. Non-motor symptoms in patients with Parkinson's disease – correlations with inflammatory cytokines in serum. PLoS One. 2012;7:e47387.
37. Marttila RJ, Eskola J, Soppi E, Rinne UK. Immune functions in Parkinson's disease lymphocyte subsets, concanavalin A-induced suppressor cell activity and in vitro immunoglobulin production. J Neurol Sci. 1985;69:121–31.
38. Saunders JA, Estes KA, Kosloski LM, Allen HE, Dempsey KM, Torres-Russotto DR, et al. $CD4^+$ regulatory and effector/memory T cell subsets profile motor dysfunction in Parkinson's disease. J Neuroimmune Pharmacol. 2012;7:927–38.
39. Fiszer U, Mix E, Fredrikson S, Kostulas V, Link H. Parkinson's disease and immunological abnormalities: increase of HLA-DR expression on monocytes in cerebrospinal fluid and of $CD45RO^+$ T cells in peripheral blood. Acta Neurol Scand. 1994;90:160–6.
40. Fiszer U, Mix E, Fredrikson S, Kostulas V, Olsson T, Link H. Gamma delta+ T cells are increased in patients with Parkinson's disease. J Neurol Sci. 1994;121:39–45.
41. Bas J, Calopa M, Mestre M, Molleví DG, Cutillas B, Ambrosio S, et al. Lymphocyte populations in Parkinson's disease and in rat models of parkinsonism. J Neuroimmunol. 2001;113: 146–52.
42. Chiba S, Matsumoto H, Saitoh M, Kasahara M, Matsuya M, Kashiwagi M. A correlation study between serum adenosine deaminase activities and peripheral lymphocyte subsets in Parkinson's disease. J Neurol Sci. 1995;132:170–3.

43. Hisanaga K, Asagi M, Itoyama Y, Iwasaki Y. Increase in peripheral CD4 bright+ CD8 dull+ T cells in Parkinson disease. Arch Neurol. 2001;58:1580–3.
44. Baba Y, Kuroiwa A, Uitti RJ, Wszolek ZK, Yamada T. Alterations of T-lymphocyte populations in Parkinson disease. Parkinsonism Relat Disord. 2005;11:493–8.
45. Luo XG, Zhang JJ, Zhang CD, Liu R, Zheng L, Wang XJ, et al. Altered regulation of CD200 receptor in monocyte-derived macrophages from individuals with Parkinson's disease. Neurochem Res. 2010;35:540–7.
46. Villaran RF, Espinosa-Oliva AM, Sarmiento M, De Pablos RM, Argüelles S, Delgado-Cortés MJ, et al. Ulcerative colitis exacerbates lipopolysaccharide-induced damage to the nigral dopaminergic system: potential risk factor in Parkinson's disease. J Neurochem. 2010;114: 1687–700.
47. Pott Godoy MC, Ferrari CC, Pitossi FJ. Nigral neurodegeneration triggered by striatal AdIL-1 administration can be exacerbated by systemic IL-1 expression. J Neuroimmunol. 2010; 222:29–39.
48. Pott Godoy MC, Tarelli R, Ferrari CC, Sarchi MI, Pitossi FJ. Central and systemic IL-1 exacerbates neurodegeneration and motor symptoms in a model of Parkinson's disease. Brain. 2008;131:1880–94.
49. Castano A, Herrera AJ, Cano J, Machado A. The degenerative effect of a single intranigral injection of LPS on the dopaminergic system is prevented by dexamethasone, and not mimicked by rh-TNF-alpha, IL-1beta and IFN-gamma. J Neurochem. 2002;81:150–7.
50. Skelly DT, Hennessy E, Dansereau MA, Cunningham C. A systematic analysis of the peripheral and CNS effects of systemic LPS, IL-1beta, TNF-alpha and IL-6 challenges in C57BL/6 mice. PLoS One. 2013;8:e69123.
51. Engler H, Doenlen R, Riether C, Engler A, Niemi MB, Besedovsky HO, et al. Time-dependent alterations of peripheral immune parameters after nigrostriatal dopamine depletion in a rat model of Parkinson's disease. Brain Behav Immun. 2009;23:518–26.
52. Seok J, Warren HS, Cuenca AG, Mindrinos MN, Baker HV, Xu W, et al. Genomic responses in mouse models poorly mimic human inflammatory diseases. Proc Natl Acad Sci U S A. 2013;110:3507–12.
53. Granger GA, Kolb WP. Lymphocyte in vitro cytotoxicity: mechanisms of immune and non-immune small lymphocyte mediated target L cell destruction. J Immunol. 1968;101: 111–20.
54. Granger GA, Williams TW. Lymphocyte cytotoxicity in vitro: activation and release of a cytotoxic factor. Nature. 1968;218:1253–4.
55. Kolb WP, Granger GA. Lymphocyte in vitro cytotoxicity: characterization of human lymphotoxin. Proc Natl Acad Sci U S A. 1968;61:1250–5.
56. Williams TW, Granger GA. Lymphocyte in vitro cytotoxicity: lymphotoxins of several mammalian species. Nature. 1968;219:1076–7.
57. Carswell EA, Old LJ, Kassel RL, Green S, Fiore N, Williamson B. An endotoxin-induced serum factor that causes necrosis of tumors. Proc Natl Acad Sci U S A. 1975;72:3666–70.
58. Green S, Dobrjansky A, Carswell EA, Kassel RL, Old LJ, Fiore N, et al. Partial purification of a serum factor that causes necrosis of tumors. Proc Natl Acad Sci U S A. 1976;73:381–5.
59. Ricciardi-Castagnoli P, Pirami L, Righi M, Sacerdote P, Locatelli V, Bianchi M, et al. Cellular sources and effects of tumor necrosis factor-alpha on pituitary cells and in the central nervous system. Ann N Y Acad Sci. 1990;594:156–68.
60. Sawada M, Kondo N, Suzumura A, Marunouchi T. Production of tumor necrosis factor-alpha by microglia and astrocytes in culture. Brain Res. 1989;491:394–7.
61. Hetier E, Ayala J, Bousseau A, Prochiantz A. Modulation of interleukin-1 and tumor necrosis factor expression by beta-adrenergic agonists in mouse ameboid microglial cells. Exp Brain Res. 1991;86:407–13.
62. Kinouchi K, Brown G, Pasternak G, Donner DB. Identification and characterization of receptors for tumor necrosis factor-alpha in the brain. Biochem Biophys Res Commun. 1991; 181:1532–8.

63. Locksley RM, Killeen N, Lenardo MJ. The TNF and TNF receptor superfamilies: integrating mammalian biology. Cell. 2001;104:487–501.
64. Watts TH. TNF/TNFR family members in costimulation of T cell responses. Annu Rev Immunol. 2005;23:23–68.
65. Hehlgans T, Mannel DN. The TNF–TNF receptor system. Biol Chem. 2002;383:1581–5.
66. Dopp JM, Mackenzie-Graham A, Otero GC, Merrill JE. Differential expression, cytokine modulation, and specific functions of type-1 and type-2 tumor necrosis factor receptors in rat glia. J Neuroimmunol. 1997;75:104–12.
67. Bradley JR, Pober JS. Tumor necrosis factor receptor-associated factors (TRAFs). Oncogene. 2001;20:6482–91.
68. MacEwan DJ. TNF receptor subtype signalling: differences and cellular consequences. Cell Signal. 2002;14(6):477–92.
69. MacEwan DJ. TNF ligands and receptors—a matter of life and death. Br J Pharmacol. 2002;135:855–75.
70. McFarlane SM, Pashmi G, Connell MC, Littlejohn AF, Tucker SJ, Vandenabeele P, et al. Differential activation of nuclear factor-kappaB by tumour necrosis factor receptor subtypes. TNFR1 predominates whereas TNFR2 activates transcription poorly. FEBS Lett. 2002;515: 119–26.
71. Mohamed AA, Jupp OJ, Anderson HM, Littlejohn AF, Vandenabeele P, MacEwan DJ, et al. Tumour necrosis factor-induced activation of c-Jun N-terminal kinase is sensitive to caspase-dependent modulation while activation of mitogen-activated protein kinase (MAPK) or p38 MAPK is not. Biochem J. 2002;366:145–55.
72. Rothe M, Sarma V, Dixit VM, Goeddel DV. TRAF2-mediated activation of NF-kappa B by TNF receptor 2 and CD40. Science. 1995;269:1424–7.
73. Chan FK. The pre-ligand binding assembly domain: a potential target of inhibition of tumour necrosis factor receptor function. Ann Rheum Dis. 2000;59 Suppl 1:50–3.
74. Chan FK, Chun HJ, Zheng L, Siegel RM, Bui KL, Lenardo MJ. A domain in TNF receptors that mediates ligand-independent receptor assembly and signaling. Science. 2000;288: 2351–4.
75. Deng GM, Zheng L, Chan FK, Lenardo M. Amelioration of inflammatory arthritis by targeting the pre-ligand assembly domain of tumor necrosis factor receptors. Nat Med. 2005;11: 1066–72.
76. Boka G, Anglade P, Wallach D, Javoy-Agid F, Agid Y, Hirsch EC. Immunocytochemical analysis of tumor necrosis factor and its receptors in Parkinson's disease. Neurosci Lett. 1994;172:151–4.
77. Mogi M, Togari A, Kondo T, Mizuno Y, Komure O, Kuno S, et al. Caspase activities and tumor necrosis factor receptor R1 (p55) level are elevated in the substantia nigra from Parkinsonian brain. J Neural Transm. 2000;107:335–41.
78. Duke DC, Moran LB, Pearce RK, Graeber MB. The medial and lateral substantia nigra in Parkinson's disease: mRNA profiles associated with higher brain tissue vulnerability. Neurogenetics. 2007;8:83–94.
79. Mogi M, Harada M, Riederer P, Narabayashi H, Fujita K, Nagatsu T. Tumor necrosis factor-alpha (TNF-alpha) increases both in the brain and in the cerebrospinal fluid from Parkinsonian patients. Neurosci Lett. 1994;165(1–2):208–10.
80. Scalzo P, Kümmer A, Cardoso F, Teixeira AL. Increased serum levels of soluble tumor necrosis factor-alpha receptor-1 in patients with Parkinson's disease. J Neuroimmunol. 2009;216:122–5.
81. Reale M, Iarlori C, Thomas A, Gambi D, Perfetti B, Di Nicola M, et al. Peripheral cytokines profile in Parkinson's disease. Brain Behav Immun. 2009;23:55–63.
82. Bongioanni P, Castagna M, Maltinti S, Boccardi B, Dadone F. T-lymphocyte tumor necrosis factor-alpha receptor binding in patients with Parkinson's disease. J Neurol Sci. 1997;149: 41–5.
83. Koziorowski D, Tomasiuk R, Szlufik S, Friedman A. Inflammatory cytokines and NT-proCNP in Parkinson's disease patients. Cytokine. 2012;60:762–6.

84. Menza M, Dobkin RD, Marin H, Mark MH, Gara M, Bienfait K, et al. The role of inflammatory cytokines in cognition and other non-motor symptoms of Parkinson's disease. Psychosomatics. 2010;51:474–9.
85. Wahner AD, Sinsheimer JS, Bronstein JM, Ritz B. Inflammatory cytokine gene polymorphisms and increased risk of Parkinson disease. Arch Neurol. 2007;64:836–40.
86. Wilson AG, Symons JA, McDowell TL, McDevitt HO, Duff GW, et al. Effects of a polymorphism in the human tumor necrosis factor alpha promoter on transcriptional activation. Proc Natl Acad Sci U S A. 1997;94:3195–9.
87. Bialecka M, Klodowska-Duda G, Kurzawski M, Slawek J, Gorzkowska A, Opala G, et al. Interleukin-10 (IL10) and tumor necrosis factor alpha (TNF) gene polymorphisms in Parkinson's disease patients. Parkinsonism Relat Disord. 2008;14:636–40.
88. Kruger R, Hardt C, Tschentscher F, Jäckel S, Kuhn W, Müller T, et al. Genetic analysis of immunomodulating factors in sporadic Parkinson's disease. J Neural Transm. 2000;107: 553–62.
89. Ross OA, O'Neill C, Rea IM, Lynch T, Gosal D, Wallace A, et al. Functional promoter region polymorphism of the proinflammatory chemokine IL-8 gene associates with Parkinson's disease in the Irish. Hum Immunol. 2004;65:340–6.
90. Pascale E, Passarelli E, Purcaro C, Vestri AR, Fakeri A, Guglielmi R, et al. Lack of association between IL-1beta, TNF-alpha, and IL-10 gene polymorphisms and sporadic Parkinson's disease in an Italian cohort. Acta Neurol Scand. 2011;124:176–81.
91. Nishimura M, Mizuta I, Mizuta E, Yamasaki S, Ohta M, Kaji R, et al. Tumor necrosis factor gene polymorphisms in patients with sporadic Parkinson's disease. Neurosci Lett. 2001;311: 1–4.
92. Wu YR, Feng IH, Lyu RK, Chang KH, Lin YY, Chan H, et al. Tumor necrosis factor-alpha promoter polymorphism is associated with the risk of Parkinson's disease. Am J Med Genet B Neuropsychiatr Genet. 2007;144B:300–4.
93. Sriram K, Matheson JM, Benkovic SA, Miller DB, Luster MI, O'Callaghan JP. Mice deficient in TNF receptors are protected against dopaminergic neurotoxicity: implications for Parkinson's disease. FASEB J. 2002;16:1474–6.
94. Rousselet E, Callebert J, Parain K, Joubert C, Hunot S, Hartmann A, et al. Role of TNF-alpha receptors in mice intoxicated with the Parkinsonian toxin MPTP. Exp Neurol. 2002;177: 183–92.
95. Leng A, Mura A, Feldon J, Ferger B. Tumor necrosis factor-alpha receptor ablation in a chronic MPTP mouse model of Parkinson's disease. Neurosci Lett. 2005;375:107–11.
96. Ferger B, Leng A, Mura A, Hengerer B, Feldon J. Genetic ablation of tumor necrosis factor-alpha (TNF-alpha) and pharmacological inhibition of TNF-synthesis attenuates MPTP toxicity in mouse striatum. J Neurochem. 2004;89:822–33.
97. McCoy MK, Martinez TN, Ruhn KA, Szymkowski DE, Smith CG, Botterman BR, et al. Blocking soluble tumor necrosis factor signaling with dominant-negative tumor necrosis factor inhibitor attenuates loss of dopaminergic neurons in models of Parkinson's disease. J Neurosci. 2006;26:9365–75.
98. De Lella Ezcurra AL, Chertoff M, Ferrari C, Graciarena M, Pitossi F. Chronic expression of low levels of tumor necrosis factor-alpha in the substantia nigra elicits progressive neurodegeneration, delayed motor symptoms and microglia/macrophage activation. Neurobiol Dis. 2010;37:630–40.
99. Chertoff M, Di Paolo N, Schoeneberg A, Depino A, Ferrari C, Wurst W, et al. Neuroprotective and neurodegenerative effects of the chronic expression of tumor necrosis factor alpha in the nigrostriatal dopaminergic circuit of adult mice. Exp Neurol. 2011;227:237–51.
100. Barger SW, Hörster D, Furukawa K, Goodman Y, Krieglstein J, Mattson MP. Tumor necrosis factors alpha and beta protect neurons against amyloid beta-peptide toxicity: evidence for involvement of a kappa B-binding factor and attenuation of peroxide and Ca^{2+} accumulation. Proc Natl Acad Sci U S A. 1995;92:9328–32.
101. Li R, Yang L, Lindholm K, Konishi Y, Yue X, Hampel H, et al. Tumor necrosis factor death receptor signaling cascade is required for amyloid-beta protein-induced neuron death. J Neurosci. 2004;24:1760–71.

102. Chao CC, Hu S. Tumor necrosis factor-alpha potentiates glutamate neurotoxicity in human fetal brain cell cultures. Dev Neurosci. 1994;16:172–9.
103. Gelbard HA, Dzenko KA, DiLoreto D, del Cerro C, del Cerro M, Epstein LG. Neurotoxic effects of tumor necrosis factor alpha in primary human neuronal cultures are mediated by activation of the glutamate AMPA receptor subtype: implications for AIDS neuropathogenesis. Dev Neurosci. 1993;15:417–22.
104. Floden AM, Li S, Combs CK. Beta-amyloid-stimulated microglia induce neuron death via synergistic stimulation of tumor necrosis factor alpha and NMDA receptors. J Neurosci. 2005;25:2566–75.
105. Akiyama H, Barger S, Barnum S, Bradt B, Bauer J, Cole GM, et al. Inflammation and Alzheimer's disease. Neurobiol Aging. 2000;21:383–421.
106. Chao CC, Hu S, Sheng WS, Peterson PK. Tumor necrosis factor-alpha production by human fetal microglial cells: regulation by other cytokines. Dev Neurosci. 1995;17:97–105.
107. Combs CK, Bates P, Karlo JC, Landreth GE. Regulation of beta-amyloid stimulated proinflammatory responses by peroxisome proliferator-activated receptor alpha. Neurochem Int. 2001;39:449–57.
108. Gimsa U, Peter SV, Lehmann K, Bechmann I, Nitsch R. Axonal damage induced by invading T cells in organotypic central nervous system tissue in vitro: involvement of microglial cells. Brain Pathol. 2000;10:365–77.
109. Ravizza T, Rizzi M, Perego C, Richichi C, Velísková J, Moshé SL, et al. Inflammatory response and glia activation in developing rat hippocampus after status epilepticus. Epilepsia. 2005;46 Suppl 5:113–7.
110. Tchelingerian JL, Quinonero J, Booss J, Jacque C. Localization of TNF alpha and IL-1 alpha immunoreactivities in striatal neurons after surgical injury to the hippocampus. Neuron. 1993;10:213–24.
111. Yin L, Ohtaki H, Nakamachi T, Dohi K, Iwai Y, Funahashi H, et al. Expression of tumor necrosis factor alpha (TNFalpha) following transient cerebral ischemia. Acta Neurochir Suppl. 2003;86:93–6.
112. Beattie EC, Stellwagen D, Morishita W, Bresnahan JC, Ha BK, Von Zastrow M, et al. Control of synaptic strength by glial TNFalpha. Science. 2002;295:2282–5.
113. Stellwagen D, Malenka RC. Synaptic scaling mediated by glial TNF-alpha. Nature. 2006;440:1054–9.
114. Romera C, Hurtado O, Botella SH, Lizasoain I, Cárdenas A, Fernández-Tomé P, et al. In vitro ischemic tolerance involves upregulation of glutamate transport partly mediated by the TACE/ADAM17-tumor necrosis factor-alpha pathway. J Neurosci. 2004;24:1350–7.
115. Watters O, Pickering M, O'Connor JJ. Preconditioning effects of tumor necrosis factor-alpha and glutamate on calcium dynamics in rat organotypic hippocampal cultures. J Neuroimmunol. 2011;234:27–39.
116. Ogoshi F, Yin HZ, Kuppumbatti Y, Song B, Amindari S, Weiss JH. Tumor necrosis-factor-alpha (TNF-alpha) induces rapid insertion of Ca^{2+}-permeable alpha-amino-3-hydroxyl-5-methyl-4-isoxazole-propionate (AMPA)/kainate (Ca-A/K) channels in a subset of hippocampal pyramidal neurons. Exp Neurol. 2005;193:384–93.
117. Rainey-Smith SR, Andersson DA, Williams RJ, Rattray M. Tumour necrosis factor alpha induces rapid reduction in AMPA receptor-mediated calcium entry in motor neurones by increasing cell surface expression of the GluR2 subunit: relevance to neurodegeneration. J Neurochem. 2010;113:692–703.
118. He P, Liu Q, Wu J, Shen Y. Genetic deletion of TNF receptor suppresses excitatory synaptic transmission via reducing AMPA receptor synaptic localization in cortical neurons. FASEB J. 2012;26:334–45.
119. Bliss RM, Finckbone VL, Trice J, Strahlendorf H, Strahlendorf J. Tumor necrosis factor-alpha (TNF-alpha) augments AMPA-induced Purkinje neuron toxicity. Brain Res. 2011;1386:1–14.
120. Combs CK, Karlo JC, Kao SC, Landreth GE. Beta-Amyloid stimulation of microglia and monocytes results in TNFalpha-dependent expression of inducible nitric oxide synthase and neuronal apoptosis. J Neurosci. 2001;21:1179–88.

121. Jara JH, Singh BB, Floden AM, Combs CK. Tumor necrosis factor alpha stimulates NMDA receptor activity in mouse cortical neurons resulting in ERK-dependent death. J Neurochem. 2007;100:1407–20.
122. Leonoudakis D, Zhao P, Beattie EC. Rapid tumor necrosis factor alpha-induced exocytosis of glutamate receptor 2-lacking AMPA receptors to extrasynaptic plasma membrane potentiates excitotoxicity. J Neurosci. 2008;28:2119–30.
123. Yang L, Lindholm K, Konishi Y, Li R, Shen Y. Target depletion of distinct tumor necrosis factor receptor subtypes reveals hippocampal neuron death and survival through different signal transduction pathways. J Neurosci. 2002;22:3025–32.
124. Jarosinski KW, Whitney LW, Massa PT. Specific deficiency in nuclear factor-kappaB activation in neurons of the central nervous system. Lab Invest. 2001;81:1275–88.
125. Listwak SJ, Rathore P, Herkenham M. Minimal NF-kappaB activity in neurons. Neuroscience. 2013;250:282–99.
126. Massa PT, Aleyasin H, Park DS, Mao X, Barger SW. NFkappaB in neurons? The uncertainty principle in neurobiology. J Neurochem. 2006;97:607–18.
127. Quintana A, Molinero A, Florit S, Manso Y, Comes G, Carrasco J, et al. Diverging mechanisms for TNF-alpha receptors in normal mouse brains and in functional recovery after injury: from gene to behavior. J Neurosci Res. 2007;85:2668–85.
128. Pejovic V, Soskić V, Pan W, Kastin AJ. Brain proteome of mice lacking the receptors for tumor necrosis factor alpha. Proteomics. 2004;4:1461–4.
129. Hartmann A, Mouatt-Prigent A, Faucheux BA, Agid Y, Hirsch EC. FADD: a link between TNF family receptors and caspases in Parkinson's disease. Neurology. 2002;58:308–10.
130. Tatton NA. Increased caspase 3 and Bax immunoreactivity accompany nuclear GAPDH translocation and neuronal apoptosis in Parkinson's disease. Exp Neurol. 2000;166:29–43.
131. Hunot S, Brugg B, Ricard D, Michel PP, Muriel MP, Ruberg M, et al. Nuclear translocation of NF-kappaB is increased in dopaminergic neurons of patients with Parkinson disease. Proc Natl Acad Sci U S A. 1997;94:7531–6.
132. Yamada M, Kida K, Amutuhaire W, Ichinose F, Kaneki M. Gene disruption of caspase-3 prevents MPTP-induced Parkinson's disease in mice. Biochem Biophys Res Commun. 2010;402:312–8.
133. Jellinger KA. Recent developments in the pathology of Parkinson's disease. J Neural Transm Suppl. 2002;(62):347–76.
134. Nold MF, Nold-Petry CA, Zepp JA, Palmer BE, Bufler P, Dinarello CA. IL-37 is a fundamental inhibitor of innate immunity. Nat Immunol. 2010;11:1014–22.
135. Fujita H, Inoue Y, Seto K, Komitsu N, Aihara M. Interleukin-37 is elevated in subjects with atopic dermatitis. J Dermatol Sci. 2013;69:173–5.
136. Auron PE, Webb AC, Rosenwasser LJ, Mucci SF, Rich A, Wolff SM, et al. Nucleotide sequence of human monocyte interleukin 1 precursor cDNA. Proc Natl Acad Sci U S A. 1984;81:7907–11.
137. Auron PE, Webb AC, Rosenwasser LJ, Mucci SF, Rich A, Wolff SM, et al. Nucleotide sequence of human monocyte interleukin 1 precursor cDNA. J Immunol. 2007;178:5413–7.
138. March CJ, Mosley B, Larsen A, Cerretti DP, Braedt G, Price V, et al. Cloning, sequence and expression of two distinct human interleukin-1 complementary DNAs. Nature. 1985;315: 641–7.
139. Gubler U, Chua AO, Stern AS, Hellmann CP, Vitek MP, DeChiara TM, et al. Recombinant human interleukin 1 alpha: purification and biological characterization. J Immunol. 1986;136: 2492–7.
140. Dinarello CA. Biology of interleukin 1. FASEB J. 1988;2:108–15.
141. Thornberry NA, Bull HG, Calaycay JR, Chapman KT, Howard AD, Kostura MJ, et al. A novel heterodimeric cysteine protease is required for interleukin-1 beta processing in monocytes. Nature. 1992;356:768–74.
142. Kilian PL, Kaffka KL, Stern AS, Woehle D, Benjamin WR, Dechiara TM. Interleukin 1 alpha and interleukin 1 beta bind to the same receptor on T cells. J Immunol. 1986;136:4509–14.

143. Dripps DJ, Brandhuber BJ, Thompson RC, Eisenberg SP. Interleukin-1 (IL-1) receptor antagonist binds to the 80-kDa IL-1 receptor but does not initiate IL-1 signal transduction. J Biol Chem. 1991;266:10331–6.
144. Hannum CH, Wilcox CJ, Arend WP, Joslin FG, Dripps DJ, Heimdal PL, et al. Interleukin-1 receptor antagonist activity of a human interleukin-1 inhibitor. Nature. 1990;343:336–40.
145. Eisenberg SP, Brewer MT, Verderber E, Heimdal P, Brandhuber BJ, Thompson RC. Interleukin 1 receptor antagonist is a member of the interleukin 1 gene family: evolution of a cytokine control mechanism. Proc Natl Acad Sci U S A. 1991;88:5232–6.
146. Arend WP. Interleukin 1 receptor antagonist. A new member of the interleukin 1 family. J Clin Invest. 1991;88:1445–51.
147. O'Neill LA. The interleukin-1 receptor/Toll-like receptor superfamily: 10 years of progress. Immunol Rev. 2008;226:10–8.
148. Stylianou E, O'Neill LA, Rawlinson L, Edbrooke MR, Woo P, Saklatvala J. Interleukin 1 induces NF-kappa B through its type I but not its type II receptor in lymphocytes. J Biol Chem. 1992;267:15836–41.
149. Sims JE, Acres RB, Grubin CE, McMahan CJ, Wignall JM, March CJ, et al. Cloning the interleukin 1 receptor from human T cells. Proc Natl Acad Sci U S A. 1989;86:8946–50.
150. Greenfeder SA, Nunes P, Kwee L, Labow M, Chizzonite RA, Ju G. Molecular cloning and characterization of a second subunit of the interleukin 1 receptor complex. J Biol Chem. 1995;270:13757–65.
151. Huang J, Gao X, Li S, Cao Z. Recruitment of IRAK to the interleukin 1 receptor complex requires interleukin 1 receptor accessory protein. Proc Natl Acad Sci U S A. 1997;94: 12829–32.
152. Radons J, Gabler S, Wesche H, Korherr C, Hofmeister R, Falk W. Identification of essential regions in the cytoplasmic tail of interleukin-1 receptor accessory protein critical for interleukin-1 signaling. J Biol Chem. 2002;277:16456–63.
153. Brikos C, Wait R, Begum S, O'Neill LA, Saklatvala J. Mass spectrometric analysis of the endogenous type I interleukin-1 (IL-1) receptor signaling complex formed after IL-1 binding identifies IL-1RAcP, MyD88, and IRAK-4 as the stable components. Mol Cell Proteomics. 2007;6:1551–9.
154. Cao Z, Henzel WJ, Gao X. IRAK: a kinase associated with the interleukin-1 receptor. Science. 1996;271:1128–31.
155. Qin J, Jiang Z, Qian Y, Casanova JL, Li X. IRAK4 kinase activity is redundant for interleukin-1 (IL-1) receptor-associated kinase phosphorylation and IL-1 responsiveness. J Biol Chem. 2004;279:26748–53.
156. Ninomiya-Tsuji J, Kishimoto K, Hiyama A, Inoue J, Cao Z, Matsumoto K. The kinase TAK1 can activate the NIK-I[kappa]B as well as the MAP kinase cascade in the IL-1 signalling pathway. Nature. 1999;398:252–6.
157. Wang C, Deng L, Hong M, Akkaraju GR, Inoue J, Chen ZJ, et al. TAK1 is a ubiquitin-dependent kinase of MKK and IKK. Nature. 2001;412:346–51.
158. Dinarello CA. The interleukin-1 family: 10 years of discovery. FASEB J. 1994;8:1314–25.
159. Kampschmidt RF, Pulliam LA, Merriman CR. Further similarities of endogenous pyrogen and leukocytic endogenous mediator. Am J Physiol Cell Physiol. 1978;235:C118–21.
160. Dinarello CA. Interleukin-1. Rev Infect Dis. 1984;6:51–95.
161. Gery I, Waksman BH. Potentiation of the T-lymphocyte response to mitogens. II. The cellular source of potentiating mediator(s). J Exp Med. 1972;136:143–55.
162. Murphy PA, Simon PL, Willoughby WF. Endogenous pyrogens made by rabbit peritoneal exudate cells are identical with lymphocyte-activating factors made by rabbit alveolar macrophages. J Immunol. 1980;124:2498–501.
163. Morrissey PJ, Mochizuki DY. Interleukin-1 is identical to hemopoietin-1: studies on its therapeutic effects on myelopoiesis and lymphopoiesis. Biotherapy. 1989;1:281–91.
164. Altman LC, Snyderman R, Oppenheim JJ, Mergenhagen SE. A human mononuclear leukocyte chemotactic factor: characterization, specificity and kinetics of production by homologous leukocytes. J Immunol. 1973;110:801–10.

165. Baracos V, Rodemann HP, Dinarello CA, Goldberg AL. Stimulation of muscle protein degradation and prostaglandin E2 release by leukocytic pyrogen (interleukin-1). A mechanism for the increased degradation of muscle proteins during fever. N Engl J Med. 1983; 308:553–8.
166. Saklatvala J, Dingle JT. Identification of catabolin, a protein from synovium which induces degradation of cartilage in organ culture. Biochem Biophys Res Commun. 1980;96:1225–31.
167. Dewhirst FE, Stashenko PP, Mole JE, Tsurumachi T. Purification and partial sequence of human osteoclast-activating factor: identity with interleukin 1 beta. J Immunol. 1985; 135:2562–8.
168. Dunne A. Inflammasome activation: from inflammatory disease to infection. Biochem Soc Trans. 2011;39:669–73.
169. Leal MC, Casabona JC, Puntel M, Pitossi FJ. Interleukin-1beta and tumor necrosis factor-alpha: reliable targets for protective therapies in Parkinson's disease? Front Cell Neurosci. 2013;7:53.
170. Takao T, Tracey DE, Mitchell WM, De Souza EB. Interleukin-1 receptors in mouse brain: characterization and neuronal localization. Endocrinology. 1990;127:3070–8.
171. Mogi M, Harada M, Kondo T, Riederer P, Inagaki H, Minami M, et al. Interleukin-1 beta, interleukin-6, epidermal growth factor and transforming growth factor-alpha are elevated in the brain from Parkinsonian patients. Neurosci Lett. 1994;180:147–50.
172. Blum-Degen D, Müller T, Kuhn W, Gerlach M, Przuntek H, Riederer P. Interleukin-1 beta and interleukin-6 are elevated in the cerebrospinal fluid of Alzheimer's and de novo Parkinson's disease patients. Neurosci Lett. 1995;202:17–20.
173. Mogi M, Harada M, Narabayashi H, Inagaki H, Minami M, Nagatsu T. Interleukin (IL)-1 beta, IL-2, IL-4, IL-6 and transforming growth factor-alpha levels are elevated in ventricular cerebrospinal fluid in juvenile parkinsonism and Parkinson's disease. Neurosci Lett. 1996;211:13–6.
174. Griffin WS, Stanley LC, Ling C, White L, MacLeod V, Perrot LJ, et al. Brain interleukin 1 and S-100 immunoreactivity are elevated in Down syndrome and Alzheimer disease. Proc Natl Acad Sci U S A. 1989;86:7611–5.
175. Minami M, Kuraishi Y, Yabuuchi K, Yamazaki A, Satoh M. Induction of interleukin-1 beta mRNA in rat brain after transient forebrain ischemia. J Neurochem. 1992;58:390–2.
176. Liu T, McDonnell PC, Young PR, White RF, Siren AL, Hallenbeck JM, et al. Interleukin-1 beta mRNA expression in ischemic rat cortex. Stroke. 1993;24:1746–50. discussion 1750–1.
177. Buttini M, Sauter A, Boddeke HW. Induction of interleukin-1 beta mRNA after focal cerebral ischaemia in the rat. Brain Res Mol Brain Res. 1994;23:126–34.
178. Wang X, Yue TL, Barone FC, White RF, Gagnon RC, Feuerstein GZ. Concomitant cortical expression of TNF-alpha and IL-1 beta mRNAs follows early response gene expression in transient focal ischemia. Mol Chem Neuropathol. 1994;23:103–14.
179. Hillhouse EW, Kida S, Iannotti F. Middle cerebral artery occlusion in the rat causes a biphasic production of immunoreactive interleukin-1beta in the cerebral cortex. Neurosci Lett. 1998;249:177–9.
180. Davies CA, et al. The progression and topographic distribution of interleukin-1beta expression after permanent middle cerebral artery occlusion in the rat. J Cereb Blood Flow Metab. 1999;19:87–98.
181. Taupin V, Toulmond S, Serrano A, Benavides J, Zavala F. Increase in IL-6, IL-1 and TNF levels in rat brain following traumatic lesion. Influence of pre- and post-traumatic treatment with Ro5 4864, a peripheral-type (p site) benzodiazepine ligand. J Neuroimmunol. 1993;42:177–85.
182. Sandhir R, Gregory E, He YY, Berman NE. Upregulation of inflammatory mediators in a model of chronic pain after spinal cord injury. Neurochem Res. 2011;36:856–62.
183. Stammers AT, Liu J, Kwon BK. Expression of inflammatory cytokines following acute spinal cord injury in a rodent model. J Neurosci Res. 2012;90:782–90.

184. Minami M, Kuraishi Y, Yamaguchi T, Nakai S, Hirai Y, Satoh M. Convulsants induce interleukin-1β messenger RNA in rat brain. Biochem Biophys Res Commun. 1990;171: 832–7.
185. Yabuuchi K, Minami M, Katsumata S, Satoh M. In situ hybridization study of interleukin-1 beta mRNA induced by kainic acid in the rat brain. Brain Res Mol Brain Res. 1993;20:153–61.
186. Bagetta G, Corasaniti MT, Berliocchi L, Nisticó R, Giammarioli AM, Malorni W, et al. Involvement of interleukin-1β in the mechanism of human immunodeficiency virus type 1 (HIV-1) recombinant protein gp120-induced apoptosis in the neocortex of rat. Neuroscience. 1999;89:1051–66.
187. Hunot S, Dugas N, Faucheux B, Hartmann A, Tardieu M, Debré P, et al. FcepsilonRII/CD23 is expressed in Parkinson's disease and induces, in vitro, production of nitric oxide and tumor necrosis factor-alpha in glial cells. J Neurosci. 1999;19:3440–7.
188. McGeer PL, Yasojima K, McGeer EG. Association of interleukin-1 beta polymorphisms with idiopathic Parkinson's disease. Neurosci Lett. 2002;326:67–9.
189. Schulte T, Schöls L, Müller T, Woitalla D, Berger K, Krüger R. Polymorphisms in the interleukin-1 alpha and beta genes and the risk for Parkinson's disease. Neurosci Lett. 2002;326: 70–2.
190. Mattila KM, Rinne JO, Lehtimäki T, Röyttä M, Ahonen JP, Hurme M. Association of an interleukin 1B gene polymorphism (–511) with Parkinson's disease in Finnish patients. J Med Genet. 2002;39:400–2.
191. Arman A, Isik N, Coker A, Candan F, Becit KS, List EO. Association between sporadic Parkinson disease and interleukin-1 beta –511 gene polymorphisms in the Turkish population. Eur Cytokine Netw. 2010;21:116–21.
192. Chu K, Zhou X, Luo BY. Cytokine gene polymorphisms and Parkinson's disease: a meta-analysis. Can J Neurol Sci. 2012;39:58–64.
193. Nishimura M, Mizuta I, Mizuta E, Yamasaki S, Ohta M, Kuno S. Influence of interleukin-1beta gene polymorphisms on age-at-onset of sporadic Parkinson's disease. Neurosci Lett. 2000;284:73–6.
194. Nishimura M, Kuno S, Kaji R, Yasuno K, Kawakami H. Glutathione-S-transferase-1 and interleukin-1beta gene polymorphisms in Japanese patients with Parkinson's disease. Mov Disord. 2005;20:901–2.
195. Liu GJ, Feng RN, Luo C, Bi S. Lack of association between interleukin-1 alpha, beta polymorphisms and Parkinson's disease. Neurosci Lett. 2010;480:158–61.
196. Mogi M, Togari A, Ogawa M, Ikeguchi K, Shizuma N, Fan D, et al. Effects of repeated systemic administration of 1-methyl-4-phenyl-1,2,3,6-tetrahydropyridine (MPTP) to mice on interleukin-1β and nerve growth factor in the striatum. Neurosci Lett. 1998;250:25–8.
197. Depino AM, Earl C, Kaczmarczyk E, Ferrari C, Besedovsky H, del Rey A, et al. Microglial activation with atypical proinflammatory cytokine expression in a rat model of Parkinson's disease. Eur J Neurosci. 2003;18:2731–42.
198. Giulian D, Lachman LB. Interleukin-1 stimulation of astroglial proliferation after brain injury. Science. 1985;228:497–9.
199. Saura J, Parés M, Bové J, Pezzi S, Alberch J, Marin C, et al. Intranigral infusion of interleukin-1β activates astrocytes and protects from subsequent 6-hydroxydopamine neurotoxicity. J Neurochem. 2003;85:651–61.
200. Nakao N, Itakura T, Uematsu Y, Nakai M, Komai N, Furukawa S. Pretreatment with interleukin-1 enhances survival of sympathetic ganglionic neuron grafts. Neurol Med Chir. 1994;34:407–11.
201. Heese K, Hock C, Otten U. Inflammatory signals induce neurotrophin expression in human microglial cells. J Neurochem. 1998;70:699–707.
202. Koprich JB, Reske-Nielsen C, Mithal P, Isacson O. Neuroinflammation mediated by IL-1beta increases susceptibility of dopamine neurons to degeneration in an animal model of Parkinson's disease. J Neuroinflammation. 2008;5:8.

203. Klevenyi P, Andreassen O, Ferrante RJ, Schleicher Jr JR, Friedlander RM, Beal MF. Transgenic mice expressing a dominant negative mutant interleukin-1beta converting enzyme show resistance to MPTP neurotoxicity. Neuroreport. 1999;10:635–8.
204. Ferrari CC, Pott Godoy MC, Tarelli R, Chertoff M, Depino AM, Pitossi FJ. Progressive neurodegeneration and motor disabilities induced by chronic expression of IL-1beta in the substantia nigra. Neurobiol Dis. 2006;24:183–93.
205. Loddick SA, Wong ML, Bongiorno PB, Gold PW, Licinio J, Rothwell NJ. Endogenous interleukin-1 receptor antagonist is neuroprotective. Biochem Biophys Res Commun. 1997;234:211–5.
206. Hailer NP, Vogt C, Korf HW, Dehghani F. Interleukin-1beta exacerbates and interleukin-1 receptor antagonist attenuates neuronal injury and microglial activation after excitotoxic damage in organotypic hippocampal slice cultures. Eur J Neurosci. 2005;21:2347–60.
207. Allan SM, Tyrrell PJ, Rothwell NJ. Interleukin-1 and neuronal injury. Nat Rev Immunol. 2005;5:629–40.
208. Carvey PM, Punati A, Newman MB. Progressive dopamine neuron loss in Parkinson's disease: the multiple hit hypothesis. Cell Transplant. 2006;15:239–50.
209. Sulzer D. Multiple hit hypotheses for dopamine neuron loss in Parkinson's disease. Trends Neurosci. 2007;30:244–50.
210. Ferrari CC, Tarelli R. Parkinson's disease and systemic inflammation. Parkinsons Dis. 2011;2011:436813.
211. Deleidi M, Gasser T. The role of inflammation in sporadic and familial Parkinson's disease. Cell Mol Life Sci. 2013;70:4259–73.

Cell Culture Models of Inflammation in Parkinson's Disease

Patrick Flood

Introduction

Parkinson's disease (PD) is a progressive degenerative disorder of the central nervous system (CNS) that leads to impairment of motor skills and speech, as well as other functions. The etiology of PD is primarily characterized by the chronic loss of dopamine production by a subset of neurons (DA neurons) within the substantia nigra (SN) and striatum. While it is postulated that a multitude of different factors, including genetic, environmental, and intrinsic mechanisms, can ultimately cause or contribute to dopaminergic neurodegeneration in PD, it is now clear that the progressive nature of PD is characterized or accompanied by chronic inflammation-induced neurodegeneration of dopamine-producing neurons [1–4]. The levels of a number of proinflammatory mediators, including TNF-α, IL-1β, IL-6, eicosanoids, as well as reactive oxygen species (ROS), are elevated in the brains and peripheral blood mononuclear cells (PBMCs) of patients with PD [5, 6]. Nitrite in the cerebrospinal fluid and increased expression of inducible nitric oxide synthase (iNOS) within the SN have been found in PD patients [7]. All of these findings lend strong support to the association of inflammation and PD. Many of these inflammatory mediators have been demonstrated to have strong neurotoxic effects on DA neurons [2, 8–10]. This evidence, and those detailed in other chapters within this book, all point to the microglial cell as central to the initiation, execution, and regulation of the inflammatory responses within the CNS leading to dopaminergic degeneration [2, 11, 12].

In order to study the role of inflammation, particularly microglial-mediated inflammation, on the production of dopamine by DA neurons, investigators have developed a number of in vitro cell culture models that measure the effects of inflammatory cells and mediators on the viability and functional dopamine production by

P. Flood, Ph.D. (✉)
Department of Faculty of Medicine and Dentistry, University of Alberta, Katz Group Centre for Pharmacy and Health Research, Edmonton, AB, Canada

M. Thomas (ed.), *Inflammation in Parkinson's Disease: Scientific and Clinical Aspects*, DOI 10.1007/978-3-319-08046-8_7,

DA neurons in vitro. These models include the use of DA-neuronal cell lines, primary DA-producing cells, as well as the generation of primary cultures of mesencephalic neuron-glial cultures, to measure the effects of inflammatory cells and mediators on the viability, function, and dopamine production of DA neurons. Each culture system has its own unique advantages in studying the molecular and cellular mechanisms associated with DA neurodegeneration, and in measuring the effects of different inflammatory triggers, anti-inflammatory cytokines, cells, and therapeutics, as well as the role of genetic, molecular, and cellular abnormalities in DA neurons that initiate or contribute to the chronic inflammatory-mediated degeneration as seen in PD. In this chapter, we will detail several different in vitro cell culture models that are currently being used to measure the inflammatory-based etiology of PD.

Use of Cell Lines in Inflammatory Cell Culture Systems

Dopamine-Producing Cells Lines

One of the major in vitro approaches used by investigators seeking to investigate the mechanisms of dopamine loss during progressive is the use of dopamine-producing cell lines. These cell lines are either continuously growing cell lines developed from in vitro cultures or immortalized by cellular fusion or isolated from patients or animals with neuroblastomas that produce dopamine and express markers indicative of dopaminergic neurons. The most commonly used cell lines currently being studied include the human cell line BG01V2 [13], the murine cell line MN9D [14], or the rat cell lines PC-12 [15] and 1RB3AN27 [16]. A number of neuroblastomas cell lines have been isolated that express markers of DA neurons, as well as a high production of dopamine, which include the human cell lines SK-N-SH, SK-N-MC, and SK-N-BE [17], a subclone of the SK-N-SH cell line SH-SY5Y [18], and the murine cell line CATH.a [19]. A list of these cell lines, along with their derivation date and number of references utilizing these cells since 2005 (along with the number of times used for in vitro assays as a model for the study of PD), are shown in Table 1.

The BG01V2 human dopamine-producing cell line was derived from the embryonic stem cell line BG01 by co-culturing these hESC with the PA6 mouse stromal cell line as previously described [13]. These cells express Pax5, Otx2, and Msx1, as well as tyrosine hydroxylase (TH) and the dopamine transporter (DAT), strongly suggesting they arise from dopaminergic neurons. Although it appears this cell line has significant potential for investigating the function of DA neurons, it appears that neuroblastoma cell lines are more commonly used to study the biology and sensitivity of DA neurons to inflammatory signals. These neuroblastoma cell lines include the most commonly studied SK-N-SH, SK-N-MC, and SK-N-BE (1) and (2) neuroblastoma lines [17]. The SK-N-SH, MC, and BE neuroblastoma cell lines are pheochromocytoma cell lines that were isolated from distinct neuroblastoma patients and have been extensively used to study neuronal biology both for their

Table 1 Cell lines regularly used in in vitro models of Parkinson's disease

Dopamine-producing cell lines	Species	Reference	Year of origin	References since 2000
BG01V2	Human	[13]	2008	1 (1)
MN9D	Murine	[14]	1991	120 (80)
PC-12	Rat	[15]	1976	8,645 (39)
1RB3AN27	Rat	[16]	1996	7 (6)
DA-neuroblastoma				
SH-SY5Y	Human	[18]	1978	13,301 (686)
SK-N-MC	Human	[17]	1973	390 (32)
SK-N-SH	Human	[17]	1973	751 (54)
SK-N-BE 1/2	Human	[17]	1973	200 (11)
CATH.a	Murine	[19]	1993	105 (20)
Neuro2A (N2A)	Murine	[20]	1970	468 (15)
Microglial cell lines				
CHME-5	Human	[21]	1995	16 (1)
N9	Human	[22]	1989	36 (13)
HAPI	Rat	[23]	2001	103 (4)
BV-2	Murine	[24]	1990	454 (29)
Macrophage/monocyte cell lines				
THP-1	Human	[25]	1980	4,704 (17)
RAW 264.7	Murine	[26]	1977	3,763 (4)

high production of dopamine and also for their distinct genetic makeup, biological properties, and marker expression. A subclone of the SK-N-SH cell line, SH-SY5Y [18], has been extensively used to study neuronal differentiation, including ability to differentiate into functionally distinct cells when stimulated with a number of different stimuli, including retinoic acid, TPA, cAMP, and neurological growth factors NGF and BDNF [27]. The SH-SY5Y cultures include both adherent and cells that grow in suspension, leading to potentially different results depending on the state of the cells being investigated. In addition, even closed populations of SH-SY5Y cells may contain two distinct phenotypes: neuroblast-like cells and epithelial-like cells [28]. These two phenotypes may best be reflected in the "N" and "S" types of SH-SY5Y by [29]. This may also lead to a dichotomy of results, as it has been reported that the "N" cells, which exhibit neuroblast-like morphology, produce dopamine and express TH, while the "S" cells exhibit epithelial-like counterpart cells that lacked these enzymatic activities [28]. Despite these characteristics, these cell lines have been extensively studied for the biological characteristics of DA neurons and can easily be used in cell cultures to measure the effects of inflammatory mediators and cells.

Rodent in vitro models of PD are also used extensively to study the role of inflammation in dopaminergic neurotoxicity. Like the human in vitro models, a number of rodent cell lines have been developed that allow investigators to measure the effects of inflammatory mediators and cells on the biology of dopamine-producing neurons. A cell line that has been extensively studied as a target for inflammatory mediators is the rat pheochromocytoma PC12 cell line [15]. This line was derived from a transplantable rat adrenal pheochromocytoma, and it differentiates into a neuronal phenotype upon exposure to NGF when plated on collagen IV-coated culture flasks. These cells produce large amounts of dopamine and DAT upon differentiation and are sensitive to a number of DA-specific neurotoxins that have been implicated in the pathogenesis of PD, including MPP^+ and 6-OHDA. Another rat cell line that serves as an in vitro model for DA neurons is 1RB3AN27 [16], an SV-40 immortalized cell line derived from fetal rat mesencephalic cells that produces a high level of dopamine in culture. Treatment of 1RB3AN27 with a cAMP-stimulating agent increases levels of TH and DAT, these cells express the neuron marker nestin but not GFAP, and these cells are likewise sensitive to 6-OHDA [30]. In contrast, the most popular murine DA-producing cell lines used in in vitro cultures are the CATH.a (Central Adrenergic TH-expressing) and N2A (Neuro2A) cell lines. The CATH.a was derived from a brain cell culture of TH-positive tumors in transgenic mice carrying the SV40 T antigen oncogene under the transcriptional control of the rat TH gene [19]. The CATH.a line expresses the SV-40 T antigen, as well as displays neuronal properties such as neurofilaments and synaptophysin. CATH.a cells are sensitive to the neurotoxic effects of MPTP and 6-OHDA, as well as to ROS-induced apoptosis. The N2A cell line is a mouse neural crest-derived cell line [20] that can be induced to produce high levels of TH and dopamine upon stimulation with dibutyryl cAMP [31]. N2A cells have been extensively used because they are both sensitive to apoptosis in the presence of inflammatory mediators TNFα and ROS, and they themselves express mRNA for the inflammatory mediators IL-1β, IL-6, TNF-α, NF-κB, and iNOS when stimulated with LPS [32].

Microglial Cell Lines

The first postmortem report of high levels of activated inflammatory cells within the SN of PD patients came over two decades ago [33], and these cells were identified as activated microglial cells. Since that time, the microglial cells have been the major focus of study as the source of inflammatory damage that leads to chronic DA neurodegeneration. Products of microglial cells, including TNF-α, IL-1β, and IL-6, have been found in high concentrations within the SN of PD patients [34, 35] as well as inflammatory mediators such as PGE2, NO, and ROS [36–40]. This indicates that the cell that is predominantly implicated in the pathology of PD is the microglial cell, and most of the in vitro cultures used as models to study inflammation in PD utilize the microglial cell. However, unlike the previously described DA-neuronal cell lines used in vitro, a microglial cell line must be able to be activated by inflammogens in order to be useful in studying the pathogenesis of inflammation on dopaminergic neurons. In addition, because of the similarities in phenotype and function between microglial cells and systemic macrophages, many in vitro cultures utilized to study inflammation and PD utilize macrophage/monocyte cell lines rather than microglial cell lines to generate inflammatory mediators and measure the effects of these mediators and/or cells on dopamine production, apoptosis, and phenotype on dopamine-producing cells.

Table 1 also includes a list of the most common microglia and macrophage cell lines used in in vitro cultures to measure the effects of inflammation on DA-neuronal activity. In vitro cell cultures investigating the role of innate immunity in PD have utilized both microglial cell lines and macrophage/monocyte cell lines to study the effects of inflammatory activation on the production of dopamine, the viability of DA neurons, and the function of these neurons following exposure to various inflammatory mediators. The most commonly used microglial cell lines for the study of human inflammation-induced DA neurodegeneration is the CHME-5 and the N9 microglial cell lines. The CHME-5 line was generated from human fetal microglia by transfection with the large T antigen of simian virus 40 [21]. This line expresses TLR2, TLR4, and TLR9 and is responsive to activation signals by producing ROS, as well as other inflammatory mediators such as TNF-α, IL-6, and MCP-1 in response to activation [41]. N9 is a human microglial cell line derived from primary mouse embryo brain cells using new recombinants (termed 3RV) carrying the v-myc or v-mil oncogenes of the avian retrovirus MH2 [22, 42]. It is capable of producing a proinflammatory response upon activation through the production of TNF-α, IL-1β, IL-6, NO, and ROS [22, 43]. Both of these cell lines have been used to study the role of microglia in DA-neuronal cell death in in vitro models of PD. A more commonly used human cell line to study DA neurodegeneration is THP-1. THP-1 is a human leukemic cell line (THP-1) cultured from the blood of a boy with acute monocytic leukemia [25]. While it is considered a monocyte line rather than a fully differentiated macrophage, this cell line exhibits properties similar to the human monocyte-derived macrophages in that activation of THP-1 with LPS or TNF-α leads to a rapid response and production of proinflammatory mediators IL-1β, TNF-α, and IL-6, as well as the production of NO and ROS species [25].

A number of rodent microglial or macrophage cell lines have been developed and utilized to measure the effect of innate immune cells on DA neurotoxicity. HAPI (highly aggressively proliferating immortalized) were isolated from a population enriched for microglial cells, and stain for the microglial markers B4 and OX-42, but do not express A2B5 or GFAP. HAPI cells are capable of phagocytosis, and when stimulated with the inflammogen, LPS produces measureable amount of the proinflammatory cytokines IL-1β, IL-6, and TNF-α, as well as the mounting of an oxidative stress response which produces NO and ROS. HAPI cells have been used to study inflammatory mediator production, cell signaling mechanisms, and sensitivity to therapeutic intervention using in vitro models of neurodegeneration. The most widely used microglial cell line of murine origin is the BV-2 cell line. The immortalized mouse microglial cell line BV-2 was developed in the laboratory of Dr. Blasi at the University of Perugia, Italy [24]. BV-2 was generated by infecting primary microglial cell cultures with a v-raf/v-myc oncogene carrying retrovirus (J2) [24]. BV-2 cells express phagocytic ability and secrete proinflammatory cytokines TNF-α, IL-1β, and IL-6, as well as NO and ROS, upon stimulation with LPS. Phenotypically BV-2 expresses the MAC1 and MAC2 antigens, but not GFAP or galactocerebroside (GC). The BV-2 cell line is the most widely studied cell line of confirmed microglial origin and has been used to study the role of microglia in a number of different chronic neurodegenerative conditions, including PD. In addition to microglial cell lines, PD investigators have also used murine macrophage cell lines to determine the response of innate immune cells in PD. The most commonly used macrophage cell line is RAW264.7. The murine cell line RAW264.7 was established from an ascites of a tumor induced in a male mouse by intraperitoneal injection of Abelson Leukaemia Virus (A-MuLV) [26]. It is a well-established model for macrophage activation and is likely the most well-studied macrophage line currently being used to study the role of innate immunity in inflammation.

Use of Primary Mesencephalic Cultures in Inflammatory Cell Culture Systems

While the existence of pure cell lines of DA neurons and microglia/macrophages can facilitate the study of inflammation in PD, it is important to determine the biological functions of primary cells to validate and extend the findings into a system that more resembles the cellular makeup of the SN and striatum. Mesencephalic-glia cultures provide an excellent model of the cellular and architectural makeup of the midbrain, both in the distribution of the cell types expressed within the SN and also in the fact that these cells represent primary cell types whose responses to inflammatory signals or mediators are most likely to reflect those of resident cells of the brain. Mesencephalic cultures are composed primarily of four major cell types: astrocytes, neurons, microglia, and DA neurons. These cultures not only provide a relatively accurate ratio of cells to those found in the intact midbrain but also allow investigators to individually analyze the role of each major cell type in the inflammatory response by selectively depleting an individual cell type based on their unique phenotypic markers or by enriching for certain cell types by differential processing and cellular growth characteristics. These cultures include neuron-glial cultures, mixed-glial cultures, enriched microglia cultures, and reconstituted neuron-microglial cultures. Each system can serve to answer specific questions regarding the role or contribution of each cell type, the molecular mechanisms of cellular responses, and the interactions between microglia-neurons, microglia-astrocytes, and microglia themselves or the interaction between all cell types in the response of DA neurons to neurotoxins, inflammogens, or inflammatory mediators. A brief description of each is given below.

Primary Mesencephalic Neuron-Glial Cultures

Primary mesencephalic neuron-glial cultures are composed of all cells normally found within the SN. The distribution of cells is approximately 50 % $GFAP^+$ cells (astrocytes), 40 % $NeuN^+$ cells (neurons), and 10 % OX-42/$MAC\text{-}1^+$ cells (microglia). Within the 40 % $NeuN^+$ cells population, about 1–2 % are positive for tyrosine hydroxylase (TH), a unique marker for DA-producing neurons within the SN. This model is created by taking rat dams at gestational day 13–15, or mouse dams at gestational day 13–14, removing the brain area, and isolating the mesencephalic region from the rest of the brain [44]. The timing of embryo harvest, as well as the delicacy of the surgery, is critical to success, so this is a procedure that may take a great deal of trial and error before achieving the desired number and proper ratio of cells within your cultures. A highly detailed procedure for proper preparation of these cultures can be found in Chapter 21 of *Microglia, Methods and Protocols* [44]. These cells are then seeded in flasks or tissue culture plates and can be utilized within 7–10 days of seeding for analysis. Once prepared, it is important to verify by immunohistochemistry the cellular composition of your culture using antibodies to GFAP, NeuN, and OX-42/MAC-1. The critical cell for measuring inflammatory responses in these cultures is the microglia, so cultures with more than 10 % OX-42/MAC-1$^+$ cells may produce highly variable results. While cumbersome, this model most closely resembles the in vivo situation within the SN, and the major advantage of using this type of culture model is for evaluating the effects of neurotoxins, inflammogens, or immunotherapeutics in DA-neuron viability and function and to measure the effects of blocking antibodies, gene silencers, or additional protein molecules on DA-neuronal activity.

Mixed-Glial Cultures

These cultures are prepared in similar to primary mesencephalic neuron-glial cultures except that they are plated with a different medium of growth, require exchange rather than supplementation of the medium, and are maintained in culture under different conditions which favors the outgrowth of astrocytes and microglia but not neurons. The final concentration of mixed-glial cultures should be 80 % GFAP$^+$ cells and 20 %OX-42/MAC-1$^+$ cells.

Enriched Microglial Cultures

Enriched microglial cultures are obtained from the mixed-glial cultures by gently shaking the culture flasks containing 14-day-old mixed-glial cultures and collecting the cellular suspension [44]. This technique relies on the fact that only microglial cells will be released from attachment under these conditions. Suspension cells can then be collected and replated and routinely result in >95 % OX-42/MAC-1$^+$ cells.

Reconstituted Neuron-Microglial Co-cultures

Neuron-glial cultures can be rendered devoid of glial cells by treatment with ara-C (arabinofuranosyl cytidine) and LME (leucine methyl ester) at a final concentration of 5–15 μM [44]. Ara-C and LME are routinely used to remove astrocytes and microglia, respectively, from culture systems. After treatment, cells are extensively washed and then reconstituted with enriched microglial cells to determine the role or contribution of astrocytes to the in vitro inflammatory response.

Another general method for generating in vitro cultures as a model for PD has also been described [45]. This technique involves culturing postnatal SN cells and allows for the generation of mixed and chimeric neuron/glial cultures of postnatal SN cells, independent of other monoaminergic nuclei in the ventral midbrain. This approach can be used for the construction of total SNpc cultures, astrocyte cultures, or hybrid neuron-glial cultures. The advantage of this technique is that it can be performed on adult mice, thereby reducing the number of brains needed for dissection, allowing phenotypic analysis on genetically altered mice prior to harvesting, as well as the tissue(s) used in this procedure include only the specific cells lost in PD rather than a large number of unaffected cells. In addition, these cultures can be used to measure the effects of inflammogens, neurotoxins, and other potential initiators of inflammation leading to DA neurotoxicity.

Measurement of DA Neurotoxicity

Cell cultures that use DA-producing cell lines or transformed neuroblastoma cells as a model for PD can be an effective way of measuring the effects of inflammatory cells or mediators on the viability and functionality of DA neurons in vitro. This approach has been used extensively to measure the effects of inflammogens such as LPS and neurotoxins such as MPP^+ or to measure the direct effects of inflammatory mediators such as TNF-α [46, 47], IL-1β [48, 49], IL-6 [50, 51], NO [52, 53], ROS [54, 55], IFNγ [56, 57], and PGE2 [58, 59] or to measure the effect of activated microglial cells lines such as BV-2 [60, 61] or N9 [62] on DA-producing neuronal cell lines. Certainly one of the biggest advantages to using DA-producing neuronal cell lines or neuroblastoma cells, and conversely using microglial or macrophage cell lines to mimic inflammation, is the ability to molecularly manipulate these lines to alter the production or response of these lines using genetic constructs and cell signaling inhibitors.

Mesencephalic cultures have also been used extensively to study the effects of inflammogens or neurotoxins on primary DA-producing neurons. These studies show that while most inflammogens have little to no direct effect on DA-producing neurons in the absence of microglial cells [12], a number of inflammatory mediators, such as TNF-α, NO, and ROS, have strong effects on both the viability and functionality of DA neurons. The most common inflammogen used in these cultures to activate microglia is LPS, but it has been used also for measuring the inflammatory potential of alpha-synuclein, MPP^+, or other antigens proposed to be involved in PD activation. More importantly, these cultures are often generated from rodents which have been genetically manipulated to overexpress a certain protein, to express mutants of these proteins, or from animals that have had a genetic knockout of a gene of interest in the inflammatory, neuron, or astrocyte lineage. These approaches have been used to study the potential role of alpha-synuclein, LRRK2, DJ-1, Parkin, and PINK1 in DA neurodegeneration [63].

The in vitro cultures used to measure inflammatory effects on DA neurons take several experimental designs. The most common is simply adding the agent of investigation directly into cultures and measuring the effects of this agent on DA viability and/or dopamine production. In neuronal cell cultures, cellular viability can be measured using vital stains, an MTT or LDH assay [64], or by measuring apoptosis using a TUNEL (TdT-mediated dUTP nick-end labeling) assay, a Comet Assay [65], and/or by measurement of cleaved caspase-3 by Western blot [66]. This is much more difficult in mesencephalic cultures; therefore, viability of DA neurons is determined by measuring the number of cells that stain positive in immunohistochemistry for tyrosine hydroxylase (TH^+), a unique marker for DA neurons. This assay simply compares the number of TH^+ neurons in control to the experimental group and is usually accompanied by an assay to measure dopamine production.

In vitro assays to measure dopamine production are generally the most definitive tests that identify alterations in DA-neuronal biology that most closely resemble PD. These tests usually involve the differential uptake of tritiated (3H)-dopamine by DA neurons [67]. This assay relies on the observation that DA neurons will uptake radioactive dopamine, while other cells without the DAT protein will not uptake this dopamine, and allows for investigators to measure the functionality of DA neurons by the amount they take up compared to other cells within the culture system. This is especially useful for the mesencephalic cultures, as the number of TH^+ neurons is often too low to accurately count, and measurement of DA uptake provides a good quantitative measure of cell functionality. Other methods are also available to measure dopamine production in vitro, including electroanalytical methods [68], plasmon resonance biosensors [69], nanofibers [70], chromatography, and various flow injection systems [71]. However, these other methods require significant time, volume, and equipment commitment for accurate measurement and do not lend themselves well to multiple sample analysis.

References

1. Bartels AL, Leenders KL. Neuroinflammation in the pathophysiology of Parkinson's disease: evidence from animal models to human in vivo studies with [11C]-PK11195 PET. Mov Disord. 2007;22:1852–6.
2. Block ML, Hong JS. Microglia and inflammation-mediated neurodegeneration: multiple triggers with a common mechanism. Prog Neurobiol. 2005;76:77–98.
3. Dauer W, Przedborski S. Parkinson's disease: mechanisms and models. Neuron. 2003;39: 889–909.
4. Gao HM, Hong JS. Why neurodegenerative diseases are progressive: uncontrolled inflammation drives disease progression. Trends Immunol. 2008;29:357–65.
5. Mogi M, Harada M, Kondo T, Riederer P, Inagaki H, Minami M, et al. Interleukin-1 beta, interleukin-6, epidermal growth factor and transforming growth factor-alpha are elevated in the brain from parkinsonian patients. Neurosci Lett. 1994;180:147–50.

6. Nagatsu T, Mogi M, Ichinose H, Togari A. Changes in cytokines and neurotrophins in Parkinson's disease. J Neural Transm Suppl. 2000;60:277–90.
7. Hunot S, Boissiere F, Faucheux B, Brugg B, Mouatt-Prigent A, Agid Y, et al. Nitric oxide synthase and neuronal vulnerability in Parkinson's disease. Neuroscience. 1996;72:355–63.
8. Qian L, Flood PM. Microglial cells and Parkinson's disease. Immunol Res. 2008;41:155–64.
9. McCoy MK, Tansey MG. TNF signaling inhibition in the CNS: implications for normal brain function and neurodegenerative disease. J Neuroinflammation. 2008;5:45.
10. Zielasek J, Hartung HP. Molecular mechanisms of microglial activation. Adv Neuroimmunol. 1996;6:191–222.
11. Czlonkowska A, Kohutnicka M, Kurkowska-Jastrzebska I, Czlonkowski A. Microglial reaction in MPTP (1-methyl-4-phenyl-1,2,3,6-tetrahydropyridine) induced Parkinson's disease mice model. Neurodegeneration. 1996;5:137–43.
12. Qian L, Flood PM, Hong JS. Neuroinflammation is a key player in Parkinson's disease and a prime target for therapy. J Neural Transm. 2010;117:971–9.
13. Vazin T, Chen J, Spivak CE, Amable R, Gabitzsch E, Lee CT, et al. Dopaminergic neurons derived from BG01V2, a variant of human embryonic stem cell line BG01. Restor Neurol Neurosci. 2008;26:447–58.
14. Choi HK, Won LA, Kontur PJ, Hammond DN, Fox AP, Wainer BH, et al. Immortalization of embryonic mesencephalic dopaminergic neurons by somatic cell fusion. Brain Res. 1991;552:67–76.
15. Greene LA, Tischler AS. Establishment of a noradrenergic clonal line of rat adrenal pheochromocytoma cells which respond to nerve growth factor. Proc Natl Acad Sci U S A. 1976; 73:2424–8.
16. Adams FS, La Rosa FG, Kumar S, Edwards-Prasad J, Kentroti S, Vernadakis A, et al. Characterization and transplantation of two neuronal cell lines with dopaminergic properties. Neurochem Res. 1996;21:619–27.
17. Biedler JL, Helson L, Spengler BA. Morphology and growth, tumorigenicity, and cytogenetics of human neuroblastoma cells in continuous culture. Cancer Res. 1973;33:2643–52.
18. Biedler JL, Roffler-Tarlov S, Schachner M, Freedman LS. Multiple neurotransmitter synthesis by human neuroblastoma cell lines and clones. Cancer Res. 1978;38:3751–7.
19. Suri C, Fung BP, Tischler AS, Chikaraishi DM. Catecholaminergic cell lines from the brain and adrenal glands of tyrosine hydroxylase-SV40 T antigen transgenic mice. J Neurosci. 1993; 13:1280–91.
20. Klebe RJ, Chen T, Ruddle FH. Controlled production of proliferating somatic cell hybrids. J Cell Biol. 1970;45:74–82.
21. Janabi N, Peudenier S, Heron B, Ng KH, Tardieu M. Establishment of human microglial cell lines after transfection of primary cultures of embryonic microglial cells with the SV40 large T antigen. Neurosci Lett. 1995;195:105–8.
22. Righi M, Mori L, De Libero G, Sironi M, Biondi A, Mantovani A, et al. Monokine production by microglial cell clones. Eur J Immunol. 1989;19:1443–8.
23. Cheepsunthorn P, Radov L, Menzies S, Reid J, Connor JR. Characterization of a novel brain-derived microglial cell line isolated from neonatal rat brain. Glia. 2001;35:53–62.
24. Blasi E, Barluzzi R, Bocchini V, Mazzolla R, Bistoni F. Immortalization of murine microglial cells by a v-raf/v-myc carrying retrovirus. J Neuroimmunol. 1990;27:229–37.
25. Tsuchiya S, Yamabe M, Yamaguchi Y, Kobayashi Y, Konno T, Tada K. Establishment and characterization of a human acute monocytic leukemia cell line (THP-1). Int J Cancer. 1980;26:171–6.
26. Ralph P, Nakoinz I, Raschke WC. Lymphosarcoma cell growth is selectively inhibited by B lymphocyte mitogens: LPS, dextran sulfate and PPD. Biochem Biophys Res Commun. 1974;61:1268–75.
27. Kovalevich J, Langford D. Considerations for the use of SH-SY5Y neuroblastoma cells in neurobiology. Methods Mol Biol. 2013;1078:9–21.
28. Ross RA, Spengler BA, Biedler JL. Coordinate morphological and biochemical interconversion of human neuroblastoma cells. J Natl Cancer Inst. 1983;71:741–7.

29. Encinas M, Iglesias M, Liu Y, Wang H, Muhaisen A, Cena V, et al. Sequential treatment of SH-SY5Y cells with retinoic acid and brain-derived neurotrophic factor gives rise to fully differentiated, neurotrophic factor-dependent, human neuron-like cells. J Neurochem. 2000;75: 991–1003.
30. Clarkson ED, Edwards-Prasad J, Freed CR, Prasad KN. Immortalized dopamine neurons: a model to study neurotoxicity and neuroprotection. Proc Soc Exp Biol Med. 1999;222: 157–63.
31. Tremblay RG, Sikorska M, Sandhu JK, Lanthier P, Ribecco-Lutkiewicz M, Bani-Yaghoub M. Differentiation of mouse Neuro 2A cells into dopamine neurons. J Neurosci Methods. 2010;186:60–7.
32. Yang C, Jiang RY, Shen J, Hong T, Liu N, Ding LC, et al. Ketamine attenuates the lipopolysaccharide-induced inflammatory response in cultured N2a cells. Mol Med Rep. 2013;8:217–20.
33. McGeer PL, Itagaki S, Boyes BE, McGeer EG. Reactive microglia are positive for HLA-DR in the substantia nigra of Parkinson's and Alzheimer's disease brains. Neurology. 1988;38: 1285–91.
34. Hirsch EC, Hunot S. Neuroinflammation in Parkinson's disease: a target for neuroprotection? Lancet Neurol. 2009;8:382–97.
35. Orr CF, Rowe DB, Halliday GM. An inflammatory review of Parkinson's disease. Prog Neurobiol. 2002;68:325–40.
36. Jenner P, Olanow CW. Understanding cell death in Parkinson's disease. Ann Neurol. 1998; 44:S72–84.
37. Liang X, Wu L, Wang Q, Hand T, Bilak M, McCullough L, et al. Function of COX-2 and prostaglandins in neurological disease. J Mol Neurosci. 2007;33:94–9.
38. Wang T, Pei Z, Zhang W, Liu B, Langenbach R, Lee C, et al. MPP^+-induced COX-2 activation and subsequent dopaminergic neurodegeneration. FASEB J. 2005;19:1134–6.
39. Lin MT, Beal MF. Mitochondrial dysfunction and oxidative stress in neurodegenerative diseases. Nature. 2006;443:787–95.
40. Monahan AJ, Warren M, Carvey PM. Neuroinflammation and peripheral immune infiltration in Parkinson's disease: an autoimmune hypothesis. Cell Transplant. 2008;17:363–72.
41. Dutta R, Krishnan A, Meng J, Das S, Ma J, Banerjee S, et al. Morphine modulation of toll-like receptors in microglial cells potentiates neuropathogenesis in a HIV-1 model of coinfection with pneumococcal pneumoniae. J Neurosci. 2012;32:9917–30.
42. Righi M, Pierani A, Boglia A, De Libero G, Mori L, Marini V, et al. Generation of new oncogenic murine retroviruses by cotransfection of cloned AKR and MH2 proviruses. Oncogene. 1989;4:223–30.
43. Mou YH, Yang JY, Cui N, Wang JM, Hou Y, Song S, et al. Effects of cobalt chloride on nitric oxide and cytokines/chemokines production in microglia. Int Immunopharmacol. 2012;13: 120–5.
44. Chen SH, Oyarzabal EA, Hong JS. Preparation of rodent primary cultures for neuron-glia, mixed glia, enriched microglia, and reconstituted cultures with microglia. Methods Mol Biol. 2013;1041:231–40.
45. Smeyne M, Smeyne RJ. Method for culturing postnatal substantia nigra as an in vitro model of experimental Parkinson's disease. Brain Res Brain Res Protoc. 2002;9:105–11.
46. Kwon SJ, Ahn TB, Yoon MY, Jeon BS. BV-2 stimulation by lactacystin results in a strong inflammatory reaction and apoptotic neuronal death in SH-SY5Y cells. Brain Res. 2008;1205: 116–21.
47. Soeda S, Ochiai T, Paopong L, Tanaka H, Shoyama Y, Shimeno H. Crocin suppresses tumor necrosis factor-alpha-induced cell death of neuronally differentiated PC-12 cells. Life Sci. 2001;69:2887–98.
48. Smith EL, Hainsworth AH. Acute effects of interleukin-1 beta on noradrenaline release from the human neuroblastoma cell line SH-SY5Y. Neurosci Lett. 1998;251:89–92.
49. Suzuki A. Amyloid beta-protein induces necrotic cell death mediated by ICE cascade in PC12 cells. Exp Cell Res. 1997;234:507–11.

50. Bissonnette CJ, Klegeris A, McGeer PL, McGeer EG. Interleukin 1alpha and interleukin 6 protect human neuronal SH-SY5Y cells from oxidative damage. Neurosci Lett. 2004;361: 40–3.
51. Satoh T, Nakamura S, Taga T, Matsuda T, Hirano T, Kishimoto T, et al. Induction of neuronal differentiation in PC12 cells by B-cell stimulatory factor 2/interleukin 6. Mol Cell Biol. 1988;8:3546–9.
52. Haby C, Lisovoski F, Aunis D, Zwiller J. Stimulation of the cyclic GMP pathway by NO induces expression of the immediate early genes c-fos and junB in PC12 cells. J Neurochem. 1994;62:496–501.
53. Lee HS, Park CW, Kim YS. MPP(+) increases the vulnerability to oxidative stress rather than directly mediating oxidative damage in human neuroblastoma cells. Exp Neurol. 2000;165: 164–71.
54. Junn E, Mouradian MM. Apoptotic signaling in dopamine-induced cell death: the role of oxidative stress, p38 mitogen-activated protein kinase, cytochrome c and caspases. J Neurochem. 2001;78:374–83.
55. Kruman I, Guo Q, Mattson MP. Calcium and reactive oxygen species mediate staurosporine-induced mitochondrial dysfunction and apoptosis in PC12 cells. J Neurosci Res. 1998;51: 293–308.
56. Cho SG, Yi SY, Yoo YS. IFNgamma and TNFalpha synergistically induce neurite outgrowth on PC12 cells. Neurosci Lett. 2005;378:49–54.
57. Tong HX, Lu CW, Zhang JH, Ma L, Zhang JH. Combination of gamma-interferon with TRAIL and cisplatin or etoposide induces apoptosis in human neuroblastoma cell line SH-SY5Y. Chin Med Sci J. 2007;22:38–43.
58. Hu JH, Zhu XZ. Rotenone-induced neurotoxicity of THP-1 cells requires production of reactive oxygen species and activation of phosphatidylinositol 3-kinase. Brain Res. 2007;1153: 12–9.
59. Nakamura K, Katoh H, Ichikawa A, Negishi M. Inhibition of dopamine release by prostaglandin EP3 receptor via pertussis toxin-sensitive and -insensitive pathways in PC12 cells. J Neurochem. 1998;71:646–52.
60. Hu Q, Li B, Xu R, Chen D, Mu C, Fei E, et al. The protease Omi cleaves the mitogen-activated protein kinase kinase MEK1 to inhibit microglial activation. Sci Signal. 2012;5:ra61.
61. Lee JK, Chung J, McAlpine FE, Tansey MG. Regulator of G-protein signaling-10 negatively regulates NF-kappaB in microglia and neuroprotects dopaminergic neurons in hemiparkinsonian rats. J Neurosci. 2011;31:11879–88.
62. Huber VC, Mondal T, Factor SA, Seegal RF, Lawrence DA. Serum antibodies from Parkinson's disease patients react with neuronal membrane proteins from a mouse dopaminergic cell line and affect its dopamine expression. J Neuroinflammation. 2006;3:1.
63. Lee Y, Dawson VL, Dawson TM. Animal models of Parkinson's disease: vertebrate genetics. Cold Spring Harb Perspect Med. 2012;2.
64. Wu FJ, Xue Y, Tang QJ, Xu J, Du L, Xue CH, et al. The protective effects of cerebrosides from sea cucumber and starfish on the oxidative damage in PC12 cells. J Oleo Sci. 2013;62: 717–27.
65. Tice RR, Agurell E, Anderson D, Burlinson B, Hartmann A, Kobayashi H, et al. Single cell gel/comet assay: guidelines for in vitro and in vivo genetic toxicology testing. Environ Mol Mutagen. 2000;35:206–21.
66. Bureau G, Longpre F, Martinoli MG. Resveratrol and quercetin, two natural polyphenols, reduce apoptotic neuronal cell death induced by neuroinflammation. J Neurosci Res. 2008; 86:403–10.
67. Liu B, Du L, Kong LY, Hudson PM, Wilson BC, Chang RC, et al. Reduction by naloxone of lipopolysaccharide-induced neurotoxicity in mouse cortical neuron-glia co-cultures. Neuroscience. 2000;97:749–56.
68. Hasanzadeh M, Shadjou N, Omidinia E. A novel electroanalytical method for simultaneous detection of two neurotransmitter dopamine and serotonin in human serum. J Neurosci Methods. 2013;219:52–60.

69. Kumbhat S, Shankaran DR, Kim SJ, Gobi KV, Joshi V, Miura N. Surface plasmon resonance biosensor for dopamine using D3 dopamine receptor as a biorecognition molecule. Biosens Bioelectron. 2007;23:421–7.
70. Mo JW, Ogorevc B. Simultaneous measurement of dopamine and ascorbate at their physiological levels using voltammetric microprobe based on overoxidized poly(1,2-phenylenediamine)-coated carbon fiber. Anal Chem. 2001;73:1196–202.
71. van Staden JF, van Staden RI. Flow-injection analysis systems with different detection devices and other related techniques for the in vitro and in vivo determination of dopamine as neurotransmitter. Talanta. 2012;102:34–43.

Clinical Aspects of Inflammation in Parkinson's Disease

Madhavi Thomas and Christopher Adams

There is consensus that inflammation is present in Parkinson's disease (PD). However, there is debate on whether the increase in inflammatory cells and the relevant markers of inflammation are a cause or consequence of PD pathogenesis. Further, there is debate regarding relative importance of inflammation as opposed to other possible mechanisms, such as mitochondrial dysfunction, oxidative stress, autophagy, and mitophagy. It is unclear whether the increased inflammation seen in PD is protective or contributory to cell death. Much of the preclinical evidence has been presented in earlier chapters. In this chapter we present translational and clinical evidence looking at the relationship between inflammation and PD.

Biological Markers

The World Health Organization has defined biomarker as "any substance, structure or process that can be measured in the body or its products and influence or predict the incidence or outcome of the disease." There are different classes of biomarkers, some are predictive and some are surrogate. Surrogate biomarkers must show consistency, accuracy and these are best used for measurement of changes in a biologic system. Clinical endpoints show changes in morbidity, mortality, and are more relevant to clinical research. Validation of these markers is an important step in clinical research. While we present evidence of various studies, none of these are widely accepted to be validated inflammatory biomarkers in current clinical practice in PD [1].

M. Thomas, M.D. (✉)
North Texas Movement Disorders Institute, Inc., Bedford, TX, USA

Department of Neurology, Baylor University Medical Center, Dallas, TX, USA

C. Adams, M.S.
North Texas Movement Disorders Institute, Inc., Bedford, TX, USA

M. Thomas (ed.), *Inflammation in Parkinson's Disease: Scientific and Clinical Aspects*,
DOI 10.1007/978-3-319-08046-8_8,

In the central nervous system (CNS) particularly in immune-mediated neurodegeneration, three mechanisms need to be reviewed: (1) Systemic response to neurodegeneration, which includes activation and transfer of immune molecules from the periphery to CNS, via the blood–brain barrier, propagation of secondary factors, and diffusion via circumventricular organs. (2) CNS autonomous mechanisms intrinsic to the neurons are immune responses within the extra-neuronal brain tissue and systemic responses to neurodegeneration. Within the neurons, cellular responses include important pathways that activate caspases. (3) Outside the neurons, there are responses initiated by glial cells [2].

T-Cell Markers

Many investigators looked specifically at peripheral T-cell-mediated response in patients with PD. In a cardiovascular health cohort, specific biomarkers including albumin, WBC count, fibrinogen, CRP (C-reactive protein), and IL-6 were measured in those who had PD. In women higher levels of IL-6 seem to correlate with higher risk of prevalent PD, while in men elevated total WBC count seemed to indicate higher risk of prevalent PD, while no biomarker could be identified for incident PD [3]. A more specific approach looking at chronic induction of T-cell stimulation as a peripheral response was taken by Saunders et al. [4]. They studied changes in phenotype of CD4 T cells and correlated with UPDRS to identify those markers that are associated with increased severity of disease. In $CD4^+$ T cells, specific patterns were noted in T Reg (regulatory T cells) and Tem (memory T cells). Higher UPDRS scores were associated with increased $CD45R0^+$ and Fas^+ CD4 T cells and decreased $\alpha 4\beta 7^+$ and $CD31^+$ $CD4^+$ T cells. This demonstration of predominant expression of memory T cells in association with higher UPDRS scores suggests a chronic inflammatory state [4]. When compared to patients with other neurological diseases, there is a higher expression of HLA-DR in CSF monocytes. There is increase in memory T-cell subset and decrease in naïve T cells in the peripheral blood. There is no change in suppressor T cells ($CD8^+$ and $CD11b^+$), supporting once again the theory of chronic immune state in PD [5]. There are also changes in hematopoietic stem cells in PD patients. Interactions between CCR2 and other interleukins can lead to further clues as to the exact mechanisms or pathways of peripheral response. In a colony-forming cell assay study from blood samples, upregulation of monocyte precursors CFU-GM and CFU-M has been shown to occur. Also, there is increase in CCR2 (chemokine receptor 2) expression but decrease in percentage of $CCR2^+$ cells overall. CCR2 and fractalkine receptor (CX3CR1) are important in the recruitment of peripheral monocytes in response to inflammation [6]. Expression of TNF-α from peripheral T cells was studied in patients with PD versus healthy controls, and patients with PD had a higher number of T-cell TNF-α receptors, and this is due to peripheral response to chronic inflammation [7]. Elevated OKT 10^+ cells and proportions of IL2 $receptor^+$ and HLA DR^+ cells have been shown in PD, suggesting activation of peripheral T lymphocytes and increased adenosine deaminase activity [8].

In PD $\gamma\delta^{+}$ T cells are elevated in CSF and peripheral system of patients with PD compared to other neurologic diseases. While this finding is relevant, the key role of these activated T cells in PD is not established [9]. Circulating CD4^{+} or CD8^{+} when they are concomitantly expressed in the same cell represents immaturity. Activation of these cells as measured by CD4 bright^{+} CD8 dull^{+} lymphocytes occurs in PD [10]. Similar findings have been reported in other immunological disorders of the nervous system [11, 12].

Many changes occur in T-cell subtypes in PD. In a study with 88 patients, looking at peripheral T-cell subtypes, there were no changes in cell counts of sampled cells labeled for CD14^{+} (monocytes), CD8^{+} (cytotoxic T cells), CD56^{+} (natural killer cells), TCR$\gamma\delta^{+}$, or CD4^{+} CD8^{+} cells in patients with PD. A decrease in TCR$\alpha\beta^{+}$, CD4^{+} (T helpers), and CD19^{+} (B) cells was noted in PD compared to controls. A reduction in CD4^{+} T-helper and CD19^{+} B cells in PD patients was noted, and there was variability with the stage of disease [13]. Specific subtyping of B-cell activity using microarray analysis is interesting, but the evidence is not conclusive [14].

Peripheral blood mononuclear cells (PBMC) are easy to study due to the fact that they are an integral part of the cytokine network in vivo. Several discrete cytokines are secreted by them when activated using mitogens in a cell culture system. Production of IL-2 and the mitogen response were significantly lower in PD patients, whereas the secretion of IL-1β, IL-6, and TNF-α was significantly enhanced. Secretion of IL-1β and IL-2 was not affected by levodopa, demonstrating a pure effect on the cytokines due to the disease pathology [15]. TNF-a, IL-1a, IL-1b, and IL-6 production by unstimulated PBMC and PBMC stimulated with mitogens LPS or Con A was significantly lower in PD than those in normal controls. IFN-c production by LPS-stimulated PBMC in PD was significantly lower than that in normal controls [16].

Immune responsiveness of PBMC in a whole-blood assay by quantification of IL-2, soluble IL-2 receptor (sIL-2R), IFN-γ, and IL-6 in T-lymphocyte subsets of patients with idiopathic PD showed selective IL-2 deficiency [17]. TNF-α, IL-1a, IL-1b, and IL-6 production by unstimulated PBMC and PBMC stimulated with mitogens was lower in PD than in normal controls [18]. In a separate study, the cytokine-producing capacity of whole-blood cultures was determined in de novo patients with idiopathic PD before and after treatment with amantadine [19].

Cytokine Markers

Multiple studies have found that CSF cytokines are increased in PD patients as compared to controls. TNF-α is a potent cytokine produced primarily by activated macrophages and elicits various biological and cytotoxic effects, including hemorrhagic necrosis, endotoxic shock, and inflammatory, proliferative, and antiviral responses, in addition to immunoregulatory effects. The first evidence of measurement of TNF-α was provided by Mogi et al. [22] in 1994. They measured TNF-α both in the CSF and brain. Elevated levels of this cytokine were found in patients with PD versus controls [20].

IFN-γ has been shown to initiate cell death in in vitro mixed mouse microglia/midbrain neuron cultures. Mice deficient in IFN-γ are protected from rotenone-induced cell death in vivo [21]. IFN-γ-stimulated human monocytes/macrophages secrete neopterin during activation. IFN-γ induces indoleamine 2, 3-dioxygenase, which breaks down l-tryptophan to kynurenine. Elevated kynurenine/tryptophan ratio (kyn/trp-ratio) reflects induction of monocyte macrophage system via IFN-γ. Neopterin concentrations and kyn/trp-ratios were increased both in the serum and CSF of PD patients, while serum tryptophan was lower [22, 23]. IL-6 is upregulated in order to protect or regenerate neurons in PD [24]. IL-1 to 3, IL-2, IL-4, and IL-6 epidermal growth factor (EGF) and transforming growth factor (TGF)-α were measured in ventricular CSF, which has higher concentration of cytokines than lumbar CSF. It is important to note that there was upregulation of IL-6 in PD patients. The concentrations of IL-l, IL-2, IL-4, and TGF-α in IL-6 were higher in PD than those from control patients [25]. Similar studies reported elevations of IL-6 in Alzheimer's and PD [26]. Nitric oxide released by active microglia is triggered by pro-inflammatory cytokines to signal apoptosis in neurons. Qureshi et al. [27] found that nitrite, a product of nitric oxide synthase (NOS), is increased in the CSF of PD patients compared to controls. Some authors reported decreased nitrate, which reflects decreased nitric oxide production in neurodegenerative disorders; this could be a methodological issue [28]. Attempts have been made to identify antibodies to dopaminergic neurons in CSF in patients with PD, confirming immune activation in CSF of patients with PD [29]. Some investigators specifically looked into viral infectious etiologies and antibody response in PD [30–32].

Increased serum IL-2, IL-10, IL-4, IL-6, TNF-α, and INF-γ concentrations were measured by cytokine assay in patients with PD and atypical PD compared to controls. However, IL-10 and IL-6 elevations were more specific to PD. This indicates peripheral immune activation in PD [33]. Elevated serum TNF-α was reported in PD [34]. Elevated serum sTNF-α Receptor I was reported in PD [35]. Colonic inflammatory pathology on biopsy has been reported in those patients who had GI Lewy body pathology [36]. C-type natriuretic peptide (CNP) is a member of the natriuretic peptide family; its amino-terminal pro-peptide (NT-pro CNP) is easy to measure in serum. NT-pro CNP localizes to many areas in the CNS. NT-pro CNP, a pro-inflammatory marker, has been found to be elevated in serum in PD patients, in addition to TNF-α indicating presence of inflammation in CNS [37]. Elevation of IL-6 is correlated with gait and balance dysfunction in one study, suggesting perhaps a variation in cytokines in subtypes of PD or association with advanced motor impairment [38]. In PD patients serum IL-6 levels do not seem to vary with levodopa usage, but higher levels of this cytokine are observed in patients with severe disease [39]. Despite a small sample size in a nested case-controlled study, of 84 patients who developed PD average 4.3 years after sample was collected, there is some evidence that IL-6 is elevated, but the other markers of inflammation were not elevated [40]. Serum IL-10 and IL-12 are also elevated, but the data need careful interpretation due to small sample size [41].

Activated microglia produce alpha- and beta-chemokines, in response to immune stimuli. Many chemokine receptors, CXCR2, CXCR3, CXCR4, CCR3, and CCR5, are associated with microglial activation in addition to RANTES. This specific activation in periphery is important to be looked at in PD. RANTES is important for activation of T lymphocytes and monocytes. One of the early studies identified increase in activity of RANTES in serum in PD compared to controls. However measurement of serum chemokines is difficult to interpret as valid biomarker [42].

Macrophage migration inhibitory factor (MIF) is a pro-inflammatory cytokine. There is elevation of MIF in serum of PD patients. The elevation in these levels does not correlate with severity of disease or MIF transcripts in blood cells implying possible origin from microglia rather than peripheral cells [43]. Other systemic inflammatory markers such as high-sensitivity C-reactive protein (hs-CRP) have been measured in PD [44, 45]. Studies have shown elevated levels of oxidized LDL (oxi-LDL), hs-CRP, and intracellular adhesion molecule (ICAM) in PD patients compared to controls [46]. Validation of these is important.

Lindqvist et al. [47, 48] studied CSF and serum inflammatory markers as a panel including CRP, IL-6, TNF-α, and IL-2 receptor in PD. Based on this evidence, there may be specific marker elevation particularly in relation to non-motor symptoms in PD such as fatigue, mood disorder, and sleep disorder as identified by them. However, before such subtype analysis for markers, all of these have to reach statistical significance. Perhaps a study of a larger number of patients would be more informative.

Epstein–Barr virus (EBV) has been studied in many autoimmune neurologic conditions. Cross-reactivity of EBV antibodies to alpha-synuclein has been demonstrated in Lewy bodies and glial cytoplasmic inclusions in PD and MSA [49]. EBV DNA by PCR was detected in CSF in a patient with postencephalitic parkinsonism and MRI brain changes [50].

Han et al. [51] used protein microarray to find ten autoantibodies that showed the highest differential expression between control ($N=40$) and PD ($N=29$) serum samples. These autoantibodies could differentiate PD from control sera with a sensitivity of 93.1 % and specificity of 100 %. The samples were from patients with early- or late-onset PD. The autoantibodies were against intercellular adhesion molecule 4 (ICAM4), pentatricopeptide repeat domain 2 (PTCD2), FERM domain containing 8 (FRMD8), recombinant human CTLA-4/Fc, myotilin (MYOT), hematopoietic SH2 domain containing (HSH2D), fibronectin 1 (FN1), tripartite motif-containing 21 (TRIM21), elongation factor 1-alpha, poly(A)-binding protein, and cytoplasmic 3 (PABPC3). Further studies are needed to establish such markers in the future as a panel.

In studies specifically focused on autoantibodies, in patients with PD there is elevation of antineuronal antibodies, anti-brain lysate antibodies, and anti-ds-DNA antibodies. Specific subtype or characterization of clinical phenotype and correlation is needed [52]. Specific immune response generated by release of neuromelanin from dying dopamine neurons into extra-neuronal space is a humoral response. Stimulation of the pro-inflammatory nuclear factor NF-κB in glial cells by extra-neuronal NM in vitro does occur. In sera of patients with PD there is elevation of antimelanin antibody [53]. When α-synuclein is released, it can cross the blood–brain barrier. Monomeric and oligomeric forms of α-synuclein are found in CSF and sera of PD patients. Various methods including ELISA and immunoblot were used in experiments to identify antibodies against α-synuclein in serum in PD patients. Elevation of antibodies to α-synuclein and its amyloid fibrillar fragments was demonstrated in serum of PD patients compared to controls [54]. In a separate study, individuals with autoantibodies for α-synuclein in their sera were found to be at increased risk for developing familial PD [55]. Other investigators have found no specific correlation between naturally occurring autoantibodies to α-synuclein in PD. This result could be due to variation in the methods of assay [56]. Anti-GM1 ganglioside antibodies have been shown to be increased in tremor-dominant PD patients [57].

Genome-Wide Association Studies

Inquiry into identification of genetics of inflammation in PD reveals involvement of several pathways and innate and adaptive immune system involvement. Genome-wide association studies show activation of leukocyte/lymphocyte activity and cytokine-mediated signaling pathways [58]. Individuals homozygous at TNF locus (−308AA) are more susceptible to PD, particularly as identified in early-onset PD [59, 60]. Of importance is the study by Wahner et al. [58] in which they studied IL-1β-511 and TNF-α-308 variant alleles together in PD. There was a threefold (OR, 2.92; 95 % CI, 1.66–5.16) increased risk of PD in carriers of a homozygous variant genotype for either or both polymorphisms compared to those carrying a homozygous wild-type genotype for both polymorphisms. Heterozygous genotype for either or both polymorphisms carried a 1.45-fold (OR, 1.45; 95 % CI, 0.97–2.16) risk, suggesting a gene-dosing effect ($p < 0.001$ for trend) [58]. Nishimura et al. [59] also found that the frequency of the TNF-1031C allele was significantly higher in early-onset PD in a Japanese population. TNF-1031C carriers homozygous for IL-1beta-511T had significantly earlier disease onset than noncarriers. IL-1beta appears to be neuroprotective, while TNF appears to increase the risk of developing PD. Consistent with a role of TNF in PD, individuals with both the TNFRSF1-609- and TNFRSF1^{+} 36-polymorphisms showed higher risk of developing PD in a German population [60].

A study of 122 Japanese PD patients found that those homozygous for IL-1beta-511* 2 showed significantly earlier disease onset, and IL-1 beta has possible neuroprotective effect on dopaminergic neurons [61]. There was no difference in the genotype or allele frequency of IL-1B-511 between PD patients and controls in Japanese patients [62]. In contrast, Schulte et al. did not find an association between IL-1β-511 polymorphism and PD. T-511 allele probably has higher frequency in the Japanese population. With regard to IL-1α-889 polymorphism a trend toward an increase of the T allele in PD was observed [63]. In the Turkish population IL-1α-889, IL-1Ra VNTR, and IL-1β +3953 polymorphisms are not associated with PD. IL-1β (−511) is associated with PD. There is protective effect of the

IL-1β-511 T allele in the development of PD [64]. Zhou et al. [65] have shown that presence of T allele of IL-1α (C-899T) is associated with reduced risk for PD. T allele of IL-1α (C-899T) has a role in modifying expression of IL-1α levels in the brain in PD, exerting a protective action thereby improving survival, regeneration, and differentiation of dopaminergic neurons. IL-1alpha-889C allele has been shown to have association with later-onset PD [66].

Cytokine gene polymorphisms such as L-17A rs8193036 and IL-10 1082G/A may be associated with higher risk for PD with cognitive impairment in the Han Chinese population [67]. IL-10 promoter -819T/C polymorphism carries a greater risk of PD in women and is associated with early-onset PD in the Han Chinese population. [68]. Polymorphisms in the genes of IFN-γ, IFN-γR2, IL-10, ICAM-1, and PAF-AH do not seem to be specific to PD. The G1082A polymorphism in the IL-10 gene promoter is related to the age at onset of PD. Based on linear regression analysis, there is significantly earlier onset of PD with more A-alleles and delayed age of onset of PD with two G-alleles compared with individuals having two A-alleles [69]. Gene polymorphisms in IL-18, a pro-inflammatory cytokine, revealed a higher risk for PD with two copies of the IL-18 –607 C alleles in a Han Chinese population [70]. In an Irish population, IL-8 (CXCL8, a chemokine) polymorphism in A-251T is associated with higher risk for PD [71]. NF-κB-mediated inflammation plays a role in the pathogenesis of PD. NOD1 (a product of CARD4 gene) and NOD2 (encoded by CARD15) are NOD (nucleotide-binding oligomerization domain) proteins. They mediate the activation of NF-κB and recognize bacterial proteins. Brain tissue is shown to have CARD15, and the action is astrocyte mediated in the setting of inflammation. Polymorphisms in CARD 15 gene are associated with higher risk of PD [72]. In another study, three SNPs in NOD 2 gene did not correlate with risk of PD [73].

The HLA-DR cell receptor is composed of an alpha- and a beta-chain coded by the HLA-DRA and HLA-DRB genes, respectively. Class II HLA-DR antigens are expressed by brain microglia and interact with T-cell receptors. Ahmed et al. [74] showed association between PD and rs660895 in the HLA-DRB1 locus compared to controls. HLA-DRB1*03 was more common in PD [75]. The International Parkinson's Disease Consortium (2011) found that the DRB5 polymorphism chr6:32588205(G) was lower in PD [76]. The HLA-DRA polymorphism rs3129882(G) was found to reduce the risk of developing PD in an Irish population, but differential effect was noted in patients from the Han Chinese and US population [77–79].

Clinical Epidemiological Studies

Traumatic brain injury can activate microglia. In 28 % cases, there were reactive microglia in patients with survival between 1 and 18 years post trauma. In the acute phase of traumatic brain injury, there are occasional microglia with amoeboid pathology; in the subacute stage there is increased activity of cr3/43 and CD

68-reactive cells, which are activated microglia. In the long-term survival group 28 % cases show extensive regions populated by amoeboid microglia [80]. The prevalence of PD in Thai boxers was 0.71, and 0.98 % in boxers older than 50 years. Incidence of PD has been studied in boxers. In a large study by Lolekha et al. [81] there is no significant difference in incidence of PD among boxers and general population. From the end of boxing career to development of PD symptoms, the time lag was 23–43 years (35.6 ± 7.9 years) [81]. There is threefold increase in risk for PD in a univariate analysis (OR, 3.0; 95 % CI, 1.2–7.6; $p=0.020$) in a study of 93 twin pairs, suggesting a greater risk for PD in closed head injuries [82]. Other studies also indicate a higher risk of PD in patients with head trauma [83].

Paraquat causes neurodegeneration via activation of microglia via dose-dependent induction of extracellular O_2 [84]. Higher incidence of PD with agricultural and other uses of pesticides such as Rotenone and Paraquat was reported in many studies [85–90]. In 110 PD cases compared to 358 controls, PD is 2.5 times more often in Rotenone and Paraquat exposure, with an odds ratio of 2.5 with 95 % CI [85]. Other studies have also shown higher risk of PD with pesticide exposure with an odds ratio 1.99 with 95 % CI [1.12–3.21], and various pesticides were studied [86]. Kamel et al. [87] showed an association between pesticides, and PD exposure and odds ration varied between 1.4 and 4.5, depending on the degree of exposure. In East Texas Firestone et al. showed increased incidence of PD with pesticides and well-water consumption [88]. Rotenone, chlorpyrifos, Paraquat, and other compounds have been associated with increased incidence of PD [89]. Plasma manganese and serum iron were found to be significantly higher in PD patients than age-matched controls in the Chinese population study [90]. Occupational exposure to copper or manganese for over 20 years has been shown to increase the risk of developing PD by over twofold [91]. Increased risk is seen with dual combinations of lead, iron, and copper [92].

Braak et al. [93] hypothesized that the stereotypic topographic expansion pattern of lesions associated with PD may be due to a pathogen capable of passing the mucosal barrier of the gastrointestinal tract and entering the central nervous system by traveling along the fibers of the postganglionic enteric neurons [93]. This increased intestinal permeability has been demonstrated in a very elegant study by Forsyth et al. [94]. Evidence for hyperpermeability of the intestinal mucosa is based on increased staining for alpha-synuclein, nitrotyrosine, *Escherichia coli*, and LPS-binding protein (LBP) in addition to elevated serum levels of LBP [94]. This correlation is critical for our understanding of external pathogens influencing development of PD and also the action of cytokines both peripherally and in the CNS. There is a higher risk for PD in patients with *Helicobacter pylori* and GI symptoms. The risk varies with severity of GI symptoms. Risk is higher in those with proton pump inhibitor use (23 %) and gastritis (22 %) [95].

Occurrence of multiple CNS infections ≥5 years prior to onset of PD has been shown to carry a higher risk for PD compared to single CNS infection [96]. A large-scale epidemiologic study has corroborated a role of inflammation in PD. Based on recorded deaths in England and Wales ($N=76{,}000$) from 1950 to 1992, individuals born around 1900 appear to have had twice the probability of dying from PD than people born around 1920 and five times the probability of dying from PD than people born around 1930 [97]. Martyn hypothesizes that the reason for the increase in PD deaths in individuals born around 1900 was due to the encephalitis lethargica, which swept the world in 1918 and 1919. In a case-control study, individuals who experienced croup, which is a common respiratory infection affecting young children, or diphtheria, which was a relatively rare condition in the first half of the twentieth century, in childhood were at greater risk of developing PD ($N=172$) compared to controls ($N=343$) [98].

Albumin was measured in cerebrospinal fluid and serum samples obtained from 73 non-demented subjects with idiopathic Parkinson's disease and 47 age-matched control subjects. The albumin ratio (AR) was calculated to assess blood–cerebrospinal fluid and blood–brain barrier function. Analysis of CSF/serum albumin ratio in 73 PD patients compared to controls shows a higher level in PD patients compared to controls. An increase of high molecular proteins in the CSF indicates blood–CSF barrier dysfunction, and the resulting BBB impairment is maintained due to possible failure of choroidal Na-K ATPase and continuing inflammation [99]. [11C]-verapamil is normally extruded from the brain by P-glycoprotein, so increased uptake would indicate a defect in the blood–brain barrier. In one PET study, advanced PD patients had increased [11C]-verapamil uptake in the frontal white matter regions compared to controls indicating a compromised blood–brain barrier [100]. On the other hand, de novo PD patients showed lower uptake in the midbrain and frontal regions compared to controls, indicating an intact blood–brain barrier. In another study, [11C]-verapamil showed elevated uptake in the midbrain of PD patients [101]. ATP-binding cassette, subfamily B, member 1 (ABCB1) gene regulates transport of endogenous molecules and exogenous toxins encoding the protein P-glycoprotein (P-gp). Single-nucleotide polymorphisms have been identified in ABCB1 gene in PD, indicating problems in BBB [102]. MDR1 is another gene that codes for P-glycoprotein. MDR1-1236C allele was found to be associated with PD. This study also found that the MDR1-1236C-2677G haplotype was associated with PD again indicating abnormalities in BBB [103]. Consistent with these results, Lee et al. [104] found that the MDR1-1236C, 2677G, and 3435C alleles significantly increased the risk of developing PD in a Chinese population (PD=206, Controls=224) [104]. These mutations may allow inflammatory cells and cytokines into the brain that are normally filtered out.

Data on Anti-inflammatory Agents in Clinical Literature

In a meta-analysis of 14 observational studies, exposure to NSAIDs or aspirin was reviewed in PD. With nonaspirin NSAIDs there is reduced risk of PD (13 %), and with ibuprofen alone, there was greater reduction in risk for PD (27 %). Important data show benefit of anti-inflammatory agents [104]. Ibuprofen use has once again been shown to decrease risk of PD in a prospective study by Gao et al. [105]. Multivariate relative risk for PD in this study is 0.62 (95 % confidence interval (CI)).

Those who used ibuprofen regularly had approximately 30 % lower PD risk compared to nonusers [105]. Another meta-analysis showed protective effect with regular use of ibuprofen, with 15 % reduction of PD risk but not aspirin [106]. In a US population recruited from subjects from the Neuro Genetics Research Consortium, smoking, caffeine, and the use of NSAIDs were all reviewed, and the combined effect of all three agents reduced the risk of PD significantly. Smoking ever in a lifetime was associated with 23 % reduction in risk, while current smokers carried 55 % reduction in risk. High coffee consumption had 25 % risk reduction. Subjects who smoked, drank high level of coffee, and used NSAIDs had 62 % lower risk [107]. Wahner et al. [108] found that nonaspirin-NSAID users showed a two-fold reduction in odds ratio for having PD. This effect was even greater for individuals who reported using nonaspirin NSAIDs for over 2 years. In contrast, Hernán et al. [109] found that nonaspirin-NSAID use increased the risk of developing PD in females and reduced the risk in males (PD = 1,258, Controls = 6,638). Further, they found that aspirin use increased the risk of PD [110]. Health Professionals Follow-up Study and the Nurses' Health Study looked at 142,902 men and women without PD, stroke, or cancer at baseline and followed up with them from 1986–2000 to 1980–1998, respectively. Both questionnaires documented NSAID use and PD diagnosis every 2 years. Chen et al. [111] found that the use of nonaspirin NSAIDs reduced the risk of PD (N=415) in this study population by twofold [111]. In a retrospective study, PD patients taking fibrates or statins showed a mean age of disease onset that was delayed by almost 9 years compared with controls [112]. Further, individuals taking statins showed a significantly smaller increase in levodopa-equivalent daily dose over 2 years. Minocycline has been shown to have anti-inflammatory properties. In a phase II placebo-controlled double-blind clinical trial, minocycline could not be rejected as futile based on the DATATOP futility threshold (Minocycline = 66, Placebo = 67) [113].

Conclusion and Future Directions

Inflammation is clearly present in PD patients based on cytological, biomarker, and comorbidity studies. Further, genome-wide association studies have uncovered multiple polymorphisms in genes involved in innate as well as acquired immunity. Epidemiological studies have also indicated that inflammation could result in PD. Based on review of current evidence, it is difficult to conclude presence of one specific biological marker for PD or a panel thereof. At this time, because of the lack of surrogate markers, be it imaging, serum, or CSF markers, and poor understanding of dynamics of the apoptotic and inflammatory pathways, it becomes difficult to postulate therapeutic options. Therapeutic targets can include anti-inflammatory agents, that work in periphery, or specific agents targeting cytokines. Further investigations are needed in the future to develop appropriate therapeutic agents that can cross the blood–brain barrier.

References

1. Strimbu K, Tavel JA. What are biomarkers? Curr Opin HIV AIDS. 2010;5:463–6.
2. Czirr E, Wyss-Coray T. The immunology of neurodegeneration. J Clin Invest. 2012;122: 1156–63.
3. Ton TG, Jain S, Biggs ML, Thacker EL, Strotmeyer ES, Boudreau R, et al. Markers of inflammation in prevalent and incident Parkinson's disease in the cardiovascular health study. Parkinsonism Relat Disord. 2012;18:274–8.
4. Saunders JA, Estes KA, Kosloski LM, Allen HE, Dempsey KM, Torres-Russotto DR, et al. $CD4^+$ regulatory and effector/memory T cell subsets profile motor dysfunction in Parkinson's disease. J Neuroimmune Pharmacol. 2012;7:927–38.
5. Fiszer U, Mix E, Fredrikson S, Kostulas V, Link H. Parkinson's disease and immunological abnormalities: increase of HLA-DR expression on monocytes in cerebrospinal fluid and of $CD45RO^+$ T cells in peripheral blood. Acta Neurol Scand. 1994;90:160–6.
6. Funk N, Wieghofer P, Grimm S, Schaefer R, Bühring HJ, Gasser T, et al. Characterization of peripheral hematopoietic stem cells and monocytes in Parkinson's disease. Mov Disord. 2013;28:392–5.
7. Bongioanni P, Castagna M, Maltinti S, Boccardi B, Dadone F. T-lymphocyte tumor necrosis factor-alpha receptor binding in patients with Parkinson's disease. J Neurol Sci. 1997;149(1): 41–5.
8. Chiba S, Matsumoto H, Saitoh M, Kasahara M, Matsuya M, Kashiwagi M. A correlation study between serum adenosine deaminase activities and peripheral lymphocyte subsets in Parkinson's disease. J Neurol Sci. 1995;132:170–3.
9. Fiszer U, Mix E, Fredrikson S, Kostulas V, Olsson T, Link H. Gamma delta+ T cells are increased in patients with Parkinson's disease. J Neurol Sci. 1994;121:39–45.
10. Hisanaga K, Asagi M, Itoyama Y, Iwasaki Y. Increase in peripheral CD4 $bright^+$ CD8 $dull^+$ T cells in Parkinson disease. Arch Neurol. 2001;58:1580–3.
11. Munschauer FE, Stewart C, Jacobs L, Kaba S, Ghorishi Z, Greenberg SJ, et al. Circulating $CD3^+$ $CD4^+$ $CD8^+$ T lymphocytes in multiple sclerosis. J Clin Immunol. 1993;13:113–8.
12. Berrih S, Gaud C, Bach MA, Le Brigand H, Binet JP, Bach JF. Evaluation of T cell subsets in myasthenia gravis using anti-T cell monoclonal antibodies. Clin Exp Immunol. 1981;45(1): 1–8.
13. Stevens CH, Rowe D, Morel-Kopp MC, Orr C, Russell T, Ranola M, et al. Reduced T helper and B lymphocytes in Parkinson's disease. J Neuroimmunol. 2012;252:95–9.
14. Kedmi M, Bar-Shira A, Gurevich T, Giladi N, Orr-Urtreger A. Decreased expression of B cell related genes in leukocytes of women with Parkinson's disease. Mol Neurodegener. 2011;6:66.
15. Reale M, Iarlori C, Thomas A, Gambi D, Perfetti B, Di Nicola M, et al. Peripheral cytokines profile in Parkinson's disease. Brain Behav Immun. 2009;23:55–63.
16. Bessler H, Djaldetti R, Salman H, Bergman M, Djaldetti M. IL-1 beta, IL-2, IL-6 and TNF-alpha production by peripheral blood mononuclear cells from patients with Parkinson's disease. Biomed Pharmacother. 1999;53:141–5.
17. Hasegawa Y, Inagaki T, Sawada M, Suzumura A. Impaired cytokine production by peripheral blood mononuclear cells and monocytes/macrophages in Parkinson's disease. Acta Neurol Scand. 2000;101:159–64.
18. Klüter H, Vieregge P, Stolze H, Kirchner H. Defective production of interleukin-2 in patients with idiopathic Parkinson's disease. J Neurol Sci. 1995;133:134–9.
19. Wandinger KP, Hagenah JM, Klüter H, Rothermundt M, Peters M, Vieregge P. Effects of amantadine treatment on in vitro production of interleukin-2 in de-novo patients with idiopathic Parkinson's disease. J Neuroimmunol. 1999;98:214–20.
20. Mogi M, Harada M, Riederer P, Narabayashi H, Fujita K, Nagatsu T. Tumor necrosis factor-alpha (TNF-alpha) increases both in the brain and in the cerebrospinal fluid from parkinsonian patients. Neurosci Lett. 1994;165:208–10.

21. Mount MP, Lira A, Grimes D, Smith PD, Faucher S, Slack R, et al. Involvement of interferon-gamma in microglial-mediated loss of dopaminergic neurons. J Neurosci. 2007; 27:3328–37.
22. Widner B, Leblhuber F, Fuchs D. Increased neopterin production and tryptophan degradation in advanced Parkinson's disease. J Neural Transm. 2002;109:181–9.
23. Fujishiro K, Hagihara M, Takahashi A, Nagatsu T. Concentrations of neopterin and biopterin in the cerebrospinal fluid of patients with Parkinson's disease. Biochem Med Metab Biol. 1990;44:97–100.
24. Müller T, Blum-Degen D, Przuntek H, Kuhn W. Interleukin-6 levels in cerebrospinal fluid inversely correlate to severity of Parkinson's disease. Acta Neurol Scand. 1998;98:142–4.
25. Mogi M, Harada M, Narabayashi H, Inagaki H, Minami M, Nagatsu T. Interleukin (IL)-1 beta, IL-2, IL-4, IL-6 and transforming growth factor-alpha levels are elevated in ventricular cerebrospinal fluid in juvenile parkinsonism and Parkinson's disease. Neurosci Lett. 1996; 211:13–6.
26. Blum-Degen D, Müller T, Kuhn W, Gerlach M, Gerlach M, Przuntek H, Riederer P. Interleukin-1 beta and interleukin-6 are elevated in the cerebrospinal fluid of Alzheimer's and de novo Parkinson's disease patients. Neurosci Lett. 1995;202:17–20.
27. Qureshi GA, Baig S, Bednar I, Södersten P, Södersten P, Forsberg G, Siden A. Increased cerebrospinal fluid concentration of nitrite in Parkinson's disease. Neuroreport. 1995;6: 1642–4.
28. Kuiper MA, Visser JJ, Bergmans PL, Scheltens P, Wolters EC. Decreased cerebrospinal fluid nitrate levels in Parkinson's disease, Alzheimer's disease and multiple system atrophy patients. J Neurol Sci. 1994;121:46–9.
29. McRae Degueurce A, Gottfries CG, Karlsson I, Svennerholm L, Dahlström A. Antibodies in the CSF of a Parkinson patient recognizes neurons in rat mesencephalic regions. Acta Physiol Scand. 1986;126:313–5.
30. Marttila RJ, Rinne UK, Tiilikainen A. Virus antibodies in Parkinson's disease. Herpes simplex and measles virus antibodies in serum and CSF and their relation to HLA types. J Neurol Sci. 1982;54:227–38.
31. Marttila RJ, Kalimo KO, Ziola BR, Halonen PE, Rinne UK. Herpes simplex virus subunit antibodies in patients with Parkinson's disease. Arch Neurol. 1978;35:668–71.
32. Elizan TS, Madden DL, Noble GR, Herrmann KL, Gardner J, Schwartz J, et al. Viral antibodies in serum and CSF of Parkinsonian patients and controls. Arch Neurol. 1979;36:529–34.
33. Brodacki B, Staszewski J, Toczyłowska B, Kozłowska E, Drela N, Chalimoniuk M, et al. Serum interleukin (IL-2, IL-10, IL-6, IL-4), TNFalpha, and INFgamma concentrations are elevated in patients with atypical and idiopathic parkinsonism. Neurosci Lett. 2008;441: 158–62.
34. Dobbs RJ, Charlett A, Purkiss AG, Dobbs SM, Weller C, Peterson DW. Association of circulating TNF-alpha and IL-6 with ageing and parkinsonism. Acta Neurol Scand. 1999;100: 34–41.
35. Scalzo P, Kümmer A, Cardoso F, Teixeira AL. Increased serum levels of soluble tumor necrosis factor-alpha receptor-1 in patients with Parkinson's disease. J Neuroimmunol. 2009;216: 122–5.
36. Devos D, Lebouvier T, Lardeux B, Biraud M, Rouaud T, Pouclet H, et al. Colonic inflammation in Parkinson's disease. Neurobiol Dis. 2013;50:42–8.
37. Koziorowski D, Tomasiuk R, Szlufik S, Friedman A. Inflammatory cytokines and NT-proCNP in Parkinson's disease patients. Cytokine. 2012;60(3):762–6.
38. Scalzo P, Kümmer A, Cardoso F, Teixeira AL. Serum levels of interleukin-6 are elevated in patients with Parkinson's disease and correlate with physical performance. Neurosci Lett. 2010;468:56–8.
39. Hofmann KW, Schuh AF, Saute J, Townsend R, Fricke D, Leke R, et al. Interleukin-6 serum levels in patients with Parkinson's disease. Neurochem Res. 2009;34:1401–4.
40. Chen H, O'Reilly EJ, Schwarzschild MA, Ascherio A. Peripheral inflammatory biomarkers and risk of Parkinson's disease. Am J Epidemiol. 2008;167:90–5.

41. Rentzos M, Nikolaou C, Andreadou E, Paraskevas GP, Rombos A, Zoga M, et al. Circulating interleukin-10 and interleukin-12 in Parkinson's disease. Acta Neurol Scand. 2009;119: 332–7.
42. Rentzos M, Nikolaou C, Andreadou E, Rentzos M, Nikolaou C, Andreadou E, et al. Circulating interleukin-15 and RANTES chemokine in Parkinson's disease. Acta Neurol Scand. 2007;116:374–9.
43. Nicoletti A, Fagone P, Donzuso G, Mangano K, Dibilio V, Caponnetto S, et al. Parkinson's disease is associated with increased serum levels of macrophage migration inhibitory factor. Cytokine. 2011;55:165–7.
44. Song IU, Kim JS, Chung SW, Lee KS. Is there an association between the level of high-sensitivity C-reactive protein and idiopathic Parkinson's disease? A comparison of Parkinson's disease patients, disease controls and healthy individuals. Eur Neurol. 2009;62: 99–104.
45. Song IU, Chung SW, Kim JS, Lee KS. Association between high-sensitivity C-reactive protein and risk of early idiopathic Parkinson's disease. Neurol Sci. 2011;32:31–4.
46. Andican G, Konukoglu D, Bozluolcay M, Bayülkem K, Firtiına S, Burcak G. Plasma oxidative and inflammatory markers in patients with idiopathic Parkinson's disease. Acta Neurol Belg. 2012;112:155–9.
47. Lindqvist D, Kaufman E, Brundin L, Hall S, Surova Y, Hansson O. Non-motor symptoms in patients with Parkinson's disease – correlations with inflammatory cytokines in serum. PLoS One. 2012;7:e47387.
48. Lindqvist D, Hall S, Surovac Y. Cerebrospinal fluid inflammatory markers in Parkinson's disease – associations with depression, fatigue, and cognitive impairment. Brain Behav Immun. 2013;33:183–9.
49. Woulfe J, Hoogendoorn H, Tarnopolsky M, Muñoz DG. Monoclonal antibodies against Epstein–Barr virus cross-react with alpha-synuclein in human brain. Neurology. 2000;55: 1398–401.
50. Espay AJ, Henderson KK. Postencephalitic parkinsonism and basal ganglia necrosis due to Epstein–Barr virus infection. Neurology. 2011;76:1529–30.
51. Han M, Nagele E, DeMarshall C, Acharya N, Nagele R. Diagnosis of Parkinson's disease based on disease-specific autoantibody profiles in human sera. PLoS One. 2012;7:e32383.
52. Benkler M, Agmon-Levin N, Hassin-Baer S, Cohen OS, Ortega-Hernandez OD, Levy A, et al. Immunology, autoimmunity, and autoantibodies in Parkinson's disease. Clin Rev Allergy Immunol. 2012;42:164–71.
53. Double KL, Rowe DB, Carew-Jones FM, Hayes M, Chan DK, Blackie J, et al. Anti-melanin antibodies are increased in sera in Parkinson's disease. Exp Neurol. 2009;217:297–301.
54. Yanamandra K, Gruden MA, Casaite V, Meskys R, Forsgren L, Morozova-Roche LA, et al. α-Synuclein reactive antibodies as diagnostic biomarkers in blood sera of Parkinson's disease patients. PLoS One. 2011;6:e18513.
55. Papachroni KK, Ninkina N, Papapanagiotou A, Hadjigeorgiou GM, Xiromerisiou G, Papadimitriou A, et al. Autoantibodies to alpha-synuclein in inherited Parkinson's disease. J Neurochem. 2007;101:749–56.
56. Besong-Agbo D, Wolf E, Jessen F, Oechsner M, Hametner E, Poewe W, et al. Naturally occurring α-synuclein autoantibody levels are lower in patients with Parkinson disease. Neurology. 2013;80:169–75.
57. Zappia M, Crescibene L, Bosco D, Arabia G, Nicoletti G, Bagalà A, et al. Anti-GM1 ganglioside antibodies in Parkinson's disease. Acta Neurol Scand. 2002;106:54–7.
58. Wahner AD, Sinsheimer JS, Bronstein JM, Ritz B. Inflammatory cytokine gene polymorphisms and increased risk of Parkinson disease. Arch Neurol. 2007;64:836–40.
59. Nishimura M, Mizuta I, Mizuta E, Yamasaki S, Ohta M, Kaji R, et al. Tumor necrosis factor gene polymorphisms in patients with sporadic Parkinson's disease. Neurosci Lett. 2001;311: 1–4.
60. Krüger R, Hardt C, Tschentscher F, Jäckel S, Kuhn W, Müller T, et al. Genetic analysis of immunomodulating factors in sporadic Parkinson's disease. J Neural Transm. 2000;107: 553–62.

61. Nishimura M, Mizuta I, Mizuta E, Yamasaki S, Ohta M, Kuno S. Influence of interleukin-1beta gene polymorphisms on age-at-onset of sporadic Parkinson's disease. Neurosci Lett. 2000; 284:73–6.
62. Nishimura M, Kuno S, Kaji R, Yasuno K, Kawakami H. Glutathione-S-transferase-1 and interleukin-1beta gene polymorphisms in Japanese patients with Parkinson's disease. Mov Disord. 2005;20:901–2.
63. Schulte T, Schöls L, Müller T, Woitalla D, Berger K, Krüger R. Polymorphisms in the interleukin-1 alpha and beta genes and the risk for Parkinson's disease. Neurosci Lett. 2002; 326:70–2.
64. Arman A, Isik N, Coker A, Candan F, Becit KS, List EO. Association between sporadic Parkinson disease and interleukin-1 beta –511 gene polymorphisms in the Turkish population. Eur Cytokine Netw. 2010;21:116–21.
65. Zhou YT, Yang JF, Zhang YL, Wang XY, Chan P. Protective role of interlekin-1 alpha gene polymorphism in Chinese Han population with sporadic Parkinson's disease. Neurosci Lett. 2008;445:23–5.
66. Wu YR, Chen CM, Hwang JC, Chen ST, Feng IH, Hsu HC, et al. Interleukin-1 alpha polymorphism has influence on late-onset sporadic Parkinson's disease in Taiwan. J Neural Transm. 2007;114:1173–7.
67. Nie K, Zhang Y, Gan R, Wang L, Zhao J, Huang Z, et al. Polymorphisms in immune/inflammatory cytokine genes are related to Parkinson's disease with cognitive impairment in the Han Chinese population. Neurosci Lett. 2013;541:111–5.
68. Li D, He Q, Li R, Xu X, Chen B, Xie A. Interleukin-10 promoter polymorphisms in Chinese patients with Parkinson's disease. Neurosci Lett. 2012;513:183–6.
69. Håkansson A, Westberg L, Nilsson S, Buervenich S, Carmine A, Holmberg B, et al. Investigation of genes coding for inflammatory components in Parkinson's disease. Mov Disord. 2005;20:569–73.
70. Xu X, Li D, He Q, Gao J, Chen B, Xie A. Interleukin-18 promoter polymorphisms and risk of Parkinson's disease in a Han Chinese population. Brain Res. 2011;1381:90–4.
71. Ross OA, O'Neill C, Rea IM, Lynch T, Gosal D, Wallace A, et al. Functional promoter region polymorphism of the proinflammatory chemokine IL-8 gene associates with Parkinson's disease in the Irish. Hum Immunol. 2004;65:340–6.
72. Bialecka M, Kurzawski M, Klodowska-Duda G, Opala G, Juzwiak S, Kurzawski G, et al. CARD15 variants in patients with sporadic Parkinson's disease. Neurosci Res. 2007;57: 473–6.
73. Appenzeller S, Thier S, Papengut F, Klein C, Hagenah J, Kasten M, et al. No association between NOD2 variants and Parkinson's disease. Mov Disord. 2012;27:1191–2.
74. Ahmed I, Tamouza R, Delord M, Krishnamoorthy R, Tzourio C, Mulot C, et al. Association between Parkinson's disease and the HLA-DRB1 locus. Mov Disord. 2012;27:1104–10.
75. Saiki M, Baker A, Williams-Gray CH, Foltynie T, Goodman RS, Taylor CJ, et al. Association of the human leucocyte antigen region with susceptibility to Parkinson's disease. J Neurol Neurosurg Psychiatry. 2010;81:890–1.
76. International Parkinson Disease Genomics Consortium, Nalls MA, Plagnol V, Hernandez DG, Sharma M, Sheerin UM, Saad M, et al. Imputation of sequence variants for identification of genetic risks for Parkinson's disease: a meta-analysis of genome-wide association studies. Lancet. 2011;377:641–9.
77. Puschmann A, Verbeeck C, Heckman MG, Soto-Ortolaza AI, Lynch T, Jasinska-Myga B, et al. Human leukocyte antigen variation and Parkinson's disease. Parkinsonism Relat Disord. 2011;17:376–8.
78. Guo Y, Deng X, Zheng W, Xu H, Song Z, Liang H, et al. HLA rs3129882 variant in Chinese Han patients with late-onset sporadic Parkinson disease. Neurosci Lett. 2011;501:185–7.
79. Hamza TH, Zabetian CP, Tenesa A, Laederach A, Montimurro J, Yearout D, et al. Common genetic variation in the HLA region is associated with late-onset sporadic Parkinson's disease. Nat Genet. 2010;42:781–5.

80. Johnson VE, Stewart JE, Begbie FD, Trojanowski JQ, Smith DH, Stewart W. Inflammation and white matter degeneration persist for years after a single traumatic brain injury. Brain. 2013;136:28–42.
81. Lolekha P, Phanthumchinda K, Bhidayasiri R. Prevalence and risk factors of Parkinson's disease in retired Thai traditional boxers. Mov Disord. 2010;25:1895–901.
82. Goldman SM, Tanner CM, Oakes D, Bhudhikanok GS, Gupta A, Langston JW. Head injury and Parkinson's disease risk in twins. Ann Neurol. 2006;60:65–72.
83. Bower JH, Maraganore DM, Peterson BJ, McDonnell SK, Ahlskog JE, Rocca WA. Head trauma preceding PD: a case–control study. Neurology. 2003;60:1610–5.
84. Wu XF, Block ML, Zhang W, Qin L, Wilson B, Zhang WQ, et al. The role of microglia in paraquat-induced dopaminergic neurotoxicity. Antioxid Redox Signal. 2005;7:654–61.
85. Tanner CM, Kamel F, Ross GW, Hoppin JA, Goldman SM, Korell M, et al. Rotenone, paraquat, and Parkinson's disease. Environ Health Perspect. 2011;119:866–72.
86. Tanner CM, Ross GW, Jewell SA, Hauser RA, Jankovic J, Factor SA, et al. Occupation and risk of parkinsonism: a multicenter case–control study. Arch Neurol. 2009;66:1106–13.
87. Kamel F, Tanner C, Umbach D, Hoppin J, Alavanja M, Blair A, et al. Pesticide exposure and self-reported Parkinson's disease in the agricultural health study. Am J Epidemiol. 2007;165:364–74.
88. Firestone JA, Smith-Weller T, Franklin G, Swanson P, Longstreth Jr WT, Checkoway H. Pesticides and risk of Parkinson disease: a population-based case–control study. Arch Neurol. 2005;62:91–5.
89. Dhillon AS, Tarbutton GL, Levin JL, Plotkin GM, Lowry LK, Nalbone JT, et al. Pesticide/environmental exposures and Parkinson's disease in East Texas. J Agromedicine. 2008;13:37–48.
90. Fukushima T, Tan X, Luo Y, Kanda H. Relationship between blood levels of heavy metals and Parkinson's disease in China. Neuroepidemiology. 2010;34:18–24.
91. Gorell JM, Johnson CC, Rybicki BA, Peterson EL, Kortsha GX, Brown GG, et al. Occupational exposures to metals as risk factors for Parkinson's disease. Neurology. 1997;48:650–8.
92. Gorell JM, Johnson CC, Rybicki BA. Occupational exposure to manganese, copper, lead, iron, mercury and zinc and the risk of Parkinson's disease. Neurotoxicology. 1999;20:239–47.
93. Braak H, Rüb U, Gai WP, Del Tredici K. Idiopathic Parkinson's disease: possible routes by which vulnerable neuronal types may be subject to neuroinvasion by an unknown pathogen. J Neural Transm. 2003;110:517–36.
94. Forsyth CB, Shannon KM, Kordower JH, Voigt RM, Shaikh M, Jaglin JA, et al. Increased intestinal permeability correlates with sigmoid mucosa alpha-synuclein staining and endotoxin exposure markers in early Parkinson's disease. PLoS One. 2011;6:e28032.
95. Nielsen HH, Qiu J, Friis S, Wermuth L, Ritz B. Treatment for Helicobacter pylori infection and risk of Parkinson's disease in Denmark. Eur J Neurol. 2012;19:864–9.
96. Fang F, Wirdefeldt K, Jacks A, Kamel F, Kamel F, Ye W, Chen H. CNS infections, sepsis and risk of Parkinson's disease. Int J Epidemiol. 2012;41:1042–9.
97. Martyn CN. Infection in childhood and neurological diseases in adult life. Br Med Bull. 1997;53:24–39.
98. Martyn CN, Osmond C. Parkinson's disease and the environment in early life. J Neurol Sci. 1995;132:201–6.
99. Pisani V, Stefani A, Pierantozzi M, Pisani V, Stefani A, Pierantozzi M, et al. Increased blood-cerebrospinal fluid transfer of albumin in advanced Parkinson's disease. J Neuroinflammation. 2012;9:188.
100. Bartels AL, Willemsen AT, Kortekaas R, de Jong BM, de Vries R, de Klerk O, et al. Decreased blood–brain barrier P-glycoprotein function in the progression of Parkinson's disease, PSP and MSA. J Neural Transm. 2008;115:1001–9.
101. Kortekaas R, Leenders KL, van Oostrom JC, Vaalburg W, Bart J, Willemsen AT, et al. Blood–brain barrier dysfunction in parkinsonian midbrain in vivo. Ann Neurol. 2005;57:176–9.

102. Westerlund M, Belin AC, Anvret A, Håkansson A, Nissbrandt H, Lind C, et al. Association of a polymorphism in the ABCB1 gene with Parkinson's disease. Parkinsonism Relat Disord. 2009;15:422–4.
103. Tan EK, Chan DK, Ng PW, Woo J, Teo YY, Tang K, et al. Effect of MDR1 haplotype on risk of Parkinson disease. Arch Neurol. 2005;62:460–4.
104. Lee CG, Tang K, Cheung YB, Lee CG, Tang K, Cheung YB, et al. MDR1, the blood–brain barrier transporter, is associated with Parkinson's disease in ethnic Chinese. J Med Genet. 2004;41:e60.
105. Rees K, Stowe R, Patel S, Ives N, Breen K, Clarke CE, et al. Non-steroidal anti-inflammatory drugs as disease-modifying agents for Parkinson's disease: evidence from observational studies. Cochrane Database Syst Rev. 2011;11:CD008454.
106. Gao X, Chen H, Schwarzschild MA, Ascherio A. Use of ibuprofen and risk of Parkinson disease. Neurology. 2011;76:863–9.
107. Gagne JJ, Power MC. Anti-inflammatory drugs and risk of Parkinson disease: a meta-analysis. Neurology. 2010;74:995–1002.
108. Powers KM, Kay DM, Factor SA, Zabetian CP, Higgins DS, Samii A, et al. Combined effects of smoking, coffee, and NSAIDs on Parkinson's disease risk. Mov Disord. 2008;23:88–95.
109. Wahner AD, Bronstein JM, Bordelon YM, Ritz B. Nonsteroidal anti-inflammatory drugs may protect against Parkinson disease. Neurology. 2007;69:1836–42.
110. Hernán MA, Logroscino G, García Rodríguez LA. Nonsteroidal anti-inflammatory drugs and the incidence of Parkinson disease. Neurology. 2006;66:1097–9.
111. Chen H, Zhang SM, Hernán MA, Schwarzschild MA, Willett WC, Colditz GA, et al. Nonsteroidal anti-inflammatory drugs and the risk of Parkinson disease. Arch Neurol. 2003; 60:1059–64.
112. Mutez E, Duhamel A, Defebvre L, Bordet R, Destée A, Kreisler A. Lipid-lowering drugs are associated with delayed onset and slower course of Parkinson's disease. Pharmacol Res. 2009;60:41–5.
113. NINDS NET-PD Investigators. A randomized, double-blind, futility clinical trial of creatine and minocycline in early Parkinson disease. Neurology. 2006;66:664–71.

PET Imaging in Neuroinflammation

David J. Brooks

Introduction

Microglia are cells derived from monocyte lineage and constitute around 15 % of the brain's white cell population. Normally they are in a resting state with extended ramified processes monitoring the brain milieu and making contact with neighbouring neurones and astrocytes [1, 2]. They are protected from antigens in the plasma by the blood–brain barrier and form the natural immune defence of the brain. Exposure to plasma proteins such as fibrinogen following blood–brain barrier disruption, or to intrinsic excitotoxic agents such as raised glutamate, nitric oxide, or cytokines, or any change in brain milieu causes them to become activated taking on amoeboid or rod-like morphology. When activated the microglia express MHC class 1 and 2 antigens and release cytokines such as TNF-α, IL1-β, and IL-6 and growth factors such as TGF-β1. They become phagocytic and can strip and remodel synapses.

It is now considered that activated microglia exist as at least two primary phenotypes: the M1 phenotype is associated with the release of cidal cytokines so promoting cell damage while the M2 phenotype is associated with phagocytosis of dead tissue, synaptic stripping and remodelling, and growth factor release so promoting neurogenesis [3]. These two phenotypes and others may well be interconvertible and predominate at different disease phases. After an acute focal brain injury activated microglia act locally to wall off, remove dead tissue, and remodel connections. In chronic neurodegenerative diseases they may act to release cytokines where disease is locally active but remodel downstream connections in the brainstem and thalamus.

The 18 kDa translocator protein (TSPO) is expressed at low levels in normal brain but, if microglial cells become activated, it can be detected in their outer mitochondrial

D.J. Brooks, M.D., D.Sc., F.R.C.P. (UK) (✉)
Imperial College London, London, UK

Aarhus University, Aarhus, Denmark

Medicine ICL, Nuclear Medicine AU, Hammersmith Hospital, London, UK

M. Thomas (ed.), *Inflammation in Parkinson's Disease: Scientific and Clinical Aspects*,
DOI 10.1007/978-3-319-08046-8_9,

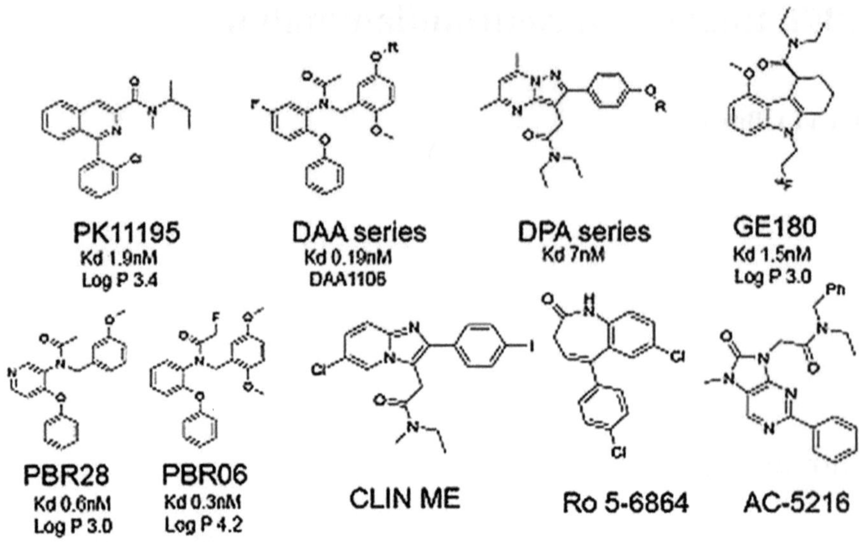

Fig. 1 Structures of PET and SPECT TSPO imaging agents

membranes. The TSPO serves a number of functions including transport of cholesterol, anions, and porphyrin, maintenance of mitochondrial membrane potential, regulation of cell apoptosis and proliferation, and immunomodulation [4]. It is present in many peripheral organs including the liver, spleen, adrenals, and myocardium [5]. TSPO was previously known as the peripheral benzodiazepine receptor (PBR) as it expresses a binding site for benzodiazepines and isoquinolines that is distinct from $GABA_A$ sites. This has enabled in vivo detection of the presence of TSPO in brain with the isoquinoline marker ^{11}C-PK11195 PET. A number of newer PET biomarkers are now available to image TSPO expression, and these include the phenoxyarylacetamides ^{11}C/^{18}F-DAA1106, ^{11}C-PBR28, ^{18}F-PBR06, and ^{18}F-PBR111, ^{18}F-FEPPA, pyrazolo-[1,5-a]-pyrimidines such as ^{11}C-DPA713 and ^{18}F-DPA714, the vinca alkaloid ^{11}C-vinpocetine, and the imidazo-[1,2a]-pyridines ^{11}C/^{18}F-CLINDE (Fig. 1) [6, 7]. While the advent of TSPO PET agents has enabled the distribution of activated microglia in the brain to be imaged in life, TSPO ligands bind to both M1 and M2 phenotypes. TSPO PET, therefore, provides a measure of total activated microglia load without providing information about the specific functional roles of these cells in different diseases and brain areas.

Imaging TSPO with PET

The radioligand that was first developed for imaging TSPO in the brain and that has seen the greatest use is the R enantiomer of the isoquinoline ^{11}C-(*R*)-PK11115. The rat unilateral facial nerve crush model results in an axonopathy, and activated microglia can be seen in the denervated ipsilateral facial nucleus. Autoradiography studies of this model have shown that ^{3}H-PK11195 binds selectively to the activated microglia rather than astrocytes [8]. These activated microglia play a role in remodelling connections to restore facial muscle function. The human equivalent of this rodent facial nerve crush model is Bell's palsy where the facial nerve becomes inflamed as it passes through the auditory canal and the local oedema results in axon compression. ^{11}C-PK11115 PET studies have demonstrated tracer uptake in the facial nerve nucleus ipsilateral to the paralysed facial muscles where connections are being remodelled [5]. Acquired limb amputations following trauma often result in a phantom limb phenomenon where the absent limb still feels as if it is present. This sensation is unpleasant, and the limb may feel as if it is compressed into the remaining stump. In these subjects one can detect thalamic inflammation contralateral to the missing limb with ^{11}C-PK11115 PET [9]. These PET studies, therefore, reveal that central microglial activation can be detected after disconnection of brain nuclei following peripheral nerve injuries. These microglia are likely to be playing a role in the remodelling of connections though it remains to be determined whether the cells express the M2 phenotype.

In brain disorders TSPO imaging reveals microglial activation both at the site of local disease activity and also due to the effects of downstream disconnection. Endothelial cells also express TSPO, and so ^{11}C-PK11115 binding can be seen in the lateral and sagittal venous sinuses. This can be problematic as the vascular ^{11}C-PK11115 signal may spill over into adjacent brain tissue—particularly the cerebellum—due to the relatively low 5-mm spatial resolution of commercial PET cameras. The result is artefactually high signals from cerebellum unless a correction is performed.

Quantitative modelling of TSPO PET can be problematic as there is no single brain region that can be guaranteed to provide a tissue reference for non-specific tracer uptake. One option is to use an arterial plasma input function to calculate brain tracer binding but ^{11}C-PK11115 sticks to plastic tubing and it can be difficult to obtain accurate wash-in and washout time activity curves (TACs) allowing measurement of peak height, delay, and dispersion. For these reasons, cluster analysis has been used to define a collection of grey matter voxels in each subject's brain that have a time activity uptake and washout curve that behaves similarly to a population of normal grey matter reference TAC in healthy controls [10]. This reference cluster can then be used to define levels of non-specific ^{11}C-PK11115 uptake in brain regions where retention is occurring in patients. At the same time signal due to vascular tracer binding, which peaks rapidly, is separated from brain parenchymal signal. Ligand binding potentials (BPs) can then be computed using a standard simple reference tissue model (SRTM) with brain-specific and non-specific compartments or standard graphical modelling approaches.

^{11}C-PK11115 PET suffers from the problem of a relatively high non-specific signal and rapid brain washout. Recently, new higher-affinity tracers have been developed with lower non-specific signal and a longer brain retention with the aim of providing more sensitive detection of microglial activation. However, binding of these new tracers has been found to be influenced to varying extents by the polymorphism of the TSPO gene being expressed by individuals; this is a minor issue with ^{11}C-PK11115 PET [11]. An Ala147Thr substitution at the rs6971 polymorphism of both TSPO genes results in homozygous subjects becoming low-affinity binders of the newer TSPO ligands and giving no specific PET signal. Heterozygotes for the Ala147Thr substitution at the rs6971 polymorphism are mixed affinity binders. In Caucasian populations around 60 % of individuals are high-, 10 % low-, and 30 % mixed affinity binders for the newer TSPO ligands. ^{11}C-PBR28 shows a 50-fold difference in affinity for TSPO between high (Kd 4nM)- and low (Kd 200nM)-affinity binders. The PET tracers ^{11}C-DAA1106, ^{11}C-DPA713, and ^{18}F-PBR111 show 4–5-fold differences in affinity for TSPO between high and low binders. Mixed affinity binders express high- and low-affinity TSPO binding sites in equal proportions. In order to use these newer TSPO PET markers subjects need to be stratified into high-, mixed, and low-affinity binders by prior genetic screening and their findings compared with appropriate control populations.

Imaging Inflammation in Parkinsonian Syndromes

Parkinson's Disease

Parkinson's disease (PD) is the second most common neurodegenerative disorder after dementia, affecting 1 % of the over sixties. It manifests as asymmetrical limb bradykinesia, rigidity, and tremor, and in 90 % of pathologically proven cases, these symptoms were responsive to levodopa. The neuronal pathology is characterized by Lewy body inclusions, which contain aggregated alpha synuclein and neurofilaments.

While the dopamine neurones of the substantia nigra compacta are primarily targeted by the Lewy body pathology, the disease process is thought to start in the medullary dorsal nucleus of the vagus at stage 1 and to then ascend the brainstem to the cortex in later stages [12]. In stage 2 the noradrenergic locus ceruleus, cholinergic pedunculopontine nucleus, and serotonergic median raphe in the pons become involved while the dopamine neurones of the substantia nigra compacta in the midbrain become targeted in stage 3 along with the cholinergic nucleus basalis. The limbic cortex and cingulate are involved at stage 4 and the association and primary neocortex in stages 5 and 6.

At postmortem microglial activation accompanies the Lewy body pathology in subcortical and cortical affected regions [13, 14]. Aggregated alpha synuclein fibrils are known to stimulate microglial activation in cell culture, but the in vivo relationship between brain inflammation and disease progression remains uncertain. The exact role of microglial activation in the degenerative process in PD is currently poorly understood. When humans and monkeys are acutely exposed to the nigral toxin MPTP, an inflammatory response results which can persist for years associated with progressively deteriorating parkinsonism [15, 16].

In an initial PET study it was reported that ten early cases of PD showed increased midbrain uptake of ^{11}C-PK11195, the levels of which correlated both with motor disability rated with the motor subscore of the Unified Parkinson's Disease Rating Scale (UPDRS) and with reductions in putamen dopamine transporter (DAT) binding measured with ^{11}C-CFT PET [17]. The authors suggested that their study provided evidence for the involvement of microglia in the loss of dopaminergic function that characterizes PD.

Subsequent ^{11}C-PK11195 PET studies, however, have failed to replicate a correlation between midbrain ^{11}C-PK11195 signals and loss of dopaminergic function in PD or indeed to consistently detect activated microglia in PD substantia nigra. In a series involving 18 more advanced PD cases, increased ^{11}C-PK11195 binding was detected in the striatum, thalamus, pons, and frontal and cingulate cortex compared to 11 age-matched controls. In this study the level and extent of regional microglial activation did not correlate with either clinical severity or striatal ^{18}F-dopa uptake. Over a 2-year follow-up period, despite ongoing clinical deterioration and loss of putamen ^{18}F-dopa storage, levels of ^{11}C-PK11195 uptake were reported to remain static in eight of these 18 PD patients [18]. These workers suggested that microglial activation is present at onset of PD and may act to drive the progression of locomotor disability.

At postmortem end-stage PD cases show widespread microglial activation which accompanies the Lewy body pathology in association cortical and subcortical regions. PET, however, allows patients with early disease to be investigated. ^{11}C-PK11195 PET is able to demonstrate the presence of cortical microglial activation in association cortical regions of early non-demented cases [18]. This suggests that cases that would be rated as Hoehn and Yahr stage 1 or 2 based on clinical criteria may well already be Braak stage 5 or 6 pathologically.

Eighty percent of PD patients will eventually develop dementia if they survive their condition for 20 years [19]. The relationship between microglia activation and cognitive status in PD has now been investigated. An inverse correlation between levels of cortical microglia activation and scores on the mini-mental state examination (MMSE) has been reported [20]. In non-demented PD cases the presence of raised levels of cortical ^{11}C-PK11195 binding correlates with an impaired performance on tests of verbal memory and visual perception [21]. These findings confirm that microglial activation is an early phenomenon in PD and suggest that it may be responsible for driving the cortical dysfunction that leads to later dementia.

Over a 2-year follow-up period, despite on-going clinical deterioration and loss of putamen ^{18}F-dopa storage, levels of cortical and subcortical ^{11}C-PK11195 uptake have been reported to remain relatively static in PD patients [18]. However, although the density of activated microglia may remain stable, these cells are still expressing cytokines at postmortem. Whether interventions should be developed to suppress microglial activity in PD is currently under debate. Clearly if they are releasing cytokines and potentially driving disease progression, switching them off would be a rational strategy; however, they also remodel connections and release growth factors, so development of drugs selectively blocking the M1 cidal or promoting the M2 restorative phenotype would be advantageous.

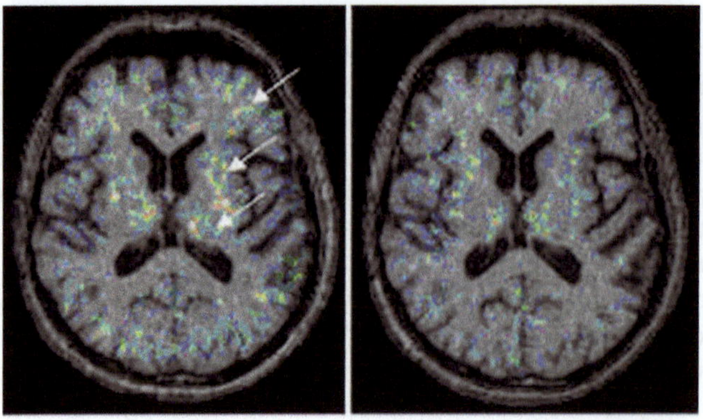

Fig. 2 ^{11}C-PK11195 PET scans in a multiple system atrophy patients before and after a 6-month course of minocycline. The microglial activation signal has fallen by 30 % in the posttreatment image [25]

Atypical Parkinsonian Disorders

Atypical Parkinsonian disorders include multiple system atrophy (MSA), progressive supranuclear palsy (PSP), and corticobasal degeneration (CBD). MSA-P is associated with asymmetric parkinsonism along with early autonomic dysfunction, postural instability, and ataxia. It is usually poorly responsive to levodopa. The pathology is characterized by argyrophilic glial cytoplasmic inclusions (GCIs) that contain alpha synuclein and target the substantia nigra, putamen, ponto-cerebellar connections, and the lateral columns of the spinal cord. At postmortem widespread microglial activation is associated with the MSA pathology [22].

An initial ^{11}C-PK11195 PET study involved five patients with multiple system atrophy (MSA-P). Activated microglia were detected in the head of caudate nucleus, putamen, substantia nigra and pons, and frontal regions in a more extensive distribution than that normally associated with PD [23].

A proteolipid protein-alpha synuclein (PLP-αSYN) overexpression transgenic mouse model of MSA has been developed [24]. This mouse shows a correlation between levels of nigral microglial activation and dopamine neurone loss. Minocycline is known to both block and reverse microglial activation in cell cultures. Its administration suppressed the inflammation present in the PLP-αSYN transgenic mouse and preserved dopamine neurones.

A human trial has been performed to determine the neuroprotective efficacy of minocycline in MSA. The drug failed to slow clinical disease progression at doses that are licensed for the treatment of acne. MSA cases receiving active medication, however, showed a 30 % reduction in brain ^{11}C-PK11195 uptake relative to placebo-treated cases (Fig. 2) [25]. This finding suggests that markers of microglial activation may be valid biomarkers when testing anti-inflammatory agents as potential neuroprotective agents.

PSP is associated with axial parkinsonism, impaired volitional eye movements, early bulbar dysfunction, and balance and gait difficulties. Dementia of a frontal type can be present, and the syndrome is poorly levodopa responsive. At postmortem cases show atrophy of the brainstem, internal globus pallidus, amygdala, frontal and parietal lobe, and nigral depigmentation. The characteristic pathology is intra-neuronal neurofibrillary tangles containing hyperphosphorylated 4-repeat tau protein and neuropil threads. Neuronal loss is seen in brainstem oculomotor nuclei, pallidum, substantia nigra, subthalamic nucleus, and frontal cortex. There is accompanying widespread brainstem, basal ganglia, and frontal microglial activation [26].

Four PSP patients who were studied with ^{11}C-PK11195 PET showed significantly increased signal in their caudate nucleus, putamen, pallidum, midbrain, substantia nigra, the frontal lobe, and the cerebellum [27]. Two of these patients were rescanned after 6–10 months, and the level of microglial activation was unchanged.

CBD is associated with asymmetrical parkinsonism, and the affected limbs are characteristically apraxic and exhibit stimulus-sensitive myoclonus and on occasion the alien limb phenomenon. Dysphasia, a supranuclear gaze palsy, and frontal dementia may all accompany the limb signs. Established cases show asymmetrical cortical atrophy targeting the superior frontal gyrus and inferior parietal areas. Microscopically ballooned achromatic neurones and astrocytic plaques containing tau are seen in affected cortical areas, the dentate nuclei, and the substantia nigra. Microglial activation is extensive in CBD, and its distribution correlates with the anatomical regions most affected [26]. The syndrome of CBD, however, can be associated with other pathologies including PSP and Pick's disease. Four patients with CBD have had ^{11}C-PK11195 PET, and they showed increased signal in caudate, putamen, substantia nigra, and frontoparietal cortex [27].

Imaging Inflammation in Dementias

Alzheimer's Disease

Dementia affects 10 % of the over sixties, the prevalence rising to one-third of the over eighties. It is characterized clinically by progressive impairment of memory along with word finding and recognition and perceptual difficulties in the absence of an altered conscious level. Personality changes occur and patients can regress a state of total dependency. At postmortem 60 % of dementia cases have Alzheimer pathology with fibrillar extracellular amyloid plaques and intra-neuronal neurofibrillary tangles of hyperphosphorylated tau. Activated microglia are seen surrounding the amyloid plaques, which target association cortex, cingulate, and striatum [28, 29]. They are also found in brain areas with dense tau pathology but sparse amyloid plaques, such as the entorhinal cortex and hippocampus.

^{11}C-PK11195 PET detects raised levels of microglial activation in patients with probable Alzheimer's disease (AD), binding potentials being raised by around 30 %

in frontal, temporal, and parietal association cortical areas [30, 31]. The newer TSPO ligand ^{11}C-DAA1106 has also been reported to show a 33 % increase in cortical uptake in AD [32]. The cortical distribution of inflammation in AD, like that of amyloid deposition, targets association areas when imaged with PET [33]. Interestingly, while levels of cortical ^{11}C-PK11195 and ^{11}C-DAA1106 uptake in AD correlate with the degree of cognitive impairment rated with the MMSE, this is not true of amyloid load [31, 34]. This suggests that it may be the cortical microglial activation rather than amyloid plaques in AD that is detrimental to cognitive function, possibly due to cytokine release by these cells. In AD activated microglia can also be detected in the thalamus, cerebellum, and brainstem as well as the association cortex; areas are not targeted by plaque or tangle pathology. The TSPO expression detected by PET is likely to reflect microglial activation in response to cortical disconnection, the cells probably acting to strip synapses and remodel connections.

Subjects with amnestic mild cognitive impairment (MCI) have isolated recall problems that are not severe enough to interfere with activities of daily living. 60 % of these cases progress to develop Alzheimer's disease over 5 years, and amnestic MCI can be regarded as a transitional state between normality and dementia [35]. ^{11}C-PK11195 and ^{11}C-DAA1106 PET have both been reported to detect microglial activation in MCI when present. In one series ^{11}C-PK11195 PET revealed increased cortical microglial activation in 40 % of amnestic MCI cases while 60 % showed evidence of amyloid plaque deposition with ^{11}C-PIB PET [36]. In another group of seven MCI cases studied with ^{11}C-DAA1106 PET there was a significant mean 27 % increase in tracer uptake across brain regions, two cases individually showing significantly elevated levels of microglial activation [37]. Five of the seven MCI subjects with ^{11}C-DAA1106 uptake raised more than 0.5 standard deviations above the normal mean progressed to dementia over a 2-year follow-up period.

Frontotemporal Dementia/Amyotrophic Lateral Sclerosis

Frontotemporal dementias are now though to be largely genetic in origin and account for around 10 % of dementia cases. Clinically they present as progressive personality change, dysphasia, and apraxia, with memory difficulties developing later. Semantic dementia where subjects recognize objects but cannot recall their function, progressive aphasias, and apraxias are all variants of FTD. There are three main pathological causes of FTD, all associated with abnormal protein aggregation: Pick's disease is associated with Pick bodies containing aggregated three-repeat hyperphosphorylated tau. A second variant is characterized by the presence of TDP-43 protein inclusions and spongiform degeneration targeting the frontal and inferior temporal lobes. These inclusions are associated with mutations of the progranulin gene. Abnormal aggregation of FUS protein represents a third type of FTD. A PET series of five clinically diagnosed FTD cases reported raised frontotemporal uptake of ^{11}C-PK11195 as would be predicted [38].

There is a clinical and pathological overlap between frontotemporal dementia and motor neurone disease (amyotrophic lateral sclerosis). The neuropathology of both can be associated with cortical TDP-43 inclusions and spongiform degeneration, and neuropsychological and imaging studies have indicated that cortical dysfunction is present in many cases of ALS. In one series ten clinically probable ALS patients on El Escorial criteria and 14 healthy controls were studied with ^{11}C-PK11195 PET [39]. Significantly increased microglial activation was seen in the motor cortex, brainstem, thalamus, dorsolateral prefrontal cortex, and occipital lobes of the ALS patients. There was a significant correlation between ^{11}C-PK11195 uptake in motor cortex and severity of upper motor neuron signs clinically.

Detection of Preclinical Microglial Activation

Huntington's disease is an autosomal dominant inherited progressive neurodegenerative disorder associated with motor, cognitive, and psychiatric symptoms. It is associated with an abnormal CAG triplet repeat expansion of the huntingtin gene on chromosome 4, which leads to an elongated polyglutamine chain at the terminus of the huntingtin protein. The effect of this is to cause intranuclear aggregations of huntingtin to form resulting in progressive loss of medium spiny striatal GABAergic neurones [40]. These neurones express either dopamine D1 or D2 receptors, and subclinical striatal dysfunction can be detected as a loss of availability of these sites for ligand binding [41].

Loss of striatal neurones in HD is associated with microglial activation [42], which can be detected with ^{11}C-PK11195 PET. Levels of striatal microglial activation correlate with loss of D2 binding measured with ^{11}C-raclopride PET and also with locomotor disability rated with the Unified Huntington's Disease Rating Scale (UHDRS) [43]. This suggests, again, that microglial activation may play a role in driving the disease process. In support of this, ^{11}C-PK11195 PET studies have reported raised microglial activation in a majority of asymptomatic adult HD gene carriers [44]. Those carriers with active disease also showed reduced dopamine D2 binding with ^{11}C-raclopride PET. Cortical microglial activation can also be detected in pre-manifesting HD carriers confirming that this is not a purely basal ganglia disorder [45]. Levels of striatal ^{11}C-PK11195 uptake have been shown to correlate with the predicted time of clinical disease onset [44, 45].

Conclusion

Microglial activation is a non-specific reaction to all forms of neurodegeneration and can be detected with PET. In chronic neurodegenerative diseases, the role of activated microglia remains uncertain. Initially, these cells could act to ingest misfolded proteins and release growth factors, but this process appears to fail in later disease. Local release of cytokines by microglia with the M1 phenotype may lead to neuronal death and disease progression. Conversely, in downstream disconnected areas, microglia could have a beneficial action leading to synaptic stripping and remodelling of connections as an adaptive response.

Currently, PET imaging of activated microglia is based on the use of TSPO substrate radioligands. While these provide a valuable in vivo tool for detecting disease activity and tracking the progression of neuroinflammation, binding of the newest ligands with lower non-specific background signals is influenced by the TSPO polymorphism expressed, and 40 % of the Caucasian population are either non- or mixed affinity binders. As TSPO polymorphism has only a small effect on ^{11}C-PK11195 binding, despite its lower affinity and higher non-specific signal, ^{11}C-PK11195 PET still provides a pragmatic approach for measuring brain inflammation. The early detection of microglia using PET provides a potential biomarker for measuring the efficacy of neuroprotective strategies designed to suppress the inflammatory response to neurodegenerative processes. In the future hopefully there will be development of both TSPO tracers uninfluenced by the genotype along with other markers of microglial activation, such as cannabinoid CB2 expression, allowing us to improve our understanding of the role of activated microglia in CNS disease.

References

1. Kreutzberg GW. Microglia: a sensor for pathological events in the CNS. Trends Neurosci. 1996;19:312–8.
2. Ransohoff RM, Perry VH. Microglial physiology: unique stimuli, specialized responses. Annu Rev Immunol. 2009;27:119–45.
3. Varnum MM, Ikezu T. The classification of microglial activation phenotypes on neurodegeneration and regeneration in Alzheimer's disease brain. Arch Immunol Ther Exp (Warsz). 2012;60:251–66.
4. Papadopoulos V, Baraldi M, Guilarte TR, Knudsen TB, Lacapere JJ, Lindemann P, et al. Translocator protein (18kDa): new nomenclature for the peripheral-type benzodiazepine receptor based on its structure and molecular function. Trends Pharmacol Sci. 2006;27: 402–9.
5. Banati RB. Visualising microglial activation in vivo. Glia. 2002;40:206–17.
6. Doorduin J, de Vries EF, Dierckx RA, Klein HC. PET imaging of the peripheral benzodiazepine receptor: monitoring disease progression and therapy response in neurodegenerative disorders. Curr Pharm Des. 2008;14:3297–315.
7. Dolle F, Luus C, Reynolds A, Kassiou M. Radiolabelled molecules for imaging the translocator protein (18 kDa) using positron emission tomography. Curr Med Chem. 2009;16:2899–923.
8. Banati RB, Myers R, Kreutzberg GW. PK ('peripheral benzodiazepine')–binding sites in the CNS indicate early and discrete brain lesions: microautoradiographic detection of [3H] PK11195 binding to activated microglia. J Neurocytol. 1997;26:77–82.
9. Banati RB. Brain plasticity and microglia: is transsynaptic glial activation in the thalamus after limb denervation linked to cortical plasticity and central sensitisation? J Physiol Paris. 2002;96:289–99.
10. Anderson AN, Pavese N, Edison P, Tai YF, Hammers A, Gerhard A, et al. A systematic comparison of kinetic modelling methods generating parametric maps for [(11)C]-(R)-PK11195. Neuroimage. 2007;36:28–37.

11. Owen DR, Yeo AJ, Gunn RN, Song K, Wadsworth G, Lewis A, et al. An 18-kDa translocator protein (TSPO) polymorphism explains differences in binding affinity of the PET radioligand PBR28. J Cereb Blood Flow Metab. 2012;32:1–5.
12. Braak H, Ghebremedhin E, Rub U, Bratzke H, Del Tredici K. Stages in the development of Parkinson's disease-related pathology. Cell Tissue Res. 2004;318:121–34.
13. McGeer P, Kawamata T, Walker DG, Akiyama H, Tooyama I, McGeer EG. Microglia in degenerative disease. Glia. 1993;7:84–92.
14. Imamura K, Hishikawa N, Sawada M, Nagatsu T, Yoshida M, Hashizume Y. Distribution of major histocompatibility complex class II-positive microglia and cytokine profile of Parkinson's disease brains. Acta Neuropathol. 2003;106:518–26.
15. Vingerhoets FJG, Snow BJ, Langston JW, Tetrud JM, Schulzer M, Calne DB. Positron emission tomographic evidence for progression of human MPTP-induced dopaminergic lesions. Ann Neurol. 1994;36:765–70.
16. Langston JW, Forno LS, Tetrud J, Reeves AG, Kaplan JA, Karluk D. Evidence of active nerve cell degeneration in the substantia nigra of humans years after 1-methyl-4-phenyl-1,2,3,6-tetrahydropyridine exposure. Ann Neurol. 1999;46:598–605.
17. Ouchi Y, Yoshikawa E, Sekine Y, Futatsubashi M, Kanno T, Ogusu T, et al. Microglial activation and dopamine terminal loss in early Parkinson's disease. Ann Neurol. 2005;57:168–75.
18. Gerhard A, Pavese N, Hotton G, Turkheimer F, Es M, Hammers A, et al. In vivo imaging of microglial activation with [(11)C](R)-PK11195 PET in idiopathic Parkinson's disease. Neurobiol Dis. 2006;21:404–12.
19. Hely MA, Reid WG, Adena MA, Halliday GM, Morris JG. The Sydney multicenter study of Parkinson's disease: the inevitability of dementia at 20 years. Mov Disord. 2008;23:837–44.
20. Edison P, Rowe CC, Rinne J, Ahmed I, Villemagne VL, Ng S, et al. Amyloid load in Lewy body dementia (LBD), Parkinson's disease dementia (PDD) and Parkinson's disease (PD) measured with C-11-PIB PET. Neurology. 2007;68:A98–A.
21. Simpson BS, Pavese N, Ramlackhansingh AF, Breen DP, Barker RA, Brooks DJ. Clinical correlates of brain inflammation in Parkinson's disease: A PET study. Mov Disord. 2012;27 Suppl 1:775.
22. Ishizawa K, Komori T, Sasaki S, Arai N, Mizutani T, Hirose T. Microglial activation parallels system degeneration in multiple system atrophy. J Neuropathol Exp Neurol. 2004;63:43–52.
23. Gerhard A, Banati RB, Goerres GB, Cagnin A, Myers R, Gunn RN, et al. [(11)C](R)-PK11195 PET imaging of microglial activation in multiple system atrophy. Neurology. 2003;61:686–9.
24. Stefanova N, Reindl M, Neumann M, Kahle PJ, Poewe W, Wenning GK. Microglial activation mediates neurodegeneration related to oligodendroglial alpha-synucleinopathy: implications for multiple system atrophy. Mov Disord. 2007;22:2196–203.
25. Dodel R, Spottke A, Gerhard A, Reuss A, Reinecker S, Schimke N, et al. Minocycline 1-year therapy in multiple-system-atrophy: effect on clinical symptoms and [(11)C] (R)-PK11195 PET (MEMSA-trial). Mov Disord. 2010;25:97–107.
26. Ishizawa K, Dickson DW. Microglial activation parallels system degeneration in progressive supranuclear palsy and corticobasal degeneration. J Neuropathol Exp Neurol. 2001;60: 647–57.
27. Gerhard A, Trender-Gerhard I, Turkheimer F, Quinn NP, Bhatia KP, Brooks DJ. In vivo imaging of microglial activation with [(11)C](R)-PK11195 PET in progressive supranuclear palsy. Mov Disord. 2006;21:89–93.
28. Dickson DW. The pathogenesis of senile plaques. J Neuropathol Exp Neurol. 1997;56: 321–39.
29. Braak H, Braak E. Frequency of stages of Alzheimer-related lesions in different age categories. Neurobiol Aging. 1997;18:351–7.
30. Cagnin A, Brooks DJ, Kennedy AM, Gunn RN, Myers R, Turkheimer FE, et al. In-vivo measurement of activated microglia in dementia. Lancet. 2001;358:461–7.
31. Edison P, Archer HA, Gerhard A, Hinz R, Pavese N, Turkheimer FE, et al. Microglia, amyloid, and cognition in Alzheimer's disease: An [11C](R)PK11195-PET and [11C]PIB-PET study. Neurobiol Dis. 2008;32:412–9.

32. Yasuno F, Ota M, Kosaka J, Ito H, Higuchi M, Doronbekov TK, et al. Increased binding of peripheral benzodiazepine receptor in Alzheimer's disease measured by positron emission tomography with [11C]DAA1106. Biol Psychiatry. 2008;64:835–41.
33. Edison P, Archer HA, Gerhard A, Hinz R, Pavese N, Turkheimer FE, Hammers A, et al. Microglia, amyloid, and cognition in Alzheimer's disease: An [11C](R)PK11195-PET and [11C]PIB-PET study. Neurobiol Dis. 2008;32(3):412–9.
34. Yokokura M, Mori N, Yagi S, Yoshikawa E, Kikuchi M, Yoshihara Y, et al. In vivo changes in microglial activation and amyloid deposits in brain regions with hypometabolism in Alzheimer's disease. Eur J Nucl Med Mol Imaging. 2011;38:343–51.
35. Petersen RC, Doody R, Kurz A, Mohs RC, Morris JC, Rabins PV, et al. Current concepts in mild cognitive impairment. Arch Neurol. 2001;58:1985–92.
36. Okello A, Edison P, Archer HA, Turkheimer FE, Kennedy J, Bullock R, et al. Microglial activation and amyloid deposition in mild cognitive impairment: a PET study. Neurology. 2009;72:56–62.
37. Yasuno F, Kosaka J, Ota M, Higuchi M, Ito H, Fujimura Y, et al. Increased binding of peripheral benzodiazepine receptor in mild cognitive impairment-dementia converters measured by positron emission tomography with [(11)C]DAA1106. Psychiatry Res. 2012;203:67–74.
38. Cagnin A, Rossor M, Sampson EL, Mackinnon T, Banati RB. In vivo detection of microglial activation in frontotemporal dementia. Ann Neurol. 2004;56:894–7.
39. Turner MR, Cagnin A, Turkheimer FE, Miller CC, Shaw CE, Brooks DJ, et al. Evidence of widespread cerebral microglial activation in amyotrophic lateral sclerosis: an [11C](R)-PK11195 positron emission tomography study. Neurobiol Dis. 2004;15:601–9.
40. Sapp E, Schwarz C, Chase K, Bhide PG, Young AB, Penney J, et al. Huntingtin localization in brains of normal and Huntington's disease patients. Ann Neurol. 1997;42:604–12.
41. Andrews TC, Weeks RA, Turjanski N, Gunn RN, Watkins LHA, Sahakian B, et al. Huntington's disease progression PET and clinical observations. Brain. 1999;122:2353–63.
42. Sapp E, Kegel KB, Aronin N, Hashikawa T, Uchiyama Y, Tohyama K, et al. Early and progressive accumulation of reactive microglia in the Huntington disease brain. J Neuropathol Exp Neurol. 2001;60:161–72.
43. Pavese N, Gerhard A, Tai YF, Ho AK, Turkheimer F, Barker RA, et al. Microglial activation correlates with severity in Huntington disease: a clinical and PET study. Neurology. 2006;66:1638–43.
44. Tai YF, Pavese N, Gerhard A, Tabrizi SJ, Barker RA, Brooks DJ, et al. Microglial activation in presymptomatic Huntington's disease gene carriers. Brain. 2007;130:1759–66.
45. Politis M, Pavese N, Tai YF, Kiferle L, Mason SL, Brooks DJ, et al. Microglial activation in regions related to cognitive function predicts disease onset in Huntington's disease: a multimodal imaging study. Hum Brain Mapp. 2011;32:258–70.

Index

A
Adaptive immune system, 77, 87–89, 93–94
Advanced glycation end products (AGEs), 38
ALP. *See* Autophagy–lysosomal pathway (ALP)
ALS. *See* Amyotrophic lateral sclerosis (ALS)
Alzheimer's disease, 130, 211–212
Amantadine, 14–15
Amyotrophic lateral sclerosis (ALS), 212–213
Animal models, 53–54
  astrocytes in, 133–135
  interleukin-1β in, 160–161
  passive immunization in, 91
Antibodies, 85–87. *See also* Autoantibodies
Anticholinergics, 14–15
Anti-inflammatory factors, 115–116, 197–198
Apokyn. *See* Apomorphine
Apomorphine, 12
Aquaporin-4, 127–128
Astrocytes
  in animal models, 133–135
  assessment of, 135–138
  importance of, 128
  protoplasmic, 127, 135
  response in neurodegenerative diseases, 130–132
  role in PD, 132–133
  structure and function of, 127–130
Astrogliosis, 128, 130, 134
Atypical Parkinsonian disorders, 210–211
Autoantibodies, 193, 194
Autologous T cells, 92
Autophagy–lysosomal pathway (ALP), 36

B
Bacterial artificial chromosome (BAC) mouse model, 31
Basal ganglia model, 43
Basal ganglia–thalamocortical circuitry, 44
BBB. *See* Blood–brain barrier (BBB)
B cell, 80, 86
Bell's palsy, 207
Biological markers, 189–190
Blood–brain barrier (BBB), 86, 197
  diapedesis across, 84
  permeability, 79
B lymphocytes, 85–87
Bone marrow-derived macrophages (BMDMs), mouse, 89
Braak hypothesis, 75–77
Braak staging, for PD, 37, 38
Bradykinesia, 1

C
Carbidopa/levodopa (CD/LD), 11
Catechol-O-methyltransferase (COMT) inhibitor, 10, 13–14
CBD. *See* Corticobasal degeneration (CBD)
CD200/CD200 receptor, 116–117
Cell lines
  dopamine-producing, 176–178
  microglia, 178–180
  neuroblastomas, 176
Cerebral mechanisms model, 45
Chronic neuroinflammation, 9, 78, 79, 86
Clonazepam, 17
Coenzyme Q10, 17
Cognitive deficits, 47, 48

M. Thomas (ed.), *Inflammation in Parkinson's Disease: Scientific and Clinical Aspects*, DOI 10.1007/978-3-319-08046-8, © Springer International Publishing Switzerland 2014

Cognitive impairment, 50
Comtan. *See* Entacapone
COMT inhibitor. *See* Catechol-O-methyltransferase (COMT) inhibitor
Copaxone, 91
Cortical microglial activation, 213
Corticobasal degeneration (CBD), 211
Counter-regulation pathways, in microglia, 114
COX inhibitors. *See* Cyclooxygenase (COX) inhibitors
Creutzfeldt–Jakob disease, 8
Cyclooxygenase (COX) inhibitors, 107
Cytokines, 107
  gene polymorphisms, 195
  marker, 191–194
  in PD, 151
  pro-inflammatory, 112, 179

D

Damage-associated molecular patterns (DAMPs), 111
DaT. *See* Dopamine transporter (DaT)
Deep brain stimulation (DBS), 18
Deep sequencing techniques, 84
Dementias, 2
  frontotemporal, 212–213
  imaging inflammation in, 211–213
  semantic, 212
Dementia with Lewy bodies (DLB), 49–50
Dihydropyridine calcium channel blocker (DiCCB), 9
Disease-modifying effect, 91
DJ-1 mutations, 6, 7
DLB. *See* Dementia with Lewy bodies
Dominant-negative inhibitor of TNF (DN-TNF), 91
Dopamine agonists, 11–12
Dopamine-producing cell lines, 176–178
Dopaminergic neuronal death, neuroinflammation in, 105
Dopaminergic neurotoxicity measurement, 182–183
Dopaminergic receptors, hyperstimulation of, 45
Dopamine transporter (DaT)
  levels in striatum, 2–3
  scan, 2
Dysautonomia, 2
Dyskinesia, management of, 15–16
Dysphasia, 211

E

EAE. *See* Experimental autoimmune encephalomyelitis (EAE)
EBV. *See* Epstein–Barr virus (EBV)
Eldepryl. *See* Selegiline
Enriched microglial cultures, 181
Entacapone, 14
Environmental factors
  and microglia, 110
  and PD, 4–5
Epstein–Barr virus (EBV), 193
Essential tremor (ET), 2–3
Estrogen receptors (ERs), 114
Experimental autoimmune encephalomyelitis (EAE), 107
Experimental autoimmune neuritis (EAN) disease, 119
Extracellular α-syn, 53
Ex vivo modification, of autologous T cells, 92

F

Fas expression, 83
Fas–FasL signaling, 85
Fc receptor-expressing cells, 87
Fractalkine (CX3CL1), 116
Fractalkine Receptor (CX3CR1), 116
Frontotemporal dementias (FTD), 212–213

G

Gene–environment interactions, 7
Genetic ablation, of NADPH oxidase, 112
Genetic factors, and PD, 5–7
Genetic mutations, cause PD, 87–90
Genetic susceptibility, 51
Genome-wide association studies (GWAS), 76, 194–195
GFAP. *See* Glial fibrillary acidic protein (GFAP)
Glatiramer acetate. *See* Copaxone
Glial-derived neurotrophic factor (GDNF), 107
Glial fibrillary acidic protein (GFAP), 128, 129
  positive thorn-shaped astrocytes, 130–131
Globus pallidus internus (GPi), 18, 42, 43
Glucocorticoids (GCs) receptor, 114
Glutathione peroxidase (GPX-1)-positive microglia, 35
GPi. *See* Globus pallidus internus (GPi)
Granulocyte-colony stimulating factor (G-CSF), 116
GWAS. *See* Genome-wide association studies (GWAS)

H

Huntington's disease, 2, 213
Hyperstimulation, of dopaminergic receptors, 45

I

ICAM-1, upregulation of, 79
IL. *See* Interleukin (IL)
IL-1β. *See* Interleukin-1β (IL-1β)
ILBD. *See* Incidental Lewy body disease (ILBD)
Imaging inflammation
  in dementias, 211–213
  in Parkinsonian syndromes, 208–211
Immune-mediated neurodegeneration, 190
Immune-relevant PD pathology, 75–76
Immune system
  adaptive, 77, 87–89, 93–94
  innate, 77
Immunomodulation, 92
Immunomodulatory therapies, 75, 90–93
Incidental Lewy body disease (ILBD), 38–39
Inducible nitric oxide synthase (iNOS), 175
Inflammatory cell culture systems
  cell lines in
    dopamine-producing, 176–178
    microglial, 178–180
    neuroblastomas, 176
  enriched microglial cultures in, 181
  mixed-glial cultures in, 181
  primary mesencephalic cultures in, 180
  primary mesencephalic neuron-glial cultures, 180–181
  reconstituted neuron-microglial co-cultures, 181–182
Inflammatory mediators, 106
Innate immunity, 77
iNOS. *See* Inducible nitric oxide synthase (iNOS)
Interferon gamma (IFN-γ), 192
Interleukin (IL), 115–116, 190
Interleukin-1β (IL-1β), 157–159
  in animal models, 160–161
  in neurodegeneration, 160–161
  polymorphisms, 159–160
  signaling mechanism of, 161–162
Intranuclear inclusions, 35
Intravenous immunoglobulin (IVIG), 92
In vitro assays, 183
In vitro models, 177
Isradipine, 9
IVIG. *See* Intravenous immunoglobulin (IVIG)

J

Japanese encephalitis virus (JEV), 82

L

LBs. *See* Lewy bodies (LBs)
Levodopa, 10, 11
Lewy bodies (LBs), 105, 133
  classic and cortical type, 32–34
  dementia with, 49–50
  disease, 38–39
    hypothetic progression pathways and stages, 40
    neuropathological staging, 39–40
  pathobiological role of, 35–36
  structure and molecular components of, 32–34
  in substantia nigra, 33
  types, 32
Lewy neurites, 133
Lewy pathology
  development of, 30–32
  guidelines for, 39–40
  multiorgan distribution of, 29–30
  staging, 36–38
Lipopolysaccharide (LPS)
  and microglia, 111
  models, 78
LRRK2 gene, 6–7
  mutations in, 89

M

Macrophage antigen complex 1 (MAC1) receptor, 111
Macrophages, 80, 85
Major Histocompatibility Class (MHC)
  expression, 82
  in PD, 80–82
Major Histocompatibility Class II (MHC-II) molecules, 80
MAO-B inhibitors. *See* Monoamine oxidase type B (MAO-B) inhibitors
Marinesco bodies, 35
Markers
  biological, 189–190
  T-cell, 190–191
MCI. *See* Mild cognitive impairment (MCI)
Mediators, inflammatory, 106
Medications
  mechanism of action of PD, 10–11
    anticholinergics and amantadine, 14–15
    COMT inhibitors, 13–14
    dopamine agonists, 11–12

Medications (*cont.*)
levodopa, 11
MAO inhibitors, 13
Memory T cells, 83
Mesencephalic cultures, primary, 180
neuron-glial, 180–181
1-Methyl-4-phenyl-1,2,3,6-tetrahydropyridine (MPTP), 7, 9, 76, 77, 84
and microglia, 111
MHC. *See* Major Histocompatibility Class
Microglia, 9, 80, 106–107
activation of, 109
alternative, 117–118
classical, 117
detection of preclinical, 213
in PD, 80–82, 145–146
activation states of, 117–118
"bad", 106–109, 111–112
cell lines, 178–180
counter-regulation pathways in, 114
cultures, enriched, 181
deactivation of, 118
effectors of, 110–113
NADPH oxidase, 112
pro-inflammatory factors, 112
ROS and superoxide, 113
expression of MHC-II molecules, 80
glutathione peroxidase-positive, 35
"good", 106–108, 113
inducers of, 109
environmental factors, 110
LPS, 111
MPTP, 111
α-synuclein aggregates, 109–110
microRNA, 117
in PD pathogenesis, 106, 108
reactive, 8, 145, 195
regulatory mechanisms of, 107, 113
anti-inflammatory factors, 115–116
counter-regulation/transrepression pathways, 114
estrogen receptors, 114
glucocorticoids receptor, 114
neuron-microglia cross-talk, 116–117
Nurr1, 115
PPARs, 115
Microgliosis, 146
reactive, 105, 111, 117, 145, 146
Migration inhibitory factor (MIF), 193
Mild cognitive impairment (MCI), 47–48, 212
Mirapex. *See* Pramipexole
Mixed-glial cultures, 181
Monoamine oxidase (MAO) inhibitors, 13
Monoamine oxidase type B (MAO-B) inhibitors, 10, 11
Motor fluctuations, management of, 15–16
MPTP. *See* 1-Methyl-4-phenyl-1,2,3,6-tetrahydropyridine
MSA. *See* Multiple system atrophy (MSA)
Multiorgan distribution, of α-synuclein and Lewy pathology, 29–30
Multiple genetic polymorphisms, 76
Multiple system atrophy (MSA), 132, 210
Mutations
DJ-1, 6, 7
genetic, cause PD, 87–90
LRRK2 gene, 89

N

NADPH oxidase, and microglia, 112
NBM. *See* Nucleus basalis of Meynert (NBM)
Neupro. *See* Rotigotine
Neuroblastomas cell lines, 176
Neurodegeneration, 76, 86
immune-mediated, 190
interleukin-1β in, 160–161
MPTP-induced, 84, 85
tumor necrosis factor-α in, 153–156
Neurodegenerative diseases, astrocytes response in, 130–132
Neurodegenerative lesions, 28
Neuroinflammation
chronic, 78
in DA neuronal death, 105
and PD, 78, 79, 105–106
Neuronal cell death, 3, 80
Neuronal dysfunction mechanism, 77–78
Neuronal vulnerability, 28–29
Neuron-glial cultures, primary mesencephalic, 180–181
Neuron-microglia cross-talk, 116–117
Neuron-microglial co-cultures, reconstitute, 181–182
Neurotoxicity, measurement of DA, 182–183
Nigrostriatal system degeneration, 26–28
Nigrostriatal tract, selective vulnerability of, 3–4
Nitrated α-synuclein, 85, 93
Nitric oxide (NO), 175, 179, 180
Nonmotor symptoms, treatment of, 16–17
Non-steroidal anti-inflammatory drugs (NSAIDs), 106, 119
NR4A2. *See* Nurr1
Nucleus basalis of Meynert (NBM), 48
Nurr1, 115

O
Oligomerization, of α-syn, 36
Orthostatic hypotension, 17
Oxidative stress, 3, 9–10

P
PAMPs. *See* Pathogen-associated molecular patterns (PAMPs)
Parkin, 5–6
Parkin-coregulated gene (PACRG), 136–137
Parkin (PARK2) gene, 89–90
Parkinson's disease (PD)
  clinical epidemiological studies, 195–197
  clinical features, 1–2
  cognitive and psychiatric symptoms, management, 16
  etiology of, 3, 4, 50–53
    environmental factors role in, 4–5
    genetic factors in, 5–7
  evidence for inflammation in, 77–79
  hereditary forms of, 87
  histopathology of, 26
  infectious etiologies for, 8
  inflammation and, 9
  laboratory studies, 2–3
  medications (*see* Medications)
  neuropathology of, 26–29, 47
  neuroprotective strategies, 17
  pathogenesis of, 50–53
  pathophysiology of, 42–46
  surgical treatment of, 18
Parkinson's disease and dementia (PDD), 48–50
Passive immunization, in animal models, 91
Pathogen-associated molecular patterns (PAMPs), 111
Pattern recognition receptors (PRRs), 111
PD. *See* Parkinson's disease (PD)
PDD. *See* Parkinson's disease and dementia (PDD)
Peripheral benzodiazepine receptor (PBR). *See* Translocator protein (TSPO)
Peripheral blood mononuclear cells (PBMC), 191
Peripheral immune cell changes, 147–150
Peripheral inflammation, 79
Peroxisome proliferator-activated receptor gamma (PPAR-γ), 9
Peroxisome proliferator-activated receptors (PPARs), 115
PINK1, 6
PLAD. *See* Pre-ligand assembly domain
Polymorphisms
  interleukin-1β, 159–160
  multiple genetic, 76
  TNF-α, 153
Positron emission tomography (PET), TSPO with, 206–208
Postmortem analysis, of PD patients, 106
PPARs. *See* Peroxisome proliferator-activated receptors (PPARs)
Pramipexole, 11, 12
Pre-ligand assembly domain (PLAD), 151
Primary mesencephalic cultures, 180–181
Prion-like disease, PD as, 8
Progressive supranuclear palsy (PSP), 211
Pro-inflammatory cytokines, 112, 179
Pro-inflammatory factors, and microglia, 112
Protein
  interactions, 41–42
  intraneuronal aggregates of, 75
Proteinopathies, 130
  TDP-43, 130, 132
Proteolipid protein-alpha synuclein (PLP-αSYN), 210
Protoplasmic astrocytes, 127, 135
PRRs. *See* Pattern recognition receptors (PRRs)
PSP. *See* Progressive supranuclear palsy (PSP)

R
Rasagiline, 13
Reactive microglia, 8, 145, 195
Reactive microgliosis, 105, 111, 117, 145, 146
Reactive oxygen species (ROS), 113, 178–180
Reconstituted neuron-microglial co-cultures, 181–182
REM sleep behavior disorder (RBD), 38
Requip. *See* Ropinirole
Rigid–akinetic type PD, 42
Rivastigmine, 16
Robust T-cell responses, 85
Rodent in vitro models, 177
Ropinirole, 11, 12
ROS. *See* Reactive oxygen species (ROS)
Rosenthal fibers, 129
Rotenone, 9
Rotigotine, 12

S
Scavenger receptors (SRs), 111
Screening protocols, 76
Selegiline, 13
Semantic dementia, 212

Signaling mechanism
  of interleukin-1β, 161–162
  of tumor necrosis factor-α, 156–157
Sinemet, 11
Single nucleotide polymorphisms (SNPs), 81
SNc. *See* Substantia nigra pars compacta (SNc)
SNCA gene, 88
SNPs. *See* Single nucleotide polymorphisms
Sporadic Parkinson's disease, etiology of, 76–77
Standard simple reference tissue model (SRTM), 207
Substantia nigra pars compacta (SNc), 3
Subthalamic nucleus (STN), 18
α-Syn-immunoreactive glial cells, 35
α-Syn-mutants, 35–36
α-Synuclein, 5
  accumulation of, 3–4
  cell-to-cell transfer of, 53
  clearance of, 91
  cortical, 41
  disease progression, 28
  extracellular, 53
  fibrils, 208
  modification of, 41
  nitrated, 85, 93
  oligomerization of, 36
  and other proteins, interactions, 41–42
  overexpression models, 91–92
  as pathological gene, 109–110
  pathology, 8
    development, 30–32
    multiorgan distribution, 29–30
  spreading of, 26
  wild-type human, 78
Synucleinopathies, 130
α-Synuclein overexpressing adenoassociated virus (AAV-Syn) model, 82
α-Synuclein-positive inclusions, 132, 133
  accumulation of, 134
  mutations in gene encoding, 134

T
Tasmar. *See* Tolcapone
Tauopathies, 130
T-cells
  adoptive transfer of, 91
  autologous, 92
  marker, 190–191
  memory, 83
  response, 85
TDP-43 proteinopathies, 130, 132
Therapeutics, 176
TIR. *See* Toll-IL-1 receptor (TIR)
TLRs. *See* Toll-like receptors (TLRs)
T lymphocytes, 83–85
Tolcapone, 14
Toll-IL-1 receptor (TIR), 158
Toll-like receptors (TLRs), 111, 158
Transforming growth factor-β (TGF-β), 115–116
Translocator protein (TSPO), 205–206
  with PET, 206–208
    quantitative modelling, 207
  polymorphism, 214
Transrepression pathways, in microglia, 114
Tremor
  dominant type of PD, 46
  essential, 2–3
  rest, 46
TSPO. *See* Translocator protein (TSPO)
Tumor necrosis factor (TNF), 194
Tumor necrosis factor-α (TNF-α), 151–152, 190, 191
  in animal models, 153–156
  in neurodegeneration, 153–156
  polymorphisms, 153
  signaling mechanism of, 156–157

U
UCH-L1, 7
Uncoupling proteins (UCP), 137
Unified Huntington's Disease Rating Scale (UHDRS), 213
Unified Parkinson's Disease Rating Scale (UPDRS), 81, 148, 190, 209

V
Vimentin, 128, 129
Viral PD models, 54

W
Wilson's disease, 2

Z
Zelapar. *See* Selegiline

MIX
Papier aus verantwortungsvollen Quellen
Paper from responsible sources
FSC® C105338

If you have any concerns about our products,
you can contact us on
ProductSafety@springernature.com

In case Publisher is established outside the EU,
the EU authorized representative is:
Springer Nature Customer Service Center GmbH
Europaplatz 3, 69115 Heidelberg, Germany

Printed by Libri Plureos GmbH
in Hamburg, Germany